Rare Pleural Diseases

Firas Ido
Editor

Rare Pleural Diseases

Springer

Editor
Firas Ido
Department of Pulmonary and Critical Care Medicine
St. Luke's University Health Network
Bethlehem, PA, USA

ISBN 978-3-032-14872-8 ISBN 978-3-032-14873-5 (eBook)
https://doi.org/10.1007/978-3-032-14873-5

This Springer imprint is published by the registered company Springer Nature Switzerland AG
The registered company address is: Gewerbestrasse 11, 6330 Cham, Switzerland

Preface

The pleura, a delicate, thin, transparent, and seemingly negligible membranous organ, reveals remarkable complexity when examined at the ultrastructural level. It is composed of a diverse group of cell types that collectively function to facilitate respiration, regulate pleural fluid turnover, and contribute to immune defense and tissue repair. Yet, it is only within the past few decades that discoveries have linked many of these cells to the development of specific diseases.

Over the past century, the medical literature has seen an increase in the documentation of rare pleural diseases, many of which have been reported solely in case reports or small case series. Despite advances in radiology, histopathology, and pleural fluid analysis, and the establishment of diagnostic criteria for some diseases, many remain underrecognized, often due to a lack of awareness or limited clinical experience, underscoring the diagnostic and therapeutic challenges.

Although certain topics, such as malignant pleural mesothelioma, may not strictly meet the criteria for rarity, their complexity and rapidly evolving body of knowledge justify their inclusion. Likewise, conditions such as hemothorax, though not inherently rare, can arise from unusual or exceptional etiologies and therefore warrant discussion in a text devoted to uncommon and underrecognized pleural diseases.

This volume is organized into sections covering non-neoplastic, inflammatory, and neoplastic pleural disorders. The first section discusses the normal anatomy, histology, and physiology of the pleura. In the second section, rare non-neoplastic primary pleural diseases, including inflammatory entities such as pleuroparenchymal fibroelastosis and fibrothorax, are discussed. Additional chapters address disorders characterized by abnormal proliferation or accumulation of tissue components within or adjacent to the pleura, such as pulmonary lymphangiomatosis and extrapleural lipomatosis. The third section reviews uncommon causes of pleural effusion, including duropleural fistula, urinothorax, and Meigs syndrome. The final section focuses on rare primary pleural neoplasms arising from mesothelial or submesothelial connective tissue cells, both differentiated and undifferentiated mesenchymal origins, including primary pleural synovial sarcoma, epithelioid hemangioendothelioma, angiosarcoma, liposarcoma, and Erdheim–Chester disease. Benign pleural tumors, such as solitary fibrous tumor of the pleura and pleural lipomas, are also examined.

This book was compiled to address these gaps by consolidating available knowledge on rare pleural disorders into a single comprehensive resource for clinicians. While some of these topics are only briefly mentioned in other texts, this volume brings together information from a broad range of sources, integrating pathophysiology, diagnosis, and treatment from the perspectives of pulmonology, pathology, radiology, oncology, and thoracic surgery, serving as both a clinical reference and an academic resource. It is the hope and goal of this text that increased awareness of these diseases will translate into earlier recognition, reduced diagnostic delays, and the encouragement of future studies to investigate and develop therapeutics.

I dedicate this book to my parents—my mother, Leila Ido, and my father, Faysal Ido—for their sacrifices, tireless efforts, and unwavering support throughout my education and career.

Bethlehem, PA, USA Firas Ido
2025

Contents

Contributors

Kyle Admire Department of Medicine, Pulmonary & Critical Care Division, Macon & Joan Brock Virginia Health Sciences, Eastern Virginia Medical School at Old Dominion University, Norfolk, VA, USA

Danish Ahmad Interventional Pulmonology, Department of Medicine, Fox Chase Cancer Center, Philadelphia, PA, USA

Matthew Bittner Department of Thoracic Medicine and Surgery, Temple University, Philadelphia, PA, USA

Peter Boshara Department of Interventional Pulmonology, University of Illinois Chicago, Chicago, IL, USA

Livia Bratis Department of Pulmonary and Critical Care Medicine, St. Luke's University Health Network, Bethlehem, PA, USA

William Burfeind Department of Thoracic Surgery, St. Luke's University Health Network, Bethlehem, PA, USA

Leon Cedeno Department of Pulmonary and Critical Care Medicine, St. Luke's University Health Network, Bethlehem, PA, USA

Timothy Daly Department of Pulmonary and Critical Care Medicine, St. Luke's University Health Network, Bethlehem, PA, USA

Razi Even Dar Pulmonary Institute, Rambam Health Care Campus, Ruth and Bruce Rappaport Faculty of Medicine, The Technion—Israel Institute of Technology, Haifa, Israel

Christos Deamont Department of Pulmonary and Critical Care, McLaren Oakland Hospital, Pontiac, MI, USA

Ashley Dean Department of Pulmonary and Critical Care, Virginia Tech Carilion Clinic, Roanoke, VA, USA

Luis Devia Department of General Surgery, St. Luke's University Health Network, Bethlehem, PA, USA

Michael DiRico Department of Pulmonology, TriHealth Physician Partners, Cincinnati, OH, USA

Yaniv Dotan Pulmonary Institute, Rambam Health Care Campus, Ruth and Bruce Rappaport Faculty of Medicine, The Technion—Israel Institute of Technology, Haifa, Israel

Joseph Evans Department of General Surgery, St. Luke's University Health Network, Bethlehem, PA, USA

Benjamin Fleming Department of Pulmonary and Critical Care, Rochester General Hospital, Rochester, NY, USA

Douglas Frenia Department of Pulmonary and Critical Care, Saint Peter's University Hospital, New Brunswick, NJ, USA

Shameek Gayen Department of Thoracic Medicine and Surgery, Temple University, Philadelphia, PA, USA

Ahmad Ghabsha Department of Pulmonary and Critical Care, McLaren Oakland Hospital, Pontiac, MI, USA

Ronald S. Go Division of Hematology, Department of Internal Medicine, Mayo Clinic, Rochester, MN, USA

Meredith Harrison Department of Thoracic Surgery, St. Luke's University Health Network, Bethlehem, PA, USA

Truong-An Andrew Ho Department of Thoracic Medicine and Surgery, Temple University, Philadelphia, PA, USA

Firas Ido Department of Pulmonary and Critical Care Medicine, St. Luke's University Health Network, Bethlehem, PA, USA

Daniel Kapadia Interventional Pulmonology, Henry Ford Health, Detroit, MI, USA

Rohit Kumar Department of Medicine, Section of Pulmonary, Interventional & Critical Care, Fox Chase Cancer Center, Temple University Health System, Philadelphia, PA, USA

Meng-Shan Lin Department of Pulmonary and Critical Care Medicine, St. Luke's University Health Network, Bethlehem, PA, USA

Santo Longo Department of Pathology, St. Luke's University Health Network, Bethlehem, PA, USA

Dustin Manchester Department of Thoracic Surgery, St. Luke's University Health Network, Bethlehem, PA, USA

Sai Mandalapu Department of General Surgery, St. Luke's University Health Network, Bethlehem, PA, USA

Hiren J. Mehta Division of Pulmonary, Critical Care & Sleep Medicine, University of Florida, Gainesville, FL, USA

Mohamed Ayman Mohamed Department of Pulmonary and Critical Care, McLaren Oakland Hospital, Pontiac, MI, USA

William J. Moore III Pulmonary/Critical Care Service, Department of Medicine, Brooke Army Medical Center, JBSA Fort Sam, Houston, TX, USA

Michael J. Morris Pulmonary/Critical Care Service, Department of Medicine, Brooke Army Medical Center, JBSA Fort Sam, Houston, TX, USA

Kaitlin Nguyen Department of General Surgery, St. Luke's University Health Network, Bethlehem, PA, USA

Michael Nicholson Department of Pulmonary and Critical Care Medicine, Robert Wood Johnson Barnabas Health, East Brunswick, NJ, USA

Emma Oskar Department of Internal Medicine, Temple University, Philadelphia, PA, USA

Jay Pescatore Department of Pulmonary and Critical Care, Baylor University Medical Center, Dallas, TX, USA

Samantha Pettigrew Department of Thoracic Medicine and Surgery, Temple University, Philadelphia, PA, USA

Anum Qadri Department of Pulmonary and Critical Care, Washington University School of Medicine, Saint Louis, MI, USA

Jay H. Ryu Division of Pulmonary and Critical Care Medicine, Department of Internal Medicine, Mayo Clinic, Rochester, MN, USA

Joshua M. Sill Department of Medicine, Pulmonary & Critical Care Division, Macon & Joan Brock Virginia Health Sciences, Eastern Virginia Medical School at Old Dominion University, Norfolk, VA, USA

Luke Simmons Department of Pulmonary and Critical Care Medicine, St. Luke's University Health Network, Bethlehem, PA, USA

Steven Tessier Department of Internal Medicine, Mayo Clinic, Rochester, MN, USA

Mohamed Turki Department of Pulmonary and Critical Care Medicine, St. Luke's University Health Network, Bethlehem, PA, USA

Toribiong Uchel Division of Pulmonary and Critical Care, Department of Internal Medicine, Virginia Commonwealth University, Richmond, VA, USA

Shuanzeng Wei Department of Pathology, Fox Chase Cancer Center, Philadelphia, PA, USA

Thomas Zanders Department of Pulmonary and Critical Care Medicine, St. Luke's University Health Network, Bethlehem, PA, USA

Matthew Zheng Department of Pulmonary and Critical Care Medicine, St. Luke's University Health Network, Bethlehem, PA, USA

Part I

The Normal Pleura

The Anatomy, Histology, and Physiology of the Normal Pleura

1

Livia Bratis, Leon Cedeno, and Firas Ido

Anatomy of the Pleura

The pleura is a thin, transparent serous membrane that lines structures within the thoracic cavity. The membrane is comprised of two contiguous layers [1]. The visceral layer, which encapsulates the lungs and extends into the interlobar fissures, reflects on itself at the root (hilum) of the lung, forming the parietal layer [2]. The parietal layer adheres to the inner chest wall, mediastinum, and diaphragm [1]. Descriptive terminology is used to specify different regions of the parietal pleura based on adjacent anatomic structures. The costal pleura lines the inner ribs, costal cartilage, and intercostal muscles. The diaphragmatic pleura lines the thoracic surface of the diaphragm. The mediastinal pleura covers the central compartment of the thoracic cavity, which includes portions of the great vessels, fibrous pericardium, and esophagus. The cervical pleura extends up to the apex of the lung, which is slightly superior to the first rib and, therefore, considered the root of the neck [3]. Beneath the pulmonary vasculature at the hilum, the visceral pleura folds on itself, extending caudally along the medial lower lobe and horizontally, posterior to the fibrous pericardium, forming a sheath-like triangular structure termed the inferior pulmonary ligament [1, 5]. This ligament merges with the diaphragmatic parietal pleura and helps stabilize the lower lobes during respiratory motion [6]. Between the two layers lies a potential space called the pleural space, which contains a small amount of fluid [4]. The pleural fluid acts as a lubricant, providing protection by preventing frictional irritation as the lungs expand against the chest wall during respiration [10]. In humans, no anatomic connection exists between the right and left pleural spaces [4]. Under normal physiological conditions, the pleural space is not visible. However, the accumulation of fluid or air, termed a pleural effusion and a pneumothorax, respectively, leads to separation of the two layers [2, 9]. During quiet respiration, the lungs do not entirely occupy the pleural cavity, leaving two areas devoid of lung tissue, referred to as the costomediastinal and costodiaphragmatic recesses [1]. The costodiaphragmatic recess, radiographically described as the costophrenic angle, is clinically significant when obliterated, suggesting fluid accumulation [5, 8].

L. Bratis (✉) · L. Cedeno · F. Ido
Department of Pulmonary and Critical Care Medicine, St. Luke's University Health Network, Bethlehem, PA, USA
e-mail: Livia.bratis@sluhn.org; Leon.Cedeno@sluhn.org; firas.ido@sluhn.org

F. Ido (ed.), *Rare Pleural Diseases*, https://doi.org/10.1007/978-3-032-14873-5_1

Pleural Vasculature

Although the parietal and visceral layers of the pleura are continuous with one another, each possesses a distinct vascular supply. The parietal pleura derives its blood supply entirely from the systemic circulation, with regional variations depending on its anatomic location [11]. The costal pleura is supplied by the intercostal and internal mammary arteries, both of which branch from the internal thoracic artery. The mediastinal pleura receives blood from the bronchial, internal mammary, and superior diaphragmatic arteries. In contrast, the diaphragmatic pleura is perfused by branches of the internal mammary artery and the aorta, including the posterior mediastinal and inferior phrenic arteries. The cervical pleura derives its arterial supply from the subclavian artery [12]. Venous drainage from the parietal pleura occurs primarily through the internal thoracic, intercostal, and phrenic veins, which converge into the azygos and hemiazygos systems before ultimately emptying into the superior vena cava. In contrast, venous return from the diaphragmatic pleura follows a separate pathway, draining via the inferior phrenic veins into the inferior vena cava [12]. The visceral pleura receives its arterial blood supply primarily from the bronchial arteries, which arise directly from the thoracic aorta. Venous drainage from the visceral pleura occurs predominantly through the pulmonary veins, which convey oxygenated blood directly into the left atrium [4, 12].

Pleural Lymphatics

The lymphatic drainage of the pleura occurs predominantly through the parietal pleura [16]. To prevent accumulation of pleural fluid, the lymphatic system removes excess liquid from the pleural space via bulk flow through specialized openings known as lymphatic stomata, or "pores," located primarily along the ventral and caudal regions of the parietal pleura [14, 16, 17]. A smaller number of stomata are situated in the ventral-cranial regions [16]. The lymphatic vessels originating from the parietal pleura drain into the intercostal, parasternal, diaphragmatic, and mediastinal lymph nodes. From these nodal groups, efferent vessels converge into the thoracic duct, which serves as the principal conduit for lymphatic return [17]. The stomata of the parietal pleura can accommodate particles as large as erythrocytes and represent a major exit pathway for fluid clearance from the pleural cavity; after passing through the thoracic duct, pleural fluid enters the systemic venous circulation via the left subclavian vein [17]. The visceral pleura, in contrast, lacks lymphatic stomata and has no direct communication between its lymphatic network and the pleural space. The visceral lymphatics are continuous with the pulmonary interstitium and drain centripetally toward the pulmonary hilum, where they empty into the tracheobronchial lymph nodes, and subsequently into the thoracic duct on the left and the right lymphatic duct on the right. There is, however, a notable variation in the visceral lymphatic drainage of the left lung. While the left upper lobe follows the typical pattern, draining into the left thoracic duct, the left lower lobe most commonly crosses the mediastinum, draining into the right tracheobronchial lymph nodes and then into the right lymphatic duct. This cross-communication reflects a necessary anatomic adaptation in left-sided lymphatic flow and has implications for disease spread across the midline [20]. Lymphatic fluid is propelled by the muscular contraction of the vessels and extrinsic contributions from respiration [21]. The lymphatics also contain one-way valves preventing reverse flow [19].

Pleural Nerve Innervation

Both the parietal and visceral pleura receive innervation from the autonomic nervous system; however, their sensory distributions differ markedly. The parietal pleura is richly supplied with somatic sensory fibers, which are absent in the visceral pleura, accounting for its sensitivity to pain, touch, and temperature. Pain fibers to the costal and peripheral pleura arise from the intercostal nerves, explaining why pleuritic pain is often well localized and referred to the corresponding chest-wall area. The diaphragmatic pleura, innervated primarily by the phrenic nerve (C3–C5), may refer pain to the ipsilateral shoulder or neck due to shared cervical roots. In contrast, the visceral pleura lacks somatic innervation and is insensitive to pain. It is supplied by autonomic fibers via the pulmonary plexus, derived from the Vagus (parasympathetic) nerve and the sympathetic trunk. It responds only to stretch or tension, not to pain stimuli [4, 22].

Pleural Histology

The total thickness of the pleura ranges from 0.2 to 0.4 mm, with the parietal pleura constituting most of this thickness [23, 28, 30]. The parietal layer contains a fibroelastic framework capable of withstanding traction, whereas the visceral pleura is thinner, approximately 15–35 μm, and extends into the interlobar fissures. The visceral pleura cannot be separated from the lung parenchyma because of the direct integration of its elastic and fibrous tissue with the underlying alveolar interstitium. Beneath the mesothelial layer of the visceral pleura, a submesothelial connective-tissue network known as the peripheral fiber system anchors within the visceral pleura and extends through the interlobular septa into the lung parenchyma, providing structural reinforcement [28, 30]. These fibers connect to the axial fiber system of the lung, which courses centrally toward the hilum. This continuity between the visceral pleura and pulmonary connective tissue plays a vital role in elastic recoil during respiration [10, 28, 30]. Microscopically, the visceral and parietal pleura differ in both architecture and function. Each is composed of a single layer of mesothelial cells resting upon a thin basement membrane of collagen and elastin. Mesothelial cells are specialized epithelial cells capable of changing shape from flattened to cuboidal or columnar in response to local mechanical stress [23, 28]. Their apical microvilli markedly increase surface area for the absorption of fluid and electrolytes and trap hyaluronic acid, which acts as a lubricant, minimizing friction during respiratory movements [24, 25]. In addition to their mechanical role, mesothelial cells actively synthesize extracellular-matrix components, cytokines, growth factors, and chemotactic peptides [26]. Among the secreted mediators are IL-1β, IL-6, TNF-α, IL-8, and VEGF, essential to inflammation and tissue repair [27]. The cytoskeletal architecture of mesothelial cells, comprising actin and intermediate filament networks, helps balance tension and compression to maintain structural integrity [15]. This model explains how the pleura withstands repetitive stress and translates mechanical forces into biochemical signals that regulate mesothelial function [15]. Mesothelial cells are connected through tight junctions, gap junctions, and desmosomes and may overlap during quiet exhalation [28]. Tight junctions restrict paracellular permeability, preserving barrier integrity, while gap junctions permit intercellular exchange of ions and signaling molecules. Desmosomes provide robust mechanical adhesion between adjacent mesothelial cells, maintaining cohesion during respiratory motion [29]. Beneath the mesothelium lies a fibroelastic sublayer containing collagen fibers, elastic tissue, small vessels, and lymphatic channels. The visceral pleura consists of five layers: the mesothelial layer, a thin connective-tissue layer, a superficial elastic layer, a loose subpleural connective-tissue layer, and a deep fibroelastic layer (Fig. 1.1a and b) [30]. In contrast, the parietal pleura comprises two layers: the mesothelium and a thick fibroelastic connective-tissue layer (Fig. 1.1c). Development of the pleural cavity occurs between the fourth and seventh weeks of gestation. The intraembryonic coelom, arising from the lateral plate mesoderm, forms the pleural, pericardial, and peritoneal cavities; both pleural layers derive from this mesoderm [41].

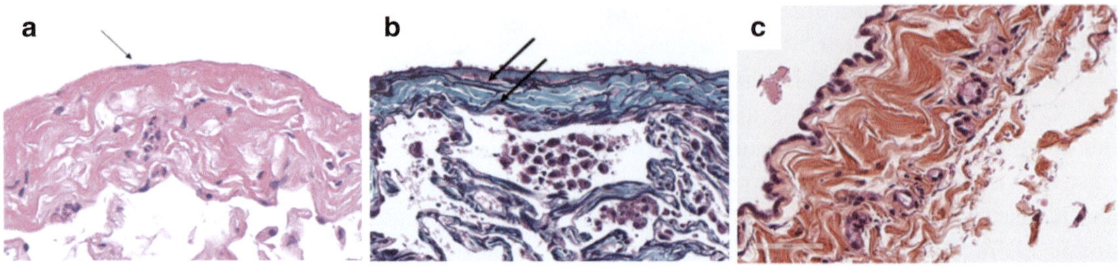

Fig. 1.1 Histologic features of the normal pleura. (**a**) Normal visceral pleura composed of a single layer of flattened mesothelial cells (arrow indicates nucleus) overlying submesothelial connective tissue (hematoxylin and eosin stain; ×500). (**b**) Normal visceral pleura demonstrating two distinct elastic layers, shown in black. The upper arrow indicates the outer elastic layer, and the lower arrow indicates the inner elastic layer (elastic trichrome stain; ×500). (**c**) Normal parietal pleura showing a single layer of mesothelial cells on the left side of the image, underlain by a thin layer of connective tissue (hematoxylin, eosin, and saffron stain; ×400)

Pleural Physiology

One of the primary functions of the pleura is to preserve lung shape and ensure smooth motion within the thoracic cavity during inspiration and expiration [7, 32]. The connective-tissue framework of both surfaces distributes mechanical stress evenly, limiting exaggerated expansion and minimizing injury. This elastic network also facilitates passive lung deflation and protects alveoli and pleural microvessels [7, 32, 33]. The pressure within the pleural cavity is consistently negative relative to atmospheric pressure, creating the gradient that drives airflow [34]. At functional residual capacity (FRC), intrapulmonary pressure approximates atmospheric pressure, while intrapleural pressure averages −5 cm H_2O; at total lung capacity (TLC), it reaches −30 cm H_2O. The difference between intrapulmonary and intrapleural pressures, termed the transpulmonary pressure, maintains airway patency and facilitates inflation. This negative pressure results from opposing elastic forces: the inward recoil of the lungs and the outward recoil of the chest wall [35]. Pleural pressure becomes more negative whenever these elastic forces intensify. In noncompliant lungs due to fibrosis, edema, or fluid accumulation, increased inward recoil further decreases pleural pressure. Similarly, enhanced chest-wall recoil, as seen in restrictive conditions such as obesity or circumferential burns, accentuates this negativity. Beyond mechanical factors, the cohesive surface tension of pleural fluid contributes significantly to maintaining negative intrapleural pressure and ensuring apposition of the visceral and parietal pleura [36]. Despite its subatmospheric pressure, the pleural space remains gas-free. Gas diffusion across pleural membranes follows partial-pressure gradients, moving from higher to lower total pressure. Because the sum of partial pressures in pleural capillaries and interstitial fluid is slightly lower than that in the pleural space, diffusion proceeds outward, maintaining a gas-free cavity [17, 37]. Another vital pleural function is the production and regulation of a thin, lubricating fluid layer, which enables frictionless gliding of the surfaces [38]. The cohesive forces of this liquid effectively "couple" the lung to the chest wall, allowing synchronous motion without shear separation. Both recoil forces and surface tension contribute to this mutual traction [17, 39]. Finally, pleural fluid homeostasis is governed by Starling forces, which balance hydrostatic and oncotic pressures across the pleural capillaries. Continuous turnover maintains equilibrium between formation and absorption, ensuring a constant fluid film and sustaining negative pressure, both of which are essential to coupling chest-wall mechanics to lung expansion [10, 40].

Pleural Fluid

The pleura plays an essential role in the production, regulation, and absorption of pleural fluid, which serves as a lubricant to minimize friction between the lung and surrounding structures such as the chest wall, diaphragm, and mediastinum. The dynamics of pleural fluid formation and absorption are complex and challenging to study directly because of the narrowness of the pleural space and its sensitivity to inflammation.

Under normal physiological conditions, pleural fluid originates predominantly from the systemic capillaries of the parietal pleura and, to a lesser extent, from the visceral pleura [42]. The parietal pleural microvessels are closer to the pleural space (10–15 μm) than the visceral bronchial microvessels (20–50 μm), facilitating more efficient transudation [43]. Fluid movement across the pleura depends on the balance between hydrostatic and oncotic pressures within the microvasculature and pleural space, a relationship governed by Starling's forces [44]. The resulting net driving pressure favors fluid movement from the capillaries into the pleural space, mainly across the parietal pleura, where filtration pressure is greater than in the visceral layer [42–44].

Pleural fluid absorption occurs primarily through lymphatic stomata located on the parietal pleural surface [45]. These openings connect directly to submesothelial lymphatic channels that actively remove protein-rich fluid and particles. Although an absorptive pressure gradient between the pleural space and lymphatic vessels (approximately −7 cm H_2O) favors drainage when pleural pressure rises, the predominant mechanism of lymphatic outflow is rhythmic contraction of lymphatic smooth muscle coupled with ventilatory and cardiac motion [45, 46]. These active contractions are critical because the intrinsic pressure gradient within the pleural cavity would otherwise favor filtration into, rather than out of, the space [47].

At functional residual capacity, pleural pressure averages approximately −4 mmHg, while interstitial pressure within pleural tissue is about −1 mmHg. This pressure differential, along with the pleural membranes' high permeability, favors slow fluid entry into the pleural cavity. The estimated turnover rate is approximately 0.01–0.02 mL/kg/h, corresponding to a flow rate of about 0.5 mL/h in and out of the pleural space [48]. Pleural pressure gradients vary slightly with height (approximately 0.5 cm H_2O per cm vertical distance), favoring the gradual downward flow of fluid from the apex to the base [48].

In healthy individuals, the pleural cavity contains approximately 10–20 mL of clear, straw-colored ultrafiltrate derived mainly from parietal pleural capillaries [49]. The fluid is rich in hyaluronic acid, a lubricating glycosaminoglycan synthesized by mesothelial cells [49]. Its electrolyte composition resembles plasma, with comparable concentrations of sodium, potassium, and glucose, but slightly higher chloride and bicarbonate levels, which account for the normal pleural pH of 7.60–7.64, marginally higher than serum [50, 51].

Normal pleural fluid contains very few cells—approximately <1000 cells/mm^3, comprising about 75% macrophages, 23% lymphocytes, and 1–2% mesothelial cells, with rare or absent neutrophils and eosinophils [52, 53]. Red blood cell counts average fewer than 40 cells/μL [52]. Total protein concentration is typically <1.5 g/dL (predominantly albumin), and LDH activity is less than 50% of serum LDH [53]. Understanding these normal biochemical parameters is essential for clinical interpretation of pleural fluid analysis.

Because normal pleural fluid is an ultrafiltrate of plasma, its biochemical composition mirrors serum values in volume-overload states, producing transudates with low protein and LDH levels. In contrast, increased vascular permeability or mesothelial injury elevates these levels, producing exudative effusions. This distinction underlies Light's criteria, a diagnostic tool that distinguishes transudates from exudates using protein and LDH ratios [54]. Recognition of these physiological principles is critical for interpreting pleural fluid findings and diagnosing pleural disease.

Acknowledgment The authors thank *Dr. Henry Tazelaar*, Pathologist, Mayo Clinic, for his contribution to the histologic images and their corresponding descriptions.

References

1. Wang NS. Anatomy of the pleura. Clin Chest Med. 1998;19(2):229–40.
2. Ilsen B, Vandenbroucke F, Beigelman-Aubry C, Brussaard C, de Mey J. Comparative interpretation of CT and standard radiography of the pleura. J Belg Soc Radiol. 2016;100(1):1–7.
3. Díaz-Jiménez JP, Rodríguez AN. Interventions in pulmonary medicine. Cham: Springer; 2023.
4. Charalampidis C, Youroukou A, Lazaridis G, Baka S, Mpoukovinas I, Karavasilis V, et al. Pleural space anatomy. J Thorac Dis. 2015;7(Suppl 1):S27–32.
5. Bertin F, Deslauriers J. Anatomy of the pleura: reflection lines and recesses. Thorac Surg Clin. 2011;21(2):165–71.
6. Rabinowitz JG, Wolf BS. Roentgen significance of the pulmonary ligament. Radiology. 1966;87(6):1013–20.
7. Choi YW, Shepard JAO, Kim J, Jeon SC, Park CK, Heo JN, et al. Left costomediastinal recess of the pleura: the potential pleural space anterior to the heart. J Comput Assist Tomogr. 2011;35(1):135–40.
8. Rudikoff JC. Early detection of pleural fluid. Chest. 1980;77(1):109–11.
9. Zarogoulidis P, Kioumis I, Pitsiou G, Porpodis K, Lampaki S, Papaiwannou A, et al. Pneumothorax: from definition to diagnosis and treatment. J Thorac Dis. 2014;6(Suppl 4):S372–6.
10. Ferreiro L, Toubes ME, Suárez-Antelo J, Rodríguez-Núñez N, Valdés L. Clinical overview of the physiology and pathophysiology of pleural fluid movement: a narrative review. ERJ Open Res. 2024;10(5):00523–2024.
11. Karpathiou G, Péoc'h M, Sundaralingam A, Rahman N, Froudarakis ME. Inflammation of the pleural cavity: pathogenesis, diagnosis, and implications in tumor pathophysiology. Cancers (Basel). 2022;14(6):1415.
12. Lee YCG, Clelland CA, Rahman NM. The pleural cavity. In: Laurent GJ, Shapiro SD, editors. Encyclopedia of respiratory diseases. Oxford: Academic Press; 2006. p. 397–402. https://doi.org/10.1016/B0-12-370879-6/00508-1.
13. Friedberg JS. Pleura: anatomy, physiology, and disorders. In: Essential practice of surgery. New York: Springer; 2003. p. 641–54. https://doi.org/10.1007/0-387-22744-X_41.
14. Albertine KH, Wiener-Kronish JP, Staub NC. The structure of the parietal pleura and its relationship to pleural liquid dynamics in sheep. Anat Rec. 1984;208(3):401–9.
15. Ingber DE, Wang N, Stamenović D. Tensegrity, cellular biophysics, and the mechanics of living systems. Rep Prog Phys. 2014;77(4):046603. https://doi.org/10.1088/0034-4885/77/4/046603.
16. Shinohara H. Distribution of lymphatic stomata on the pleural surface of the thoracic cavity. Anat Rec. 1997;249:16–23.
17. Negrini D. Pleural function and lymphatics. Acta Physiol (Oxf). 2013;209(2):244–59.
18. Ellis H. Clinical Anatomy. 11th ed. Oxford: Blackwell; 2006.
19. Okiemy G, Ele N, et al. Lymphatic drainage of intertracheobronchial lymph nodes. Mali Med. 2008;23:34–7.
20. Neef H. Anatomical pathways of lymphatic flow between lung and mediastinum. Ann Ital Chir. 1999;70(6):857–66.
21. Negrini D, Ballard ST, Benoit JN. Contribution of lymphatic myogenic activity and respiratory movements to pleural lymph flow. J Appl Physiol (1985). 1994;76(6):2267–74.
22. Brims FJ, Davies HE, Lee YC. Respiratory chest pain: diagnosis and treatment. Med Clin North Am. 2010;94(2):217–32.
23. Wang NS. Anatomy and physiology of the pleural space. Clin Chest Med. 1985;6(1):3–16.
24. Light RW, Lee YCG, editors. Textbook of pleural diseases. 3rd ed. Boca Raton: CRC Press; 2016.
25. Jantz MA, Antony VB. Pathophysiology of the pleura. Respiration. 2008;75(2):121–33. https://doi.org/10.1159/000113629.
26. Acencio MMP, Silva BR, Teixeira LR, Alvarenga VA, Rocha Silva CS, Pereira da Silva AG, et al. Evaluation of cellular alterations and inflammatory profile of mesothelial and/or neoplastic cells exposed to talc used for pleurodesis. Oncotarget. 2020;11(41):3730–6.
27. Mutsaers SE. The mesothelial cell. Int J Biochem Cell Biol. 2004;36(1):9–16. https://doi.org/10.1016/S1357-2725(03)00242-5.
28. Markov AG, Amasheh S. Tight junction physiology of pleural mesothelium. Front Physiol. 2014;5:221. https://doi.org/10.3389/fphys.2014.00221.

29. Tomashefski JF, Cagle PT. Farver CF. In: Fraire AE, editor. Dail and Hammar's pulmonary pathology. Volume 1: nonneoplastic lung disease. New York: Springer; 2008. ISBN:9780387983950.
30. Broaddus VC, Wiener-Kronish JP, Berthiaume Y, Staub NC. Removal of pleural liquid and protein by lymphatics in awake sheep. J Appl Physiol (1985). 1988;64(1):384–90.
31. Broaddus VC, Ernst JD, King TE Jr, Lazarus SC, Sarmiento KF, Schnapp LM, et al., editors. Murray & Nadel's textbook of respiratory medicine. 7th ed. Philadelphia: Elsevier; 2021.
32. Noppen M, De Waele M, Li R, Van Gucht K, D'Haese J, Gerlo E, et al. Volume and cellular content of normal pleural fluid in humans examined by pleural lavage. Am J Respir Crit Care Med. 2000;162(3 Pt 1):1023–6.
33. Feher JJ. The mechanics of breathing. In: Quantitative human physiology: an introduction. Amsterdam: Elsevier; 2012. p. 623–32.
34. Agostoni E. Mechanics of the pleural space. Physiol Rev. 1972;52(1):57–128.
35. Hills BA. The pleural interface. Thorax. 1985;40(1):1–8. https://doi.org/10.1136/thx.40.1.1.
36. Ivezić Z, Kurbel S, Škrinjarić-Cincar S, Radić R. Resorption of gas trapped in body cavities: comparison of alveolar and pleural space. Adv Physiol Educ. 2006;30(1):30–2.
37. Smith ML, Leslie KO, Wick MR. Practical pulmonary pathology: A volume in the pattern recognition series. 3rd ed. Philadelphia: Elsevier; 2022.
38. Clements JA. Lung surface tension and surfactant: the early years. In: West JB, editor. Respiratory physiology: people and ideas. New York: Springer; 1996. p. 121–38.
39. Knudsen L, Ochs M. The micromechanics of lung alveoli: structure and function of surfactant and tissue components. Histochem Cell Biol. 2018;150(6):661–76. https://doi.org/10.1007/s00418-018-1747-9.
40. Moore KL, Dalley AF, Agur AMR. Clinically oriented anatomy. 9th ed. Philadelphia: Wolters Kluwer; 2023.
41. Zocchi L. Mechanics of the pleural space. Respir Physiol Neurobiol. 2002;131(3):179–201. https://doi.org/10.1016/S1569-9048(02)00041-6.
42. Staub NC. Transport through the pleura: physiology of normal liquid and solute exchange in the pleural space. New York: Marcel Dekker; 1985.
43. Miserocchi G, Negrini D, Mariani E, Passafaro M. Reabsorption of a saline- or plasma-induced hydrothorax. J Appl Physiol (1985). 1983;54(6):1574–1578. doi:https://doi.org/10.1152/jappl.1983.54.6.1574.
44. Lai-Fook SJ. Pleural mechanics and fluid exchange. Physiol Rev. 2004;84(2):385–410. https://doi.org/10.1152/physrev.00020.2003.
45. Zocchi L. Physiology and pathophysiology of pleural fluid turnover. Eur Respir J. 2002;20(6):1545–58. https://doi.org/10.1183/09031936.02.00403202.
46. von der Weid PY, Zawieja DC. Lymphatic smooth muscle: the motor unit of lymph drainage. Int J Biochem Cell Biol. 2004;36(7):1147–53. https://doi.org/10.1016/j.biocel.2003.12.008.
47. Wiener-Kronish JP, Broaddus VC, Albertine KH, Staub NC. Pleural liquid pressure and flow during pulmonary edema. J Appl Physiol (1985). 1984;56(2):459–63. https://doi.org/10.1152/jappl.1984.56.2.459.
48. Lai YL, Wiener-Kronish JP, Staub NC. Distribution of pleural liquid thickness in dogs. J Appl Physiol (1985). 1991;70(3):967–73. https://doi.org/10.1152/jappl.1991.70.3.967.
49. Yoshino Y, Koga H, Fukuoka M, Miyazaki M, Koga T. Hyaluronic acid concentration in pleural fluid: a diagnostic aid for tuberculous pleurisy. J Clin Med Res. 2015;7(1):20–4. https://doi.org/10.14740/jocmr1948w.
50. Sahn SA. Getting the most from pleural analysis. Respir Med. 2011;105(2):186–93. https://doi.org/10.1016/j.rmed.2010.10.014.
51. Kataoka H. Electrolyte composition and pH of pleural effusions. Chest. 2018;154(4):908–16. https://doi.org/10.1016/j.chest.2018.04.013.
52. Broaddus VC, Light RW. Pleural effusion. In: Broaddus VC, Mason RJ, Ernst JD, editors. Murray & Nadel's textbook of respiratory medicine. 6th ed. Philadelphia: Elsevier; 2016. p. 1858–1879.
53. Noppen M. Normal volume and cellular contents of pleural fluid. Paediatr Respir Rev. 2004;5(Suppl 1):S335–7. https://doi.org/10.1016/j.prrv.2004.04.017.
54. Light RW. Useful tests on pleural fluid in the management of patients with pleural effusions. Curr Opin Pulm Med. 1999;5(4):245–9. https://doi.org/10.1097/00063198-199907000-00006.

Part II

Non-neoplastic Rare Pleural Diseases

2 Fibrothorax

Sai Mandalapu, Dustin Manchester, and Firas Ido

Introduction

Fibrothorax is the replacement or obliteration of the pleural space by scar tissue. It is considered the most severe form of pleural fibrosis. The condition can occur due to undrained infected or non-infected pleural fluid, or direct pleural injury that leads to the deposition of dense connective tissue within the pleural space [1]. Over time, the healing process leads to chronic progressive pleural fibrosis and eventual fusion of the visceral and parietal pleura. Subsequently, this results in contracture and loss of volume of the affected lung, which translates clinically to restrictive lung disease [2, 3]. The exact definition of a fibrothorax is somewhat unclear. However, one proposed definition includes a pleural thickness greater than 5 mm that spans contiguously at least 8 cm vertically and 5 cm laterally. Another definition is the presence of pleural thickening involving at least 25% of the pleura in bilateral cases, or 50% when only one hemithorax is affected [4].

Epidemiology, Risk Factors, and Associated Disease

The causes of fibrothorax are numerous and include infection, pleural irritants, autoimmune diseases, systemic illnesses, specific medications, and environmental exposures (Table 2.1).

Given the vast number of etiologies, compiling epidemiologic data is challenging. Two of the most frequently cited causes of fibrothorax include chronic empyema and hemothorax [20, 21]. In the 19th and early 20th centuries, fibrothorax was primarily associated with chronic tuberculous (TB) empyema, especially in untreated cases [22]. Tuberculous pleural involvement has been estimated to occur in 3–5% of cases in the US, but up to 30% in resource-poor endemic areas. Pleural thickening or fibrothorax as a complication of TB pleural involvement ranges between 5% and 50% [24, 25]. Despite completing treatment, radiologic evidence of pleural fibrosis or pleural thickening was still present in about 23% and 20%, respectively [26]. The overall prevalence of fibrothorax following an empyema occurs in about 8% of cases [27]. In cases of retained hemothorax, the occurrence of fibrothorax ranges from 1% to 30%, with a higher inci-

S. Mandalapu
Department of General Surgery, St. Luke's University Health Network, Bethlehem, PA, USA
e-mail: sai.mandalapu@sluhn.org

D. Manchester (✉)
Department of Thoracic Surgery, St. Luke's University Health Network, Bethlehem, PA, USA
e-mail: Dustin.manchester@sluhn.org

F. Ido
Department of Pulmonary and Critical Care Medicine, St. Luke's University Health Network, Bethlehem, PA, USA
e-mail: firas.ido@sluhn.org

F. Ido (ed.), *Rare Pleural Diseases*, https://doi.org/10.1007/978-3-032-14873-5_2

Table 2.1 Etiologies of Fibrothorax

Infectious	Empyema [5], tuberculosis [6], paragonimiasis [7]
Pleural irritants	Pleural effusion [8], hemothorax, chylothorax, pneumothorax [7], therapeutic pleurodesis [9], ventriculopleural shunt [10], foreign body [11]
Autoimmune	Rheumatoid arthritis [12], systemic lupus erythematosus [13], IgG-4 related [14], familial Mediterranean fever [15]
Systemic	Uremia [7], malignancy (e.g., non-small-cell lung adenocarcinoma) [16], Erdheim-Chester disease [17], nephrogenic systemic fibrosis [18]
Drug-related	Ergot alkaloids bromocriptine [7], dasatinib [19], methysergide [20], pergolide [21]
Environmental	Asbestosis [7], silicosis [22]
Other	Idiopathic [7], pleuroparenchymal fibroelastosis [23]

dence in cases that fail tube thoracostomy drainage [3, 28].

Pathophysiology

Following damage to the pleura, the release of a potent chemokine, such as interleukin-8 (IL-8), recruits macrophages and neutrophils to the site of injury [29, 30]. Other cytokines, such as TNF-α and IFN-γ, also stimulate the expression of cell adhesion molecules, which facilitate the translocation of pro-inflammatory immune cells into the pleural space [29, 31]. A procoagulant, tissue factor, is also released into the pleural space, driving the cascade that leads to fibrin formation and deposition [31]. As the inflammatory process progresses, the expression of VEGF enables the onset of angiogenesis. This, along with TGF-β, a potent chemoattractant for fibroblasts, plays a key role in the repair process and promotes the deposition of a collagen matrix within the pleural space [7, 29].

The encircling pleural scar, which fuses the visceral and parietal pleura, may cause contracture of the affected lung, limit movement of the diaphragm, and thus impair expansion during respiration. These changes result in physiologic changes that can be observed on pulmonary function testing as a proportional reduction in the forced expiratory volume during the first second (FEV1) and forced vital capacity (FVC). In addition, the vital capacity (VC) and total lung capacity (TLC) are also significantly reduced, all of which signify the presence of restrictive lung disease [30]. The diffusion capacity for carbon monoxide (DLco) is often decreased; however, this may be normal when corrected for the reduction in lung volume, suggesting an extrapulmonary restrictive nature to the disease [31]. The flow-volume loop will typically appear diminished in size in all dimensions while maintaining a normal shape [32].

The external compression on the lung parenchyma by the thickened scar may also be transmitted to the pulmonary vasculature, resulting in decreased lung perfusion and precapillary pulmonary hypertension, although this is not well documented [33]. Severe or bilateral disease can result in hypoxia, hypercarbia, pulmonary hypertension, and cor pulmonale [34].

Clinical Features

The symptoms of fibrothorax are nonspecific. The most common complaint is chronic dyspnea. Additional symptoms include chest tightness, chest pain, nonproductive cough, and fatigue [4]. Exam findings include limited excursion of the affected hemithorax, dullness to percussion, and diminished breath sounds [35].

Diagnosis

Imaging

Radiological evaluation is very helpful in diagnosing a fibrothorax. A chest x-ray can reveal pleural thickening, decreased unilateral volume of the affected hemithorax, and elevation of the

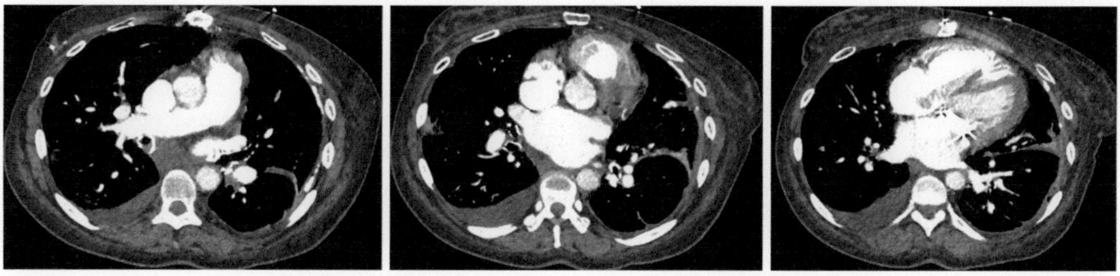

Fig. 2.1 Axial computed tomography images of the chest demonstrating a chronic fibrothorax of the left hemithorax that developed years after a retained hemothorax following coronary artery bypass grafting. The multilevel axial sections (left, middle, and right panels) show circumferential pleural thickening with scattered calcifications and hemithoracic contracture. A small right-sided pleural effusion is also visible

ipsilateral diaphragm. In contrast to apical caps, fibrothorax tends to involve the lower lateral chest wall, the diaphragmatic surface, and the obliteration of the costophrenic sulcus, reflecting areas of prior fluid accumulation. The pleural thickening typically appears as uniform, dependent radiodensities [36]. In more severe cases, the pleural thickening can extend superiorly.

Computed tomography (CT) of the thorax can accurately detect the presence of a fibrothorax. Findings include a regular uniform, circumferential pleural thickening with soft-tissue attenuation. This is in contrast to the irregular thickening that is often associated with mesothelioma. Additionally, CT can also help differentiate fibrothorax from pleural plaques, with the latter typically demonstrating focal pleural thickening that may be calcified and occasionally associated with adjacent rounded atelectasis (Fig. 2.1) [36, 37]. A "split pleura" sign refers to thickening of the visceral and parietal pleura separated by an area of fluid seen on contrast-enhanced CT and is suggestive of an empyema. This can also serve as an early indicator for the future development of a fibrothorax [38]. In cases of severe fibrothorax, additional CT findings include marked reduction in lung volume, elevation of the diaphragm, mediastinal shift toward the affected hemithorax, and extensive, scattered, or complete calcifications. Occasionally, despite complete pleural fluid drainage, the contracted lung due to a fibrothorax may fail to re-expand, termed a trapped lung [13, 39].

Treatment

Evacuation of hemothorax, empyema, or large pleural effusions allows the underlying lung to expand. This approach is paramount in preventing the development of fibrothorax. At times, chest tube thoracostomy may not fully drain pleural effusions, especially if loculated [40]. In addition, despite noninvasive pleural fluid drainage, a trapped lung may still occur [48]. Failure of thoracentesis or tube thoracostomy to achieve complete evacuation of the pleural fluid should prompt early thoracoscopy or video-assisted thoracic surgery (VATS) drainage, which enables drainage and debridement of the pleural space [41, 42].

Surgery

The mainstay treatment for fibrothorax is decortication. This surgical procedure can be performed via VATS or open thoracotomy to strip the fibrinous peel from the pleural surface. Currently, there is limited information regarding the exact indications and timing for decortication. In general, the procedure is mainly indicated in the case of significant symptoms and evidence of impaired lung function and restrictive lung disease [43, 44]. Data regarding pleural tuberculosis and traumatic hemothorax have shown that a vital capacity $\leq 70\%$ predicted can be considered a cut-off indicator for necessitating decortication [44].

Surgery consists of bluntly dissecting the peel in the plane between the endothoracic fascia and the parietal pleura. The thickened parietal peel is then incised to enter the pleural cavity, which is evacuated of fluid and debris. For visceral decortication, the plane of dissection is between the visceral pleura and the fibrous peel [45].

Nonsurgical Treatments

Minimal nonsurgical options exist for the treatment of fibrothorax. A single case of percutaneous intercostal percutaneous cryoneurolysis to treat symptoms of dyspnea and chronic chest pain in a poor surgical candidate has been documented [46]. Many ongoing studies are exploring novel targets for interventional therapy to prevent and even reverse pleural fibrosis, with targets under investigation including GSK-3β (glycogen synthase kinase 3β), DOCK2 (dedicator of cytokinesis 2), myocardin, EPCR (endothelial protein C receptor), NOX1 (NADPH oxidase 1), uPAR (urokinase plasminogen activator receptor), αβ crystallin, CSP7 (caveolin spanning peptide seven amino acid deletion fragment), and mTOR (mechanistic target of rapamycin) [47–59].

Prognosis

Untreated fibrothorax will result in persistent restrictive lung physiology. Progression is dependent on the underlying etiology and whether inflammation recurs [60]. Though there is no data on whether fibrothorax itself reduces life expectancy, there is evidence that its sequelae, such as restrictive lung disease and cor pulmonale, significantly shorten lifespan [61].

Several months following decortication, TLC and DLco have been shown to improve by an average of 10%. Vital capacity also improves by an average of 15% [60]. FEV1 can increase by up to 50–60% within the first year [62]. Both ventilation and perfusion of the affected lung have shown improvements following decortication of 30% and 20%, respectively [63]. Long-lasting improvements in dyspnea have been documented following decortication; however, lung function often does not return to predicted normal values [64].

The best predictor of improved pulmonary function after decortication is the absence of underlying parenchymal lung disease [60, 65, 66]. A shorter duration of pleural disease prior to intervention is also associated with improved results [65, 67]. Early decortication has been associated with a shorter postoperative course, a lower incidence of recurrence, and fewer complications [68, 69]. However, pulmonary function may still improve even when decortication has been performed years after the development of a fibrothorax [68, 70, 71].

Post-decortication 30-day mortality is estimated at 3–5% [72, 73]. In contrast to open thoracotomy, VATS has shown similar clinical outcomes but is associated with decreased morbidity and hospital length of stay [74, 75].

Attribution Original image courtesy of *Dr. Firas Ido*. This figure has not been previously published and is reproduced here with permission of the author.

References

1. Stefano E, Claudio S, Giampietro M, Stefano N, Natalia B. Chapter 12 – pneumonia and volume overload complicating chronic Fibrothorax with persistent fluid collection. In: Sorino C, Feller-Kopman D, Marchetti G, editors. Pleural Diseases. Philadelphia: Elsevier; 2022. p. 113–22.
2. Silva CIS, Müller NL. The teaching files: Chest. Saunders/Elsevier; 2010.
3. Zeiler J, Idell S, Norwood S, Cook A. Hemothorax: a review of the literature. Clin Pulm Med. 2020;27(1):1–12.
4. Sorino C, Feller-Kopman D, Marchetti G. Pleural diseases: clinical cases and real-world Discussions. Elsevier; 2021.
5. Søgaard M, Nielsen RB, Nørgaard M, Kornum JB, Schønheyder HC, Thomsen RW. Incidence, length of stay, and prognosis of hospitalized patients with pleural empyema: a 15-year Danish nationwide cohort study. Chest. 2014;145(1):189–92.
6. Choi JA, Hong KT, Oh YW, Chung MH, Seol HY, Kang EY. CT manifestations of late sequelae in patients with tuberculous pleuritis. AJR Am J Roentgenol. 2001;176(2):441–5.
7. Light RW, Lee YCG. 81 – Pneumothorax, Chylothorax, Hemothorax, and Fibrothorax. In: Broaddus VC,

Mason RJ, Ernst JD, King TE, Lazarus SC, Murray JF, et al., editors. Murray and Nadel's textbook of respiratory medicine. 6th ed. Philadelphia: W.B. Saunders; 2016. p. 1439–60.e10.
8. Karkhanis VS, Joshi JM. Pleural effusion: diagnosis, treatment, and management. Open Access Emerg Med. 2012;4:31–52.
9. Mierzejewski M, Korczynski P, Krenke R, Janssen JP. Chemical pleurodesis – a review of mechanisms involved in pleural space obliteration. Respir Res. 2019;20(1):247.
10. Khan TA, Khalil-Marzouk JF. Fibrothorax in adulthood caused by a cerebrospinal fluid shunt in the treatment of hydrocephalus. J Neurosurg. 2008;109(3):478–9.
11. Levine RL, Allen TC, Cartwright J Jr, Cagle PT. Silicone thorax due to a ruptured breast implant. Chest. 2005;127(5):1854–7.
12. Patel IA, Vahil N, Albrektson K, Griffin L. A 69-year-old man with rheumatoid arthritis and pleural effusion. CHEST Pulmonary. 2024;2(2):100057.
13. Alhassan S, Fasanya A, Thirumala R. Extensive calcified Fibrothorax. Am J Respir Crit Care Med. 2017;195(4):e25–e6.
14. Muller R, Ebbo M, Habert P, Daniel L, Briantais A, Chanez P, et al. Thoracic manifestations of IgG4-related disease. Respirology. 2023;28(2):120–31.
15. Ariad S, Sandbank J, Lupu L. Bronchoalveolar carcinoma in a patient with recurrent familial Mediterranean attacks, fibrothorax, and treatment with colchicine. Isr Med Assoc J. 1999;1(2):121–2.
16. Cesario A, Onorati D, Cardaci V, Margaritora S, Porziella V, Piraino A, et al. Symptom-free T4 lung cancer with bilateral pulmonary artery infiltration. Lancet Oncol. 2005;6(1):64.
17. Das JP, Xie L, Riedl CC, Hayes SA, Ginsberg MS, Halpenny DF. Cardiothoracic manifestations of Erdheim-Chester disease. Br J Radiol. 2019;92(1104):20190473.
18. Mansour J, Coleman C, Mendoza F, Lammi M, Saketkoo LA. Nephrogenic systemic fibrosis-related pulmonary restriction: an under-appreciated manifestation potentially reversible with imatinib therapy. J Scleroderma Relat Disord. 2022;7(3):Np7–np11.
19. Adrianza AM, Jimenez CA, Aldana GL, Pozo L, Cortes JE, Sagar AES. Tyrosine kinase inhibitor-associated Fibrothorax. Am J Respir Crit Care Med. 2019;199(11):1432.
20. V Courtney Broaddus Mason R. Murray & Nadel's textbook of respiratory medicine. 6th ed: Elsevier Saunders; 2016.
21. Bleumink GS, van der Molen-Eijgenraam M, Strijbos JH, Sanwikarja S, van Puijenbroek EP, Stricker BH. Pergolide-induced pleuropulmonary fibrosis. Clin Neuropharmacol. 2002;25(5):290–3.
22. Hoy RF, Chambers DC. Silica-related diseases in the modern world. Allergy. 2020;75(11):2805–17.
23. Watanabe K. Pleuroparenchymal Fibroelastosis: its clinical characteristics. Curr Respir Med Rev. 2013;9(4):299–37.
24. Vorster MJ, Allwood BW, Diacon AH, Koegelenberg CF. Tuberculous pleural effusions: advances and controversies. J Thorac Dis. 2015;7(6):981–91.
25. Barbas CS, Cukier A, de Varvalho CR, Barbas Filho JV, Light RW. The relationship between pleural fluid findings and the development of pleural thickening in patients with pleural tuberculosis. Chest. 1991;100(5):1264–7.
26. Tandon R, Agarwal A, Nirala P, Sinha A. Evaluation of radiological sequelae after treatment completion in new cases of pulmonary and pleural tuberculosis. Int J Mycobacteriol. 2021;10(4):398–404.
27. Alfageme I, Muñoz F, Peña N, Umbría S. Empyema of the thorax in adults. Etiology, microbiologic findings, and management. Chest. 1993;103(3):839–43.
28. Sherman RT, Pate JW. The role of intrapleural blood in fibrothorax. Am Surg. 1965;31:1–5.
29. Huggins JT, Sahn SA. Causes and management of pleural fibrosis. Respirology. 2004;9(4):441–7.
30. Liu CT, Cellerino A, Baldi S, Huang NQ, Tian YL, Rapellino M, et al. Pulmonary function in patients with pleural effusion of varying magnitude and fibrothorax. Panminerva Med. 1991;33(2):86–92.
31. Autio V. The reduction of respiratory function by parenchymal and pleural lesions. A bronchospirometric study of patients with unilateral involvement. Acta Tuberc Scand. 1959;37:112–25.
32. Bolliger CT, de Kock MA. Influence of a fibrothorax on the flow/volume curve. Respiration. 1988;54(3):197–200.
33. Ahmed AE, Ibrahim AS, Elshafie SM. Pulmonary hypertension in patients with treated pulmonary tuberculosis: analysis of 14 consecutive cases. Clin Med Insights Circ Respir Pulm Med. 2011;5:1–5.
34. Robin ED, Cross CE, Kroetz F, Totten RS, Bron K. Pulmonary hypertension and unilateral pleural constriction with speculation on pulmonary Vasoconstrictive substance. Arch Intern Med. 1966;118(4):391–400.
35. Sugarbaker DJ, Bueno R, Burt BM, Groth SS, Loor G, Wolf AS, et al. Sugarbaker's adult chest surgery, 3e. New York, NY: McGraw-Hill Education; 2020.
36. Maffessanti M, Bortolotto P, Grotto M. Imaging of pleural diseases. Monaldi Arch Chest Dis. 1996;51(2):138–44.
37. Roach HD, Davies GJ, Attanoos R, Crane M, Adams H, Phillips S. Asbestos: when the dust settles an imaging review of asbestos-related disease. Radiographics. 2002;22:S167–84.
38. Kraus GJ. The split pleura sign. Radiology. 2007;243(1):297–8.
39. Barosa M, Trindade M, Marques R. Trapped lung from calcified Fibrothorax. Acta Medica Port. 2022;35:915.
40. Huang HC, Chang HY, Chen CW, Lee CH, Hsiue TR. Predicting factors for outcome of tube thoracostomy in complicated parapneumonic effusion for empyema. Chest. 1999;115(3):751–6.
41. Angelillo Mackinlay TA, Lyons GA, Chimondeguy DJ, Piedras MA, Angaramo G, Emery J. VATS

debridement versus thoracotomy in the treatment of loculated postpneumonia empyema. Ann Thorac Surg. 1996;61(6):1626–30.
42. Cassina PC, Hauser M, Hillejan L, Greschuchna D, Stamatis G. Video-assisted thoracoscopy in the treatment of pleural empyema: stage-based management and outcome. J Thorac Cardiovasc Surg. 1999;117(2):234–8.
43. Sharma S, Smith R, Al-Hameed F. Fibrothorax and severe lung restriction secondary to lupus pleuritis and its successful treatment by pleurectomy. Can Respir J. 2002;9(5):335–7.
44. Lopez-Majano V, Joshi RC. Indications for decortication. Respiration. 1970;27(6):565–81.
45. Shields TW, LoCicero J III, Reed CE, Feins RH. General thoracic surgery. 7th ed. Lippincott Williams & Wilkins; 2009.
46. Delijani K, Wei B, Huang J. Percutaneous intercostal Cryoneurolysis in the Management of Symptomatic Fibrothorax. J Vasc Interv Radiol. 2023;34(2):305–7.
47. Tucker TA, Idell S. Update on novel targeted therapy for pleural organization and fibrosis. Int J Mol Sci. 2022;23(3):1587.
48. Logan R, Jeffers A, Qin W, Owens S, Chauhan P, Komatsu S, et al. TGF-β regulation of the uPA/uPAR axis modulates mesothelial-mesenchymal transition (MesoMT). Sci Rep. 2021;11(1):21210.
49. Tucker TA, Williams L, Koenig K, Kothari H, Komissarov AA, Florova G, et al. Lipoprotein receptor-related protein 1 regulates collagen 1 expression, proteolysis, and migration in human pleural mesothelial cells. Am J Respir Cell Mol Biol. 2012;46(2):196–206.
50. Qin W, Jeffers A, Owens S, Chauhan P, Komatsu S, Qian G, et al. NOX1 promotes mesothelial-mesenchymal transition through modulation of reactive oxygen species-mediated signaling. Am J Respir Cell Mol Biol. 2021;64(4):492–503.
51. Qian G, Adeyanju O, Roy S, Sunil C, Jeffers A, Guo X, et al. DOCK2 promotes pleural fibrosis by modulating mesothelial to mesenchymal transition. Am J Respir Cell Mol Biol. 2022;66(2):171–82.
52. Tucker T, Tsukasaki Y, Sakai T, Mitsuhashi S, Komatsu S, Jeffers A, et al. Myocardin is involved in mesothelial-mesenchymal transition of human pleural mesothelial cells. Am J Respir Cell Mol Biol. 2019;61(1):86–96.
53. Keshava S, Magisetty J, Tucker TA, Kujur W, Mulik S, Esmon CT, et al. Endothelial cell protein C receptor deficiency attenuates Streptococcus pneumoniae-induced pleural fibrosis. Am J Respir Cell Mol Biol. 2021;64(4):477–91.
54. Jeffers A, Qin W, Owens S, Koenig KB, Komatsu S, Giles FJ, et al. Glycogen synthase kinase-3β inhibition with 9-ING-41 attenuates the progression of pulmonary fibrosis. Sci Rep. 2019;9(1):18925.
55. Boren J, Shryock G, Fergis A, Jeffers A, Owens S, Qin W, et al. Inhibition of glycogen synthase kinase 3β blocks Mesomesenchymal transition and attenuates streptococcus pneumonia-mediated pleural injury in mice. Am J Pathol. 2017;187(11):2461–72.
56. Bellaye PS, Wettstein G, Burgy O, Besnard V, Joannes A, Colas J, et al. The small heat-shock protein αB-crystallin is essential for the nuclear localization of Smad4: impact on pulmonary fibrosis. J Pathol. 2014;232(4):458–72.
57. Marudamuthu AS, Bhandary YP, Fan L, Radhakrishnan V, MacKenzie B, Maier E, et al. Caveolin-1-derived peptide limits development of pulmonary fibrosis. Sci Transl Med. 2019;11(522)
58. Nagaraja MR, Tiwari N, Shetty SK, Marudamuthu AS, Fan L, Ostrom RS, et al. p53 expression in lung fibroblasts is linked to mitigation of fibrotic lung remodeling. Am J Pathol. 2018;188(10):2207–22.
59. Woodcock HV, Eley JD, Guillotin D, Platé M, Nanthakumar CB, Martufi M, et al. The mTORC1/4E-BP1 axis represents a critical signaling node during fibrogenesis. Nat Commun. 2019;10(1):6.
60. Siebens AA, Storey CF, Newman MM, Kent DC, Standard JE. The physiologic effects of fibrothorax and the functional results of surgical treatment. J Thorac Surg. 1956;32(1):53–73.
61. Syabbalo NC. How long do patients with cor pulmonale secondary to pulmonary fibrosis survive? Chest. 1991;99(1):263–4.
62. Rappaport JM, Siddiqui HU, Tang A, Thuita LW, Raja S, Bribriesco A, et al. Pleural space management after lung transplant: early and late outcomes of pleural decortication. J Heart Lung Transplant. 2021;40(7):623–30.
63. Nieminen MM, Antila P, Markkula H, Karvonen J. Effect of decortication in fibrothorax on pulmonary function. Respiration. 1985;48(1):94–6.
64. Rzyman W, Skokowski J, Romanowicz G, Lass P, Dziadziuszko R. Decortication in chronic pleural empyema – effect on lung function. Eur J Cardiothorac Surg. 2002;21(3):502–7.
65. Patton WE, Watson TR Jr, Gaensler EA. Pulmonary function before and at intervals after surgical decortication of the lung. Surg Gynecol Obstet. 1952;95(4):477–96.
66. Barker WL, Neuhaus H, Langston HT. Ventilatory improvement following decortication in pulmonary tuberculosis. Ann Thorac Surg. 1965;1:532–45.
67. Carroll D, Mc CJ, Himmelstein A, Cournand A. Pulmonary function following decortication of the lung. Am Rev Tuberc. 1951;63(3):231–51.
68. Petty TLFG, Mitchell RS. Objective functional improvement by decortication after twenty years of artificial pneumothorax for pulmonary tuberculosis. Am Reu Respir Dis. 1961;84:572.
69. Carey JA, Hamilton JR, Spencer DA, Gould K, Hasan A. Empyema thoracis: a role for open thoracotomy and decortication. Arch Dis Child. 1998;79(6):510–3.
70. Hughes RL, Jensik RJ, Faber LP, Bliss K. Evaluation of unilateral decortication. A patient successfully treated 44 years after onset of tuberculosis. Ann Thorac Surg. 1975;19(6):704–15.

71. Massard G, Rougé C, Wihlm JM, Ameur S, Dabbagh A, Kessler R, et al. Decortication is a valuable option for late empyema after collapse therapy. Ann Thorac Surg. 1995;60(4):888–95.
72. Towe CW, Carr SR, Donahue JM, Burrows WM, Perry Y, Kim S, et al. Morbidity and 30-day mortality after decortication for parapneumonic empyema and pleural effusion among patients in the Society of Thoracic Surgeons' general thoracic surgery database. J Thorac Cardiovasc Surg. 2019;157(3):1288–97.e4.
73. Zorbas KA, Abbas AE, Song KJ, Zorbas IA, Lois W, Burack JH. A simple prediction score for post-operative mortality after decortication. J Thorac Dis. 2023;15(12):6483–92.
74. Reichert M, Pösentrup B, Hecker A, Schneck E, Pons-Kühnemann J, Augustin F, et al. Thoracotomy versus video-assisted thoracoscopic surgery (VATS) in stage III empyema-an analysis of 217 consecutive patients. Surg Endosc. 2018;32(6):2664–75.
75. Shen KR. Current state of the art for the surgical management of empyema thoracis. J Thorac Cardiovasc Surg. 2019;157(3):1300–1.

3 Pleuroparenchymal Fibroelastosis

Jay Pescatore, Emma Oskar, and Shameek Gayen

Introduction

Pleuroparenchymal fibroelastosis (PPFE) is a progressive fibrotic lung disease characterized by scarring of the visceral pleura accompanied by marked deposition of elastic fibers in the adjacent subpleural parenchyma. The condition was first described in Japan by Amitani et al. in 1992, based on case reports that highlighted a distinctive pattern of predominant upper-lobe pulmonary fibrosis [1]. Subsequently, additional case reports and series consistently described similar upper-lobe-predominant fibrotic changes. In 2004, Frankel et al. formally introduced the term *pleuroparenchymal fibroelastosis* after analyzing five cases that could not be classified within any established category of interstitial lung disease (ILD). Radiographically, these cases demonstrated characteristic pleural and parenchymal involvement in the mid- to upper lung zones. Histopathological evaluation revealed uniform findings across all patients, including visceral pleural fibrosis, prominent subpleural fibroelastosis, sparing of deeper parenchymal regions distal to the pleura, and only minimal lymphoplasmacytic infiltrates or fibroblastic foci [2]. Over the following decade, as recognition of PPFE expanded, Thusthen et al. compiled and summarized all known cases, totaling 69 by 2013 [3]. That same year, the American Thoracic Society (ATS) and the European Respiratory Society (ERS) published their international, multidisciplinary classification of idiopathic interstitial pneumonias, formally designating PPFE as a distinct clinical and pathological entity [4].

Epidemiology

The true incidence and prevalence of PPFE remain unknown. This uncertainty is largely attributable to the novelty of the disease, the relatively recent establishment of formal diagnostic criteria, and the lack of uniform application across studies [5]. Although PPFE is classified by the American Thoracic Society and European Respiratory Society as a rare idiopathic interstitial pneumonia, emerging evidence suggests that its prevalence may be higher than initially recognized. In 2015, Nakatani et al. reviewed 205 surgical lung biopsies and determined that 5.9% met either definitive or consistent criteria for PPFE

J. Pescatore
Department of Pulmonary and Critical Care, Baylor University Medical Center, Dallas, TX, USA
e-mail: Jay.pescatore@bswhealth.org

E. Oskar
Department of Internal Medicine, Temple University, Philadelphia, PA, USA
e-mail: Emma.Oskar@tuhs.temple.edu

S. Gayen (✉)
Department of Thoracic Medicine and Surgery, Temple University, Philadelphia, PA, USA
e-mail: Shameek.Gayen@tuhs.temple.edu

F. Ido (ed.), *Rare Pleural Diseases*, https://doi.org/10.1007/978-3-032-14873-5_3

[6]. Similarly, in a single-center cohort of 375 patients with idiopathic interstitial pneumonia, the incidence of PPFE was reported as 7.7% [7].

The reported age at diagnosis ranges widely from 13 to 87 years, with a mean of approximately 53 years. A bimodal distribution has been described, with peaks in the third and sixth decades of life [8]. Gender distribution appears to be equal (1:1); however, female patients are often diagnosed at a younger age compared with their male counterparts [9]. These epidemiologic estimates are likely to evolve with the increasing use of high-resolution computed tomography (HRCT) and the growing recognition of PPFE as a distinct clinicopathologic entity.

Associated Diseases

PPFE has been described as either secondary to another disease process or idiopathic in the absence of any potential cause. Pleuroparenchymal fibroelastosis has been documented as a complication following hematopoietic stem cell (bone marrow) transplantation. The association was first described in 2011, when four post-transplant patients developed PPFE characterized by spontaneous pneumothoraces on imaging and subpleural fibrosis on histologic evaluation. The reported incidence in this setting was less than 1% [10, 11, 35]. PPFE has also been described following lung transplantation. In 2013, approximately 2% of lung transplant recipients were reported to exhibit upper-lobe-predominant fibrosis with histologic features consistent with PPFE. As recognition of this entity increased, subsequent studies in 2016 estimated the post-lung transplant incidence to be as high as 7.5% [11, 12].

The disease has further been associated with exposure to specific chemotherapeutic agents, particularly cyclophosphamide and carmustine [13–16]. Other proposed etiologic factors include chronic hypersensitivity pneumonitis, occupational exposure to silica, aluminum, and asbestos, as well as recurrent lower respiratory tract infections [17–19]. A strong association has also been observed with connective tissue diseases, such as systemic sclerosis and rheumatoid arthritis [20, 21]. Additionally, overlapping interstitial lung disease patterns, including fibrotic hypersensitivity pneumonitis, usual interstitial pneumonia (UIP), and nonspecific interstitial pneumonia (NSIP), are frequently identified in patients with PPFE [5, 19, 22, 23].

Familial/Genetic

There is increasing evidence to suggest a genetic predisposition in PPFE. Familial clustering has been described, including reports of siblings developing the disease. For example, two brothers were included in a seven-patient case series, and three sisters were diagnosed with PPFE across the 1980s and 1990s [24, 25]. Furthermore, individuals with a family history of ILD may be at heightened risk. In a 12-patient case study, two individuals reported a family history of ILD [19]. A separate case report described a 26-year-old man with PPFE whose father had died of idiopathic pulmonary fibrosis (IPF) [26]. Such familial patterns suggest that heritable factors may contribute to disease development and could account for the observation that some patients manifest PPFE decades earlier than typical presentations of other ILDs [27]. Genetic studies further support this hypothesis. Alrehaili et al. analyzed telomere length and genetic variants in six PPFE patients, finding that five (83%) had lymphocyte and granulocyte telomere lengths below the tenth percentile. Among these, four patients (80%) carried variants in telomere-related genes, including *telomerase reverse transcriptase* (*TERT*), *telomerase RNA component* (*TERC*), and *regulator of telomere elongation helicase 1* (*RTEL1*). In addition, one patient harbored a heterozygous *surfactant protein A2* (*SFTPA2*) variant; this same variant was also identified in a maternal first cousin diagnosed with usual interstitial pneumonia on lung biopsy rather than PPFE [28]. Another reported case described a PPFE patient with telomere length at the lower limit of normal and a pathogenic *TERT* variant [29].

Pathophysiology

Histologically, pleuroparenchymal fibroelastosis is characterized by intra-alveolar fibrosis with marked septal elastosis, a process that may be triggered by the disease associations discussed previously [8]. The condition is thought to arise as an aberrant interstitial inflammatory response to an inciting factor, leading to abnormal tissue repair marked by visceral and subpleural fibrosis, accompanied by excessive elastin deposition. The accumulation of collagen and elastic fibers results in contraction of the lung parenchyma, obliteration of distal bronchioles, and secondary post-obstructive atelectasis. The underlying mechanisms that drive this distinctive and irregular fibrotic repair process remain poorly understood [5, 31, 32].

Clinical Features

The most common presenting symptoms of pleuroparenchymal fibroelastosis include progressive dyspnea, dry cough, chest discomfort, and pleuritic chest pain. Systemic manifestations such as weight loss may also occur, though this typically represents a late finding and often develops months to years after radiographic evidence of disease has already appeared [5, 33].

On physical examination, patients frequently appear thin, with body mass index (BMI) values commonly ranging from 16 to 20 [33]. Auscultatory findings may be normal, though inspiratory crackles are occasionally detected. Digital clubbing is rare in PPFE, and its presence should prompt evaluation for alternative diagnoses. A distinctive physical feature of PPFE is platythorax, which results from a marked loss of upper-lobe volume, combined with reduced chest wall musculature and weight loss. These changes decrease the anteroposterior thoracic diameter, resulting in the flattening of the anterior chest wall. Associated findings include a deepened suprasternal notch and posterior retraction of the trachea [1, 5]. Importantly, PPFE is strongly associated with pneumothorax, which occurs in an estimated 60% of patients during their lifetime. Notably, many of these pneumothoraces are asymptomatic [34, 35].

Pulmonary function testing (PFT) can provide valuable diagnostic insights, though findings are neither highly sensitive nor specific for PPFE. Lung volumes typically demonstrate a restrictive pattern, with total lung capacity (TLC) below the lower limit of normal. A characteristic feature is an elevated residual volume (RV) to TLC ratio, attributable to several mechanisms: reduction in TLC from fibrotic remodeling of the upper lung parenchyma, increased elastic recoil secondary to abnormal elastin deposition, and a neuromuscular-like component related to sarcopenia of chest wall musculature [36]. In addition, compensatory hyperinflation of the lung bases contributes to the elevated RV/TLC ratio, with values $\geq$115% serving as a helpful discriminator between PPFE and idiopathic pulmonary fibrosis (IPF) [37]. Expected additional findings include reduced forced vital capacity (FVC) and decreased diffusion capacity for carbon monoxide (DLCO) [36, 38].

Differential Diagnoses

Pleuroparenchymal fibroelastosis shares clinical and radiographic features with several other pulmonary disorders, and careful exclusion of alternative diagnoses is essential. Idiopathic pulmonary fibrosis, for example, can mimic PPFE in the context of pleural and subpleural fibrosis. However, IPF is characterized by extensive lung remodeling with fibrosis that is heterogeneous, and primarily affects the lower lobes. Histopathologically, IPF demonstrates fibroblastic foci, marked architectural distortion with interspersed areas of preserved lung, and honeycombing [39]. IPF is also commonly associated with digital clubbing, which is rare in PPFE.

Fibrotic hypersensitivity pneumonitis (HP) may also present with upper-lobe-predominant fibrosis. Unlike PPFE, however, fibrotic HP frequently demonstrates poorly formed granulomas and bronchiocentric fibrosis extending beyond the subpleural parenchyma. Additional disorders that may mimic PPFE include asbestosis, fibrotic sarcoidosis, radiation-induced lung injury, and drug-induced lung toxicity. These conditions are distinguishable radiographically and, histologically, lack the defining intra-alveolar fibrosis with septal elastosis seen in PPFE. The presence of asbestos bodies or granulomas on histopathologic analysis should prompt consideration of an alternative diagnosis to PPFE [8].

Chronic fibrosis of organizing pneumonia (CFOP) shares some features with PPFE but is more heterogeneous, typically presenting with alveolar filling by granulation tissue plugs and patchy interstitial fibrosis. CFOP generally involves the lower lobes with a peribronchovascular distribution, whereas PPFE exhibits homogeneous subpleural fibrosis predominantly in the upper lobes [8].

Connective tissue diseases (CTDs), such as systemic sclerosis or Sjögren's disease, can also manifest with upper-lobe fibrosis on imaging. The challenge lies in the fact that CTDs may present with a variety of interstitial lung disease patterns, including PPFE itself. In CTD-associated ILDs not consistent with PPFE, imaging often reveals ground-glass opacities in a nonspecific interstitial pneumonia pattern, which is not characteristic of PPFE. Patients with PPFE also tend to be older and have a lower body mass index compared with those with CTD-related ILD [20].

Infectious processes, including *Mycobacterium avium-intracellulare* complex (MAC) and tuberculosis, may also resemble PPFE radiographically. Differentiation relies on a detailed history to identify prior mycobacterial infection and confirmatory sputum cultures. Notably, advanced PPFE itself is thought to predispose patients to MAC infection due to underlying parenchymal destruction [37].

Pulmonary apical capping (PAC) is another potential diagnostic pitfall. PAC is defined as a fibroelastotic scar affecting one or both lung apices and may occur in various conditions, including chronic bronchitis, recurrent pulmonary infections, malignancy, and sarcoidosis. Histologically, PAC is believed to arise from inflammation leading to mural thickening of pulmonary arteries and the subsequent development of wedge-shaped scarring. Distinguishing PAC in PPFE from other causes can be challenging; however, progressive radiographic changes are more typically associated with PPFE. Furthermore, PPFE usually manifests as bilateral and more extensive fibroelastosis, whereas PAC from other etiologies is often unilateral and localized [40].

Obliterative bronchiolitis (OB), commonly seen after lung or hematopoietic stem cell transplantation, may also share pathophysiologic features with PPFE. Both processes involve aberrant immune-mediated remodeling, leading to fibrosis, with OB specifically affecting the bronchioles. Some investigators have suggested that restrictive allograft dysfunction following lung transplantation and PPFE may exist along a spectrum [41]. Pulmonary function testing helps differentiate the two conditions: OB typically demonstrates fixed airflow obstruction with hyperinflation and air trapping due to small airway involvement, whereas PPFE is characterized by reduced total lung capacity and an elevated RV/TLC ratio, as discussed previously.

Diagnosis

Imaging

On chest radiography, pleuroparenchymal fibroelastosis typically demonstrates upper-lobe-predominant irregular pleural thickening of the apical portion of both lungs with subpleural reticular fibrosis. Additionally, significant volume loss of the upper lobes, accompanied by hyperinflation of the lower lobes, may be present [8].

High-resolution computed tomography provides additional detail. The disease is characterized by bilateral upper-lobe pleural thickening with subpleural reticular fibrosis with sparing of parenchyma distant from the pleural surface. Pleural thickening is confined primarily to the upper lobes, resulting in marked volume loss, along with compensatory hyperinflation of the lower lobes. Traction bronchiectasis is frequently encountered as a secondary consequence of fibrotic remodeling (Fig. 3.1a) [8]. Occasionally,

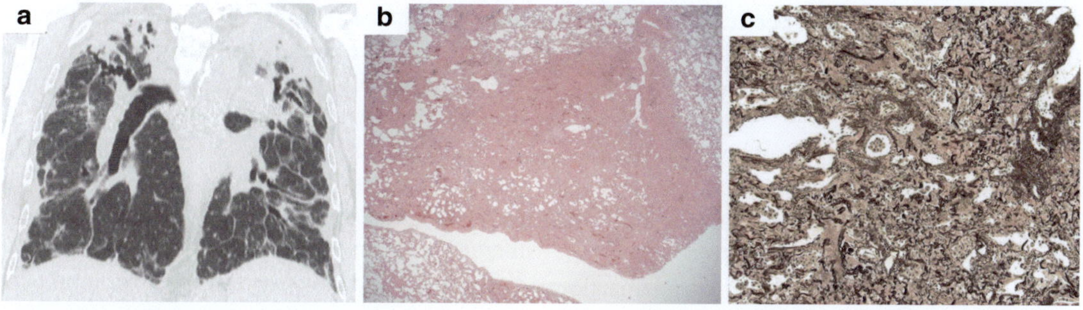

Fig. 3.1 Radiologic and histopathologic features of PPFE. (**a**) Non-contrast coronal computed tomography of the chest demonstrating upper-lobe pleural thickening with adjacent pulmonary fibrosis, architectural distortion, and traction bronchiectasis. (**b**) Histopathologic section showing extensive, dense subpleural fibrosis leading to alveolar obliteration with an abrupt transition to preserved small air spaces (hematoxylin–eosin stain, original magnification ×100). (**c**) Elastin stain (Verhoeff–Van Gieson) highlighting prominent deposition of numerous interrupted elastic fibers (black) along the alveolar septa

findings consistent with nonspecific interstitial pneumonia and usual interstitial pneumonia may be present simultaneously in the middle or lower lobes of the lung [19].

Diagnostic Criterion

Several diagnostic criteria have been proposed for pleuroparenchymal fibroelastosis. The first formal criteria were introduced by Reddy et al. in 2012, consisting of: (1) computed tomography (CT) findings of upper-lobe subpleural fibrosis with pleural thickening, and (2) histopathology demonstrating intra-alveolar fibrosis, pleural fibrosis, and alveolar septal elastosis [19]. A significant limitation of these criteria is that not all patients are candidates for surgical lung biopsy due to comorbidities or prohibitive procedural risk. Consequently, Reddy and colleagues, along with Nakatani et al., recommended a multidisciplinary diagnostic approach involving clinicians, radiologists, and pathologists [6, 19]. Critiques of these criteria noted the absence of disease progression as a component and questioned the necessity of histopathologic confirmation given the lack of effective therapies. The most widely recognized set of criteria is that of Watanabe, which stratifies patients into two groups: those diagnosed by a combination of surgical lung biopsy (SLB) and high-resolution computed tomography, and those diagnosed by HRCT alone. Enomoto et al. subsequently proposed revised criteria in 2017, comprising: (1) radiologic features consistent with PPFE, specifically bilateral dense consolidations with upper-lobe pleural thickening; (2) evidence of radiographic progression, including increasing upper-lobe consolidations, worsening pleural thickening, and/or reduction in upper-lobe volumes; and (3) exclusion of alternative causes of fibrosis or elastosis [22]. These criteria differ from Watanabe's in their emphasis on longitudinal imaging to establish disease progression and to help exclude other differential diagnoses. Importantly, none of the three proposed frameworks has been universally endorsed over the others. The lack of standardized diagnostic criteria has hindered the accurate determination of the true incidence and prevalence of PPFE.

Histology

Histologically, pleuroparenchymal fibroelastosis is classified as either *definitive* or *consistent* based on characteristic pathologic findings. A *definitive* diagnosis requires dense visceral pleural fibrosis predominantly involving the upper lobes, accompanied by homogeneous subpleural intra-alveolar fibrosis and alveolar septal elastosis (Fig. 3.1b). Additionally, there should be relative sparing of the deeper lung parenchyma distal to the pleura, with only scant lymphoplasmacytic infiltrates and a limited number of fibroblastic foci.

The *consistent* category is defined by the presence of intra-alveolar fibrosis and alveolar septal elastosis, but with one or more of the following distinctions: absence of pleural fibrosis, a distribution not primarily subpleural, or localization outside the upper lobes. Routine hematoxylin and eosin (H&E) staining typically reveals thickened visceral pleura, subpleural fibrosis, and dense collagen deposition. Elastic stains, most notably the Elastic Van Gieson method, are valuable for highlighting markedly excessive deposition of elastin fibers within the lung parenchyma adjacent to the pleural fibrosis [19, 30]. Elastic fiber staining is also valuable in the differential diagnosis. In PPFE, Van Gieson staining demonstrates abundant, dense, and well-organized elastic fibers around the alveolar walls (Fig. 3.1c). In contrast, diseases such as fibrotic hypersensitivity pneumonitis, asbestosis, radiation-induced lung injury, and usual interstitial pneumonia may also contain elastin; however, the fibers in these conditions are typically sparse, fragmented, and irregularly distributed within the fibrotic tissue [19, 32].

Treatment

The management of pleuroparenchymal fibroelastosis requires a multimodal approach, with treatment strategies largely extrapolated from other interstitial lung diseases, given the paucity of disease-specific data. Supportive care remains the cornerstone of therapy and includes pulmonary rehabilitation, nutritional optimization, and supplemental oxygen in patients with documented hypoxemia. Noninvasive positive pressure ventilation (NPPV) is generally discouraged in PPFE unless indicated for coexisting conditions such as obstructive sleep apnea. Patients with PPFE frequently develop hypercapnia as a consequence of markedly reduced lung compliance. The application of NPPV in this context is poorly tolerated, confers no proven benefit, and may increase the already heightened risk of pneumothorax, a well-recognized complication of this disease [42].

In the setting of acute clinical deterioration accompanied by new ground-glass opacities or consolidations on imaging, anti-inflammatory therapy may be considered. In such cases, management is typically approached in a manner similar to acute exacerbations of other interstitial lung diseases, following an appropriate diagnostic evaluation to exclude infection, pulmonary embolism, or other alternative causes. These therapies appear to be most effective in patients who demonstrate concurrent lower-lobe infiltrates [42]. The use of higher-dose immunomodulatory agents, including corticosteroids, azathioprine, and methotrexate, remains a topic of controversy. Current evidence is insufficient to support their routine use, and the potential benefits are outweighed in many patients by the significant risk of infectious complications [5].

Pleuroparenchymal fibroelastosis has largely been excluded from major antifibrotic randomized controlled trials. As a result, the benefits of antifibrotic agents cannot be directly extrapolated to PPFE patients [43]. Nonetheless, several groups have investigated the role of antifibrotic therapy in both idiopathic and secondary PPFE, with inconsistent outcomes. One study reported no measurable benefit of nintedanib in idiopathic PPFE [44], whereas another demonstrated a slower rate of lung function decline in patients with both idiopathic and secondary PPFE treated with antifibrotic agents [45]. The small sample sizes and study design constraints limit the interpretation of these findings.

In patients with concomitant idiopathic pulmonary fibrosis or another progressive fibrosing ILD, antifibrotic therapy is clearly indicated, consistent with the INBUILD trial results [42]. For patients with advanced or progressive PPFE who fail to respond to medical management, referral to a specialized lung transplant center for evaluation remains the definitive therapeutic option [42].

Surgical Procedures

As previously discussed, patients with advanced or rapidly progressive pleuroparenchymal fibroelastosis should be referred to a lung transplant center for evaluation, as transplantation remains the only effective therapeutic option for end-stage disease. Shiiya et al. reviewed 14 reported cases of PPFE patients who underwent lung transplantation to assess procedural tolerance and outcomes. At the time of publication in 2020, nine patients (64.2%) were alive. One patient died from complications of pulmonary hypertension following recurrence of PPFE in the transplanted lung, while outcome data were unavailable for two patients (14.2%). Postoperative complications reported among this cohort included chest wall rigidity requiring prolonged rehabilitation, secondary pulmonary hypertension, chylothorax, dysphagia, vocal cord paralysis, and pneumonia [46]. Despite these complications, lung transplantation remains a viable and potentially life-prolonging intervention for selected patients with advanced PPFE.

Prognosis

The overall prognosis of pleuroparenchymal fibroelastosis remains poor. In a cohort study of 85 patients with either idiopathic or secondary PPFE, the median survival was reported as 11 years [47]. Shioya et al. conducted a retrospective analysis of 375 patients with idiopathic interstitial pneumonia (IIP), of whom 29 were diagnosed with idiopathic pleuroparenchymal fibroelastosis (IPPFE). These patients exhibited significantly worse outcomes compared with those with idiopathic pulmonary fibrosis in advanced stages. Multiple factors have been identified as poor prognostic indicators in PPFE, including female sex, cumulative smoking history, prior pneumothorax, higher gender–age–physiology (GAP) index and stage, reduced percent predicted forced vital capacity, total lung capacity, diffusing capacity of the lungs for carbon monoxide, and DLCO/alveolar ventilation ratio. Additional predictors include an elevated alveolar–arterial oxygen gradient, coexisting pulmonary hypertension, chronic hypercapnia, elevated serum KL-6 levels, and progressive declines in FVC or TLC [7, 34, 48]. Specifically, an FVC of less than 70% predicted, a DLCO of less than 60% predicted, or a body mass index (BMI) of less than 18 were associated with a survival of less than three years [42]. A partial pressure of carbon dioxide ($PaCO_2$) greater than 50 mmHg correlated with a median survival of less than one year, compared with approximately two years in patients with $PaCO_2$ values below 50 mmHg [49].

The major causes of death among patients with PPFE include progressive respiratory failure, acute exacerbation of interstitial lung disease, and pulmonary infection [42]. In the study by Shioya et al., 11 of 29 patients (38%) died during the observation period: four from progressive disease, four from acute exacerbation, one from pneumonia, one from pulmonary embolism, and one from suicide [7]. Similarly, Suzuki et al. analyzed 62 patients with IPPFE and 323 with IPF. The IPPFE group had a median survival time of 34.6 months among clinically diagnosed cases and 47.8 months among those with pathological confirmation. Most deaths (73.8%) were due to chronic respiratory failure, and 14.3% were due to acute exacerbations. The five-year survival rate for IPPFE was 38.5%, significantly lower than that of IPF, which was 63.5% [50].

Future Direction

As pleuroparenchymal fibroelastosis remains a relatively newly recognized disease entity, multiple aspects of its pathogenesis, progression, and management warrant further investigation. Additional genetic studies are needed to clarify whether reduced telomere length and variants in the surfactant protein gene are associated with more rapid declines in forced vital capacity, shorter transplant-free survival, and other adverse clinical outcomes [28]. Moreover, large prospective studies are essential to better define the natural history and prognosis of PPFE, as most existing data are derived from retrospective analyses. Such studies would also help determine whether antifibrotic therapy confers measurable benefit in slowing disease progression [42]. Further research should also aim to establish objective physiological thresholds, such as specific FVC, residual volume to total lung capacity ratio, and body mass index cutoffs, that could guide optimal timing for lung transplant referral and listing [46]. Standardization of these criteria may improve post-transplant outcomes and patient selection. Finally, the development of a unified and universally accepted diagnostic framework for PPFE is imperative. Standardized diagnostic criteria would enhance research quality, reduce selection bias, yield more accurate epidemiologic data regarding disease prevalence and incidence, and facilitate more consistent evaluation of therapeutic interventions.

References

1. Amitani R, Niimi A, Kuse F. Idiopathic pulmonary upper lobe fibrosis (IPUF). Kokyu. 1992;11:693–9.
2. Frankel SK, Cool CD, Lynch DA, Brown KK. Idiopathic Pleuroparenchymal Fibroelastosis. Chest. 2004;126(6):2007–13.
3. Thusen J. Pleuroparenchymal Fibroelastosis: its pathological characteristics. Curr Respir Med Rev. 2014;9(4):238–47.
4. Travis WD, Costabel U, Hansell DM, King TE, Lynch DA, Nicholson AG, et al. An official American Thoracic Society/European Respiratory Society statement: update of the international multidisciplinary classification of the idiopathic interstitial pneumonias. Am J Respir Crit Care Med. 2013;188(6):733–48.
5. Chua F, Desai SR, Nicholson AG, Devaraj A, Renzoni E, Rice A, et al. Pleuroparenchymal Fibroelastosis. A review of clinical, radiological, and pathological characteristics. Ann Am Thorac Soc. 2019;16(11):1351–9.
6. Nakatani T, Arai T, Kitaichi M, Akira M, Tachibana K, Sugimoto C, et al. Pleuroparenchymal fibroelastosis from a consecutive database: a rare disease entity? Eur Respir J. 2015;45(4):1183–6.
7. Shioya M, Otsuka M, Yamada G, Umeda Y, Ikeda K, Nishikiori H, et al. Poorer prognosis of idiopathic Pleuroparenchymal Fibroelastosis compared with idiopathic pulmonary fibrosis in advanced stage. Can Respir J. 2018;13:1–7.
8. Cheng SKH, Chuah KL. Pleuroparenchymal Fibroelastosis of the lung: a review. Arch Pathol Lab Med. 2016;140(8):849–53.
9. von der Thüsen JH. Pleuroparenchymal Fibroelastosis: its pathological characteristics. Curr Respir Med Rev. 2013;9(4):238–47.
10. von der Thüsen JH, Hansell DM, Tominaga M, Veys PA, Ashworth MT, Owens CM, et al. Pleuroparenchymal fibroelastosis in patients with pulmonary disease secondary to bone marrow transplantation. Mod Pathol. 2011;24(12):1633–9.
11. Mariani F, Gatti B, Rocca A, Bonifazi F, Cavazza A, Fanti S, et al. Pleuroparenchymal fibroelastosis: the prevalence of secondary forms in hematopoietic stem cell and lung transplantation recipients. Diagn Interv Radiol. 2016;22(5):400–6.
12. Pakhale SS, Hadjiliadis D, Howell DN, Palmer SM, Gutierrez C, Waddell TK, et al. Upper lobe fibrosis: a novel manifestation of chronic allograft dysfunction in lung transplantation. J Heart Lung Transplant. 2005;24(9):1260–8.
13. Beynat-Mouterde C, Beltramo G, Lezmi G, Pernet D, Camus C, Fanton A, et al. Pleuroparenchymal fibroelastosis as a late complication of chemotherapy agents. Eur Respir J. 2014;44(2):523–7.
14. Chen F, Matsubara K, Miyagawa-Hayashino A, Tada K, Handa T, Yamada T, et al. Lung transplantation for pleuroparenchymal fibroelastosis after chemotherapy. Ann Thorac Surg. 2014;98(5):e115–7.
15. Portillo K, Guasch Arriaga I, Ruiz-Manzano J. Pleuroparenchymal fibroelastosis: is it also an idiopathic entity? Arch Bronconeumol. 2015;51(10):509–14.
16. Rodrigues Vieira AC, Monteiro Ferra JR, Vicente De Carvalho JS, Melo N, Caetano Mota P, Novais E, Bastos H, et al. Pleuroparenchymal fibroelastosis as a complication of chemotherapy: a case report. Mol Clin Oncol. 2022;16(3):71.
17. Jacob J, Odink A, Brun AL, Macaluso C, de Lauretis A, Kokosi M, et al. Functional associations of pleuroparenchymal fibroelastosis and emphysema with hypersensitivity pneumonitis. Respir Med. 2018;138:95–101.
18. Xu L, Rassaei N, Caruso C. Pleuroparenchymal Fibroelastosis with long history of Asbestos and silicon exposure. Int J Surg Pathol. 2018;26(2):190–3.
19. Reddy TL, Tominaga M, Hansell DM, von der Thusen J, Rassl D, Parfrey H, et al. Pleuroparenchymal fibro-

elastosis: a spectrum of histopathological and imaging phenotypes. Eur Respir J. 2012;40(2):377–85.
20. Enomoto Y, Nakamura Y, Colby TV, Johkoh T, Sumikawa H, Nishimoto K, et al. Radiologic pleuroparenchymal fibroelastosis-like lesion in connective tissue disease-related interstitial lung disease. PLoS One. 2017;12(6):e0180283.
21. Atienza-Mateo B, Remuzgo Martinez S, Pulito-Cueto V, Ferrer D, Blanco G, Izquierdo S, et al. Pleuroparenchymal fibroelastosis: a special clinical situation in patients with interstitial lung disease associated with connective tissue diseases. Descriptive study from a referral Centre. Ann Rheum Dis. 2023;82:781–2.
22. Enomoto Y, Nakamura Y, Satake Y, Sumikawa H, Johkoh T, Colby TV, et al. Clinical diagnosis of idiopathic pleuroparenchymal fibroelastosis: a retrospective multicenter study. Respir Med. 2017;133:1–5.
23. Oda T, Ogura T, Kitamura H, Hagiwara E, Baba T, Enomoto Y, et al. Distinct characteristics of Pleuroparenchymal Fibroelastosis with usual interstitial pneumonia compared with idiopathic pulmonary fibrosis. Chest. 2014;146(5):1248–55.
24. Shiota S, Shimizu K, Suzuki M, Nakaya Y, Sakamoto K, Iwase A, et al. Seven cases of marked pulmonary fibrosis in the upper lobe. Nihon Kokyuki Gakkai Zasshi. 1999;37(2):87–96.
25. Azoulay E, Paugam B, Heymann MF, Kambouchner M, Haloun A, Valeyre D, et al. Familial extensive idiopathic bilateral pleural fibrosis. Eur Respir J. 1999;14(4):971.
26. Kobayashi Y, Sakurai M, Kushiya M, Mizukoshi T, Nishi Y, Choo JH, et al. Idiopathic pulmonary fibrosis of the upper lobe: a case report. Nihon Kokyuki Gakkai Zasshi. 1999;37(10):812–6.
27. Ishii H, Kinoshita Y, Kushima H, Nagata N, Watanabe K. The similarities and differences between pleuroparenchymal fibroelastosis and idiopathic pulmonary fibrosis. Chron Respir Dis. 2019;16:1479973119867994.
28. Alrehaili G, Kemppainen J, Kalra S, Pinto E, Vairo F, Moua T, Yi ES, et al. Genetic testing goes beyond imaging and histological evaluation in Pleuroparenchymal Fibroelastosis. Lung. 2024;202(2):151–6.
29. Jaula H, Mattila L, Lappi-Blanco E, Salonen J, Vähänikkilä H, Ahvenjärvi L, et al. Clinical, radiological and histopathological features of patients with familial pulmonary fibrosis. Respir Res. 2024;25(1):239.
30. Kusagaya H, Nakamura Y, Kono M, Kaida Y, Kuroishi S, Enomoto N, et al. Idiopathic pleuroparenchymal fibroelastosis: consideration of a clinicopathological entity in a series of Japanese patients. BMC Pulm Med. 2012;12(1):72.
31. Tabaj GC, Fernandez CF, Sabbagh E, Leslie KO. Histopathology of the idiopathic interstitial pneumonias (<scp>IIP</scp>): a review. Respirology. 2015;20(6):873–83.
32. Hirota T, Yoshida Y, Kitasato Y, Yoshimi M, Koga T, Tsuruta N, et al. Histological evolution of pleuroparenchymal fibroelastosis. Histopathology. 2015;66(4):545–54.
33. Watanabe K, Nagata N, Kitasato Y, Wakamatsu K, Nabeshima K, Harada T, et al. Rapid decrease in forced vital capacity in patients with idiopathic pulmonary upper lobe fibrosis. Respir Investig. 2012;50(3):88–97.
34. Kono M, Nakamura Y, Enomoto Y, Yasui H, Hozumi H, Karayama M, et al. Pneumothorax in patients with idiopathic Pleuroparenchymal Fibroelastosis: incidence, clinical features, and risk factors. Respiration. 2021;100(1):19–26.
35. Nguyen HN, Das S, Gazzaneo MC, Melicoff E, Mallory GB, Eldin KW, et al. Clinico-radiologic features of pleuroparenchymal fibroelastosis in children. Pediatr Radiol. 2019;49(9):1163–70.
36. Watanabe S, Waseda Y, Takato H, Matsunuma R, Johkoh T, Egashira R, et al. Pleuroparenchymal fibroelastosis: distinct pulmonary physiological features in nine patients. Respir Investig. 2015;53(4):149–55.
37. Watanabe K, Ishii H, Kiyomi F, Terasaki Y, Hebisawa A, Kawabata Y, et al. Criteria for the diagnosis of idiopathic pleuroparenchymal fibroelastosis: a proposal. Respir Investig. 2019;57(4):312–20.
38. Lee JH, Chae EJ, Song JS, Kim M, Song JW. Pleuroparenchymal fibroelastosis in Korean patients: clinico-radiologic-pathologic features and 2-year follow-up. Korean J Intern Med. 2021;36(Suppl 1):S132–41.
39. Raghu G, Collard HR, Egan JJ, Martinez FJ, Behr J, Brown KK, et al. An official ATS/ERS/JRS/ALAT statement: idiopathic pulmonary fibrosis: evidence-based guidelines for diagnosis and management. Am J Respir Crit Care Med. 2011;183(6):788–824.
40. Lagstein A. Pulmonary apical cap-what's old is new again. Arch Pathol Lab Med. 2015;139(10):1258–62.
41. Ofek E, Sato M, Saito T, Wagnetz U, Roberts HC, Chaparro C, et al. Restrictive allograft syndrome post lung transplantation is characterized by pleuroparenchymal fibroelastosis. Mod Pathol. 2013;26(3):350–6.
42. Yamakawa H, Oda T, Sugino K, Hirama T, Komatsu M, Katano T, et al. Proposed clinical algorithm for Pleuroparenchymal Fibroelastosis (PPFE). J Clin Med. 2024;13(13)
43. Flaherty KR, Wells AU, Cottin V, Devaraj A, Walsh SLF, Inoue Y, et al. Nintedanib in progressive Fibrosing interstitial lung diseases. N Engl J Med. 2019;381(18):1718–27.
44. Kinoshita Y, Miyamura T, Ikeda T, Ueda Y, Yoshida Y, Kushima H, et al. Limited efficacy of nintedanib for idiopathic pleuroparenchymal fibroelastosis. Respir Investig. 2022;60(4):562–9.
45. Nasser M, Si-Mohamed S, Turquier S, Traclet J, Ahmad K, Philit F, et al. Nintedanib in idiopathic and secondary pleuroparenchymal fibroelastosis. Orphanet J Rare Dis. 2021;16(1):419.
46. Shiiya H, Sato M. Lung transplantation for Pleuroparenchymal Fibroelastosis. J Clin Med. 2021;10(5):957.

47. Watanabe K. Pleuroparenchymal Fibroelastosis: its clinical characteristics. Curr Respir Med Rev. 2014;9(4):229–37.
48. Muto Y, Sekine A, Hagiwara E, Komatsu S, Baba T, Oda T, et al. Clinical characteristics of pulmonary hypertension in patients with pleuroparenchymal fibroelastosis. Respir Investig. 2022;60(4):543–50.
49. Kinoshita Y, Utsunomiya T, Koide Y, Wada K, Ueda Y, Yoshida Y, et al. Partial pressure of carbon dioxide levels reflect disease severity in idiopathic pleuroparenchymal fibroelastosis. Respir Investig. 2023;61(4):379–86.
50. Suzuki Y, Fujisawa T, Sumikawa H, Tanaka T, Sugimoto C, Kono M, et al. Disease course and prognosis of pleuroparenchymal fibroelastosis compared with idiopathic pulmonary fibrosis. Respir Med. 2020;171:106078.

Extrapleural Lipomatosis

4

Ahmad Ghabsha
and Mohamed Ayman Mohamed

Introduction

Extrapleural lipomatosis is defined as an excessive accumulation of diffuse, nonencapsulated adipose tissue within the extrapleural space [1]. This space lies between the parietal pleura and the inner aspect of the thoracic cage and contains adipose tissue, loose connective tissue, lymphatic vessels, the endothoracic fascia, and the innermost layer of the intercostal muscles [2]. This entity represents a rare pleural disorder with inconsistently defined diagnostic criteria in the literature. Fat accumulation may develop beneath the chest wall or within the mediastinum, the latter referred to as mediastinal lipomatosis, which typically involves the upper anterior mediastinum [3]. Extrapleural lipomatosis is a benign process that is often identified incidentally on imaging and is usually asymptomatic. It differs from pleural lipoma, which is an encapsulated tumor, though lipomatosis may similarly appear as a mass-like lesion on chest imaging [4]. Owing to its rarity, the incidence and prevalence of extrapleural lipomatosis remain unknown, with only isolated case reports available in the literature.

A. Ghabsha (✉) · M. A. Mohamed
Department of Pulmonary and Critical Care,
McLaren Oakland Hospital, Pontiac, MI, USA

Pathophysiology

Extrapleural and mediastinal lipomatoses have been associated with corticosteroid therapy and Cushing syndrome, both of which can cause abnormal redistribution of adipose tissue to these regions [3, 4]. The condition has also been linked to systemic lipomatosis syndromes, such as Madelung's disease (multiple symmetric lipomatosis) [5]. Obesity is considered a significant predisposing factor, as generalized fat accumulation promotes increased deposition within the extrapleural compartment [6, 7]. The disorder is nonneoplastic, with no reported cases of malignant transformation. Extrapleural fat typically accumulates bilaterally along the posterolateral chest wall [3]. Mediastinal lipomatosis, by contrast, leads to mediastinal widening on imaging but typically lacks focal bulging of the mediastinal contour [1]. In some instances, the excess fat may produce a "double-cardiac contour" on chest radiographs due to superimposed mediastinal fat layers [6].

Clinical Features

Both extrapleural and mediastinal lipomatoses are slow-growing processes that are most often discovered incidentally. The majority of patients remain asymptomatic [7]. When symptoms do occur, dyspnea is the most frequent

F. Ido (ed.), *Rare Pleural Diseases*, https://doi.org/10.1007/978-3-032-14873-5_4

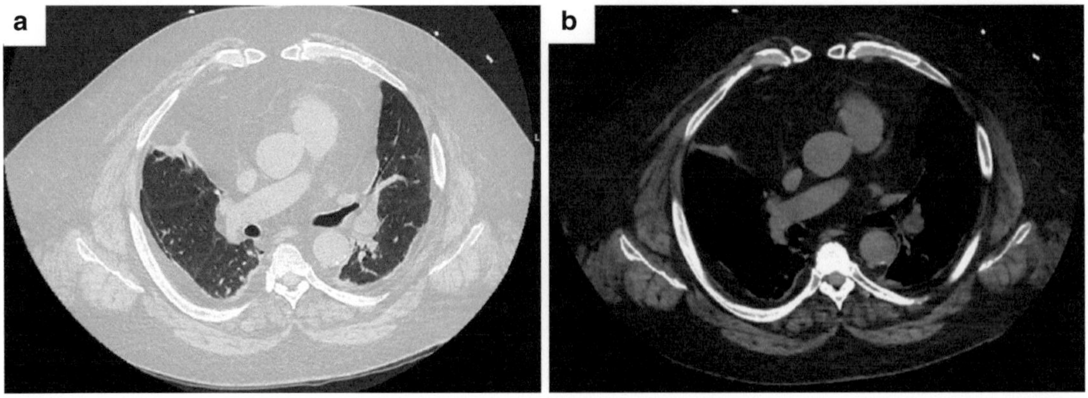

Fig. 4.1 Computed tomography of the thorax demonstrating bilateral pleural lesions with irregular contours, located in the dependent, posterolateral areas. (**a**) On lung window settings, the pleural thickening mimics pleural effusions or organized pleural fibrosis. (**b**) On abdominal (soft-tissue) window settings, the pleural lesions exhibit attenuation values consistent with fat density, confirming pleural lipomatosis. Associated mediastinal lipomatosis is also noted

complaint, usually secondary to compression of adjacent lung parenchyma or restrictive chest wall mechanics in large lesions. Because obesity is a frequent comorbidity, distinguishing whether dyspnea results from lipomatosis or reduced chest wall compliance due to subcutaneous fat accumulation can be difficult [8]. Chest discomfort may arise from irritation of adjacent intercostal nerves, and cough may occur with pleural irritation [8, 9]. Rarely, when the fatty proliferation extends superiorly toward the thoracic inlet, thoracic outlet syndrome may develop due to neurovascular compression [10].

Diagnosis

Diagnosis is primarily established via imaging, with computed tomography (CT) being the modality of choice [1, 2]. On chest radiography, findings may include mediastinal widening with smooth margins and obtuse angles [9–11]. When located laterally, extrapleural lipomatosis may mimic pleural thickening, pleural effusion, or plaques. On CT, lesions demonstrate homogeneous fat attenuation, typically ranging from −50 to −150 Hounsfield units, identical to subcutaneous fat [8]. The deposition is well delineated and confined to the extrapleural space (Fig. 4.1a, b). Because these lesions lack vascular structures, no contrast enhancement is observed [12]. If CT findings are inconclusive, magnetic resonance imaging (MRI) can be performed, which shows high signal intensity on both T1- and T2-weighted sequences [12]. Biopsy is generally unnecessary, except when differentiation from other fat-containing or infiltrative lesions is difficult.

Differential Diagnosis

The differential diagnosis of extrapleural lipomatosis includes several other fat-containing lesions [12, 13]. Pleural lipoma is a well-encapsulated adipose tumor confined to the pleura. Liposarcoma, the malignant counterpart of lipoma, is typically heterogeneous on CT due to necrosis or soft-tissue components and often infiltrates into surrounding structures [14]. Pleural plaques, indicative of asbestos exposure, can mimic lipomatosis due to pleural thickening, but are distinguishable by analyzing Hounsfield units [7]. Subpleural fat may also simulate pleural effusion, occasionally leading to unnecessary thoracentesis attempts. Extrapleural lipomatosis should be considered in obese patients, particularly those receiving corticosteroids, once other causes of dyspnea have been excluded [8].

Treatment and Prognosis

Most cases of extrapleural lipomatosis are asymptomatic, and conservative management with observation is appropriate, accompanied by periodic imaging for surveillance [16]. When associated with exogenous steroid use, discontinuation or dose reduction may result in partial regression of the fatty accumulation. Weight reduction is another effective conservative measure [13]. Surgical excision is reserved for symptomatic patients or those with evidence of compression of adjacent organs [14, 15]. Video-assisted thoracoscopic surgery (VATS) offers a minimally invasive approach with reduced morbidity compared to open thoracotomy [16]. Both pleural and mediastinal lipomatosis carry an excellent prognosis, with no documented malignant potential in the literature [17].

Attribution Original images courtesy of *Dr. Firas Ido*. These figures are unpublished and reproduced here with permission of the author.

References

1. Fisher ER, Godwin JD. Extrapleural fat collections: Pseudotumors and other confusing manifestations. AJR Am J Roentgenol. 1993;161(1):47–52.
2. Santamarina MG, Beddings I, Lermanda Holmgren GV, Opazo Sanchez H, Volpacchio MM. Multidetector CT for evaluation of the Extrapleural space. Radiographics. 2017;37(5):1352–70. https://doi.org/10.1148/rg.2017160180. Epub 2017 Aug 4. PMID: 28777699.
3. Glazer HS, Wick MR, Anderson DJ, Semenkovich JW, Molina PL, Siegel MJ, Sagel SS. CT of fatty thoracic masses. AJR Am J Roentgenol. 1992;159(6):1181–7. https://doi.org/10.2214/ajr.159.6.1442378. PMID: 1442378.
4. Gaerte SC, Meyer CA, Winer-Muram HT, Tarver RD, Conces DJ Jr. Fat-containing lesions of the chest. Radiographics. 2002;22:S61–78. https://doi.org/10.1148/radiographics.22.suppl_1.g02oc08s61. PMID: 12376601.
5. Maximiano LF, Gaspar MT, Nakahira ES. Madelung disease (multiple symmetric lipomatosis). Autops Case Rep. 2018;8(3):e2018030. https://doi.org/10.4322/acr.2018.030. PMID: 30101135; PMCID: PMC6066263.
6. Molinari F, Bankier AA, Eisenberg RL. Fat-containing lesions in adult thoracic imaging. AJR Am J Roentgenol. 2011;197(5):W795–813. https://doi.org/10.2214/AJR.11.6932. PMID: 22021525.
7. Alfudhili KM, Lynch DA, Laurent F, Ferretti GR, Dunet V, Beigelman-Aubry C. Focal pleural thickening mimicking pleural plaques on chest computed tomography: tips and tricks. Br J Radiol. 2016;89(1057):20150792. https://doi.org/10.1259/bjr.20150792. Epub 2015 Nov 5. PMID: 26539633; PMCID: PMC4985966.
8. Lim JY, KA MA, Chang CL. Dyspnoea and restrictive lung disease due to mediastinal and pleural lipomatosis in morbid obesity. Respirol Case Rep. 2019;7(5):e00421. https://doi.org/10.1002/rcr2.421. PMID: 31007928; PMCID: PMC6454808.
9. de Souza Junior AS, Zanetti G, Marchiori E. Fat-containing mediastinal lesions: computed tomography findings in a series of 18 patients. J Bras Pneumol. 2013;39(5):596–603. https://doi.org/10.1590/S1806-37132013000500015.
10. Matsumoto AH, Angle JF, Ray CE, et al. Updates in interventional radiology: new applications and techniques in 2015. J Vasc Surg Cases. 2015;1(1):1–6. https://doi.org/10.1016/j.jvsc.2015.12.002.
11. Mansour J, Raptis D, Bhalla S, Heeger AP, Abbott GF, Parkar N, Hammer MM, Kiernan J, Raptis C. Radiographics. 2022;42(2):359–78.
12. Sabri YY, Elroos MSEM, El Hinnawy YH, et al. Extra-pleural space on CT: common lesions and diagnostic approach. Egypt J Radiol Nucl Med. 2023;54:28. https://doi.org/10.1186/s43055-023-00978-2.
13. Kaur N, Singh J, Haq S, Garg S, Bhatnagar S. Pleural and mediastinal lipomatosis with Subpleural fat as a mimicker of pleural effusion- a rare case report. J Clin Diagn Res. 2017;11(7):TD03–4. https://doi.org/10.7860/JCDR/2017/26182.10156. Epub 2017 Jul 1. PMID: 28893005; PMCID: PMC5583791.
14. Thway K. Well-differentiated liposarcoma and dedifferentiated liposarcoma: an updated review. Semin Diagn Pathol. 2019;36(2):112–21. https://doi.org/10.1053/j.semdp.2019.02.006. Epub 2019 Feb 28. PMID: 30852045.
15. Karmakar S, Bhattacharya S, Thakur S, Rai DK. Pleural lipomatosis: A rare cause of pleural effusion. Lung India. 2020;37(4):344–6. https://doi.org/10.4103/lungindia.lungindia_517_19. PMID: 32643647; PMCID: PMC7507924.
16. Imperatori A, Rotolo N, Gatti M, Nardecchia E, De Monte L, Conti V, Dominioni L. Peri-operative complications of video-assisted thoracoscopic surgery (VATS). Int J Surg. 2008;6(Suppl 1):S78–81. https://doi.org/10.1016/j.ijsu.2008.12.014. Epub 2008 Dec 13. PMID: 19186114.
17. Politis J, Funahashi A, Gehlsen JA, DeCock D, Stengel BF, Choi H. Intrathoracic lipomas: report of three cases and review of the literature with emphasis on endobronchial lipoma. J Thorac Cardiovasc Surg. 1979;77(4).

Diffuse Pulmonary Lymphangiomatosis

5

Toribiong Uchel and Ashley Dean

Introduction

Lymphangiomatosis is a rare disorder of the lymphatic system characterized by the aberrant proliferation and formation of lymphatic channels, affecting an estimated 1 in 50,000 individuals [23]. The true incidence remains uncertain, as most available data are derived from isolated case reports and small series [2]. The disease can involve any region containing lymphatic structures, with potential infiltration into visceral organs, soft tissues, and even bone. While pulmonary involvement may occur in isolation, multisystem disease is also frequently reported [1].

Diffuse pulmonary lymphangiomatosis (DPL) is a localized disease limited to the lymphatics in the lungs, pleura, and mediastinum [1, 4, 5, 16]. Typically, it manifests from childhood through young adulthood; however, cases have been reported in patients as old as 80 years [1, 2, 11]. There is no reported sex predilection, with males and females equally affected [1, 2, 8, 11, 13].

T. Uchel (✉)
Division of Pulmonary and Critical Care, Department of Internal Medicine, Virginia Commonwealth University, Richmond, VA, USA
e-mail: uchelt@vcu.edu

A. Dean
Department of Pulmonary and Critical Care, Virginia Tech Carilion Clinic, Roanoke, VA, USA
e-mail: awdean@carilionclinic.org

Pathogenesis

While the full pathogenesis of this disease remains unclear, it is believed to be a congenital disorder caused by mutations in the lymphatic system that occur before the 20th week of gestation [2, 3]. Hormonal factors have been suggested as a reason for its development in adulthood [11]. Gene mutations in BCL6, located on chromosome 3, and ATM, on chromosome 11q22–23, may contribute to the development of DPL [2]. BCL6 functions as an antiapoptotic regulator in germinal center B cells, controlling genes involved in activation, differentiation, apoptosis, proliferation, and DNA damage response. Germline mutations in ATM have been linked to ataxia telangiectasia [2]. It is also hypothesized that DPL could be a hamartomatous process, supported by histological evidence showing disorganized lymphatic structures and local tissue components within the lesions [34]. Smoking does not seem to increase DPL risk, with one study indicating that up to 75% of patients with DPL have never smoked [23].

Clinical Features

The disease's natural progression involves tissues gradually becoming increasingly infiltrated with enlarging lesions. Patients often remain asymptomatic until compression of nearby structures

F. Ido (ed.), *Rare Pleural Diseases*, https://doi.org/10.1007/978-3-032-14873-5_5

occurs, leading to the development of symptoms [1]. Commonly reported symptoms include dyspnea (22–83%), chronic cough (40–78.6%), wheezing (23.8–44%), sputum production (24–58%), chest pain, recurrent respiratory infections (38.1%), and hemoptysis (4.8–58%) [2, 3, 6, 8, 10, 13, 23]. Interstitial infiltration may cause inspiratory crackles, particularly at dependent lung bases [32]. Fever is uncommon and often suggests a concurrent infection [30]. Other physical exam findings may include a low BMI and signs of malnutrition (52.4%), which can result from significant protein loss caused by recurrent or profusely draining chylothorax. These findings can also occur with lymphangioma involving the gastrointestinal tract in multisystemic disease [33]. Additionally, in multisystem disease, bone involvement is common, with lytic lesions present in 75% of cases. These lesions may be asymptomatic or may cause bone pain [17]. Since there are no lymphatic structures within the CNS, this system is the only one protected from disease [17].

Diagnosis

Recurrent, frequently bilateral pleural effusions are common, though the exact incidence is unclear [1, 2]. On physical exam, pleural effusion may be indicated by absent breath sounds and dullness to percussion. Pleural fluid studies are frequently chylous in nature, characterized by their milky appearance, absence of infectious elements, lymphocyte predominance (>80%), presence of chylomicrons, and elevated triglyceride levels (>1.1 mmol/L) [6, 18, 29]. These effusions are common in neonates and children but are less frequent in adults. When present in adults, they can be an important diagnostic clue for pulmonary lymphangiomatosis [1, 29]. A review of pediatric chylothoraxes in Beijing from 2007–2017 showed primary chylous pleural effusions in 50–61.8% of children, with DPL accounting for less than 6.5% (34). The effusions in diffuse pulmonary lymphangiomatosis may also be serosanguinous or hemorrhagic, especially if chest wall lesions rupture into the pleural space [6, 11]. Chyloptysis results from lymphatic flow stasis refluxing into the tracheobronchial tree and occurs in up to 58% of DPL patients [20, 23]. Subsequently, plastic bronchitis can develop [28]. About 20% of patients remain symptomatic throughout their disease course [2, 3].

Imaging findings are often nonspecific. Indicators suggestive of obstructed lymphatic drainage include interlobular septal thickening (70%), ground-glass opacities (80%), pleural effusion (40–67%), diffuse mediastinal infiltration (83–90%), pleural thickening (67%), and bronchial wall thickening (67%), which can all appear on non-contrast computed tomography (CT) scans of the chest (Fig. 5.1a, b). The differential diagnosis for these imaging features is broad, encompassing conditions such as pulmonary lymphangiectasia (including primary congenital lymphangiectasia and secondary forms caused by heart failure, pulmonary hypertension, or other venous obstruction causes), congenital lymphatic anomalies (CLA) like Kaposiform lymphangiomatosis (KLA), Gorham-Stout disease (GSD), generalized lymphatic anomaly (GLA), similar to DPL but involving lymphatic structures outside the thorax, as well as amyloidosis, sarcoidosis, lymphoma, and Erdheim-Chester disease. To obtain a definitive diagnosis and to distinguish between these disease processes, a biopsy is generally required [18, 20, 23, 31]. Lymphangiomas within the mediastinal soft tissue can present as mediastinal fat attenuation, mediastinal enlargement, discrete mediastinal masses, or cystic lesions [12, 13, 16, 20].

MRI of lesions typically reveals low signal intensity on T1-weighted images, high signal intensity on T2-weighted images, and usually no enhancement after contrast administration [2, 22, 28]. Non-contrast MR lymphangiography provides a noninvasive method for visualizing the entire lymphatic duct, confirming its continuity and aiding in the diagnosis of lymphatic channel anomalies. The capability for 3D projection can also support surgical planning. However, these advanced imaging techniques may only be accessible at specialized centers [19]. Positron emission tomography (PET) generally offers limited benefit; however, when performed, lesions typi-

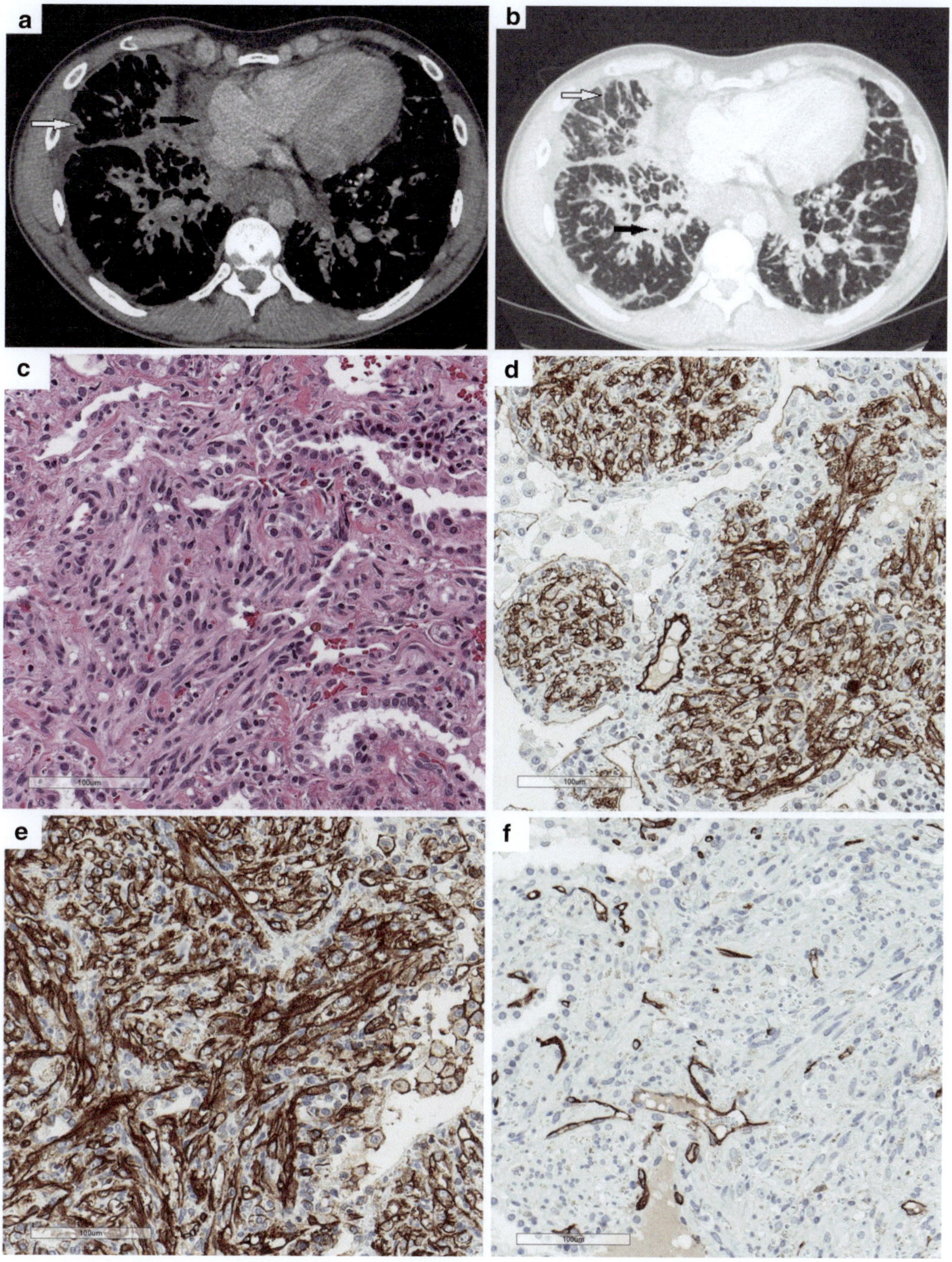

Fig. 5.1 Radiologic and histopathologic features of diffuse pulmonary lymphangiomatosis. (**a**) Contrast-enhanced computed tomography (CT) in a soft-tissue window showing diffuse mediastinal infiltration (black arrow) and pleural thickening (white arrow). (**b**) Contrast-enhanced CT in a lung window demonstrating diffuse interlobular septal thickening (white arrow) and peribronchovascular interstitial thickening (black arrow). (**c**) Hematoxylin and eosin–stained section (×200) revealing dense proliferation of numerous thin-walled vessels and spindle cells. (**d**) D2–40 immunohistochemical stain (×200) showing moderate membranous positivity in proliferating lymphatic vessels. (**e**) CD31 immunostain (×200) demonstrating strong membranous reactivity in endothelial cells of anastomosing vascular channels. (**f**) CD34 immunostain (×200) highlighting positive staining in surrounding capillaries with mostly negative staining within the lymphatic proliferation

cally show no significant uptake of fluorodeoxyglucose [7, 16, 22]. Lymphangiography is an invasive procedure that involves cannulating a lymphatic vessel and injecting an oil-based contrast agent into the lymphatic system. It can detect multiple lesions in the thoracic duct, dilated lymphatic channels throughout the lungs, and lymphangiomas within the lung tissue. Additionally, it helps rule out mediastinal tumors and distinguish lymphangiomas from hemangiomas [1, 11]. A less invasive alternative is the direct injection of contrast into a lymph node [11]. Video-assisted thoracoscopy (VATS) can be employed to biopsy suspected lymph nodes, pleural surfaces, or lung tissue [16]. If less invasive diagnostic methods fail to provide a diagnosis, surgical lung biopsy or wedge resection may be necessary [35].

Bronchoscopy can identify signs of inflammation such as bronchial narrowing, erythema, and edema (42.8%), as well as chylous secretions (14.2%) and hemorrhage (14.2%). In advanced cases, it may reveal thin-walled vesicles containing lymphatic or chylous fluid (28.5%) [10, 11, 14]. Transbronchial cryobiopsy might provide diagnostic samples, but these are smaller than those obtained through VATS or wedge biopsy, which might limit their diagnostic usefulness [22]. Complications from bronchoscopy with biopsy have been reported, including potentially life-threatening massive chyloptysis [13]. Additionally, chylothorax can occur following lung biopsy or surgical removal of mediastinal or parenchymal masses [13].

Histologically, evidence shows irregular proliferation and dilation of lymphatic vessels [16]. Unlike pulmonary lymphangiectasia, there is not only an enlargement of lymphatic structures but also an increased number of these abnormally dilated channels (Fig. 5.1c, d) [31]. The lung parenchyma remains intact, and abnormal lymphatic channels are contained within the normal pathways in the mediastinum and lung, unlike in lymphangioleiomyomatosis (LAM) [1, 10]. Key endothelial markers include Factor VIII-related antigen, D2–40 (podoplanin), CD31 (PECAM1), and Ulex europaeus I agglutinin, identified by immunohistochemical staining (Fig. 5.1e, f) [1–3, 6–8, 10, 11, 13, 15, 33]. The adjacent lung may be hypervascular and contain hemosiderin-laden macrophages [1, 8, 11, 26, 31, 33]. Ki67, which indicates cell proliferation, is low [21]. Surrounding stromal spindle cells of peripheral lymphatic smooth muscle form poorly defined fascicles and stain positive for vimentin, desmin, and smooth muscle actin, occasionally also for progesterone receptor [33]. Conversely, staining for estrogen receptor, glycoprotein gp100, and HMB-45 is negative, unlike in LAM [8, 9, 11, 16]. Serum VEGF-D, a growth factor involved in lymphangiogenesis, is elevated in patients with diffuse pulmonary lymphangiomatosis. While it holds potential as a future diagnostic biomarker, it is presently used solely for research purposes (27). Pulmonary function tests may exhibit a mixed pattern of obstruction and/or restriction, accompanied by a decreased diffusion capacity of the lung for carbon monoxide (DLCO); however, these findings are not specific to DPL [1, 10, 23, 28, 32].

Treatment

There are no standardized treatment protocols or guidelines for diffuse pulmonary lymphangiomatosis. Treatment decisions are mainly based on case reports and are tailored to the patient's symptoms. Various treatment approaches have been tried, with different levels of success. Mild or limited disease can be observed without treatment. Surgical resection may be an option for localized lung or mediastinal lesions causing compression of vital structures or exerting mass effect, but recurrence is frequent. The success of surgery often depends on the challenge of distinguishing abnormal lymphatic collections from nearby structures [1, 2, 13, 30]. In cases of complex or extensive lesions, complete excision may not be feasible, making a palliative treatment approach necessary.

Percutaneous sclerotherapy targeting localized lesions has been documented through the injection of streptococcus antigen OK-432 or doxycycline. Patients often report this procedure as painful, which is why it is not commonly used in routine practice [1, 11, 23]. Sirolimus is an mTOR inhibitor that binds to vascular endothelial growth factor receptor-3 (VEGFR-3), which is also present on lymphatic endothelial cells, disrupting downstream signaling and preventing lymphatic vessel proliferation. It is frequently used to treat diffuse pulmonary lymphangiomatosis [2, 6, 15, 21, 23]. Treatment with sirolimus has shown clinical benefits, including decreased cough, reduced sputum, improved dyspnea, partial resolution of pleural effusions, and enhanced chest imaging [6]. It also increases forced expiratory volume in 1 second (FEV1) and forced vital capacity (FVC) on posttreatment pulmonary function tests and decreases the volume of abnormal lymphatic lesions seen on imaging [2]. Dosing is individualized based on trough levels, but no standardized regimen exists. Case reports suggest maintenance doses from 5 ng/mL to 15 ng/mL, resulting in clinical stability or improvement over periods up to 4 years. Symptoms and imaging improvements generally appear around 10 weeks. The efficacy of similar drugs, such as everolimus, remains unclear [21, 23, 24]. Conditions related to generalized lymphatic anomaly and Kaposiform lymphangiomatosis also respond well to sirolimus, likely because these diseases involve similar activated signaling pathways (PI3K, AKT, mTOR, and MAPK) [27].

Bevacizumab, a monoclonal antibody targeting VEGF type A—a known mediator of lymphangiomatosis—functions similarly to sirolimus [2, 3, 7, 10, 12, 15, 21, 25]. One case report describes radiographic improvements on CT, along with increases in FEV1 (+17.5%), FVC (+4.6%), total lung capacity (TLC), and DLCO (8.9%), following treatment every three weeks over six months without significant adverse effects [7]. Although there is concern about using this treatment in patients who report hemoptysis, case reports of patients treated at 1 mg/kg every three weeks have shown no harmful effects and even improvement in hemoptysis, stabilization of hemoglobin levels, and reduced lesion size [24]. Patients remained clinically stable for at least 10 months after stopping therapy [25].

Propranolol, a nonselective beta blocker known to inhibit VEGF signaling pathways, has been frequently used to treat DPL, resulting in symptom relief and reductions in lesion size and pleural effusions visible on imaging after at least 6 months of use [2, 3, 10, 12, 15]. Additionally, there is no standardized dosing protocol, with case reports indicating doses ranging from 0.5 mg/kg/day to 20 mg daily [11, 17]. Propranolol is generally well tolerated by patients and has fewer systemic side effects compared to other chemotherapy-based treatments [17].

Corticosteroids have been effectively used alone or in combination with other agents, such as sirolimus, to improve symptoms, including productive cough and shortness of breath, after at least two months of treatment [2, 3, 10, 14, 15]. However, there is no standardized treatment protocol, no recommended strategies for tapering steroid doses, and no clear preference for a specific agent.

Chemotherapy agents, such as cyclophosphamide, tamoxifen, thalidomide, and interferon-alpha 2b, have historically been used to treat DPL. However, due to their poor safety profiles and lower patient tolerability, they are now less frequently employed [3, 10, 12, 15]. Nonetheless, case reports have documented improvements in clinical condition and imaging results [2, 3, 10, 11, 15, 33].

Sildenafil, a phosphodiesterase-5 inhibitor, has been effectively used to treat patients with GLA involving the thorax at a dose of 20 mg three times daily for up to 6 months. Case reports indicate improvements in chest imaging and clinical stability after one year [12, 28].

Localized radiation therapy can lead to regression of symptomatic disease for several months [2, 3, 10, 11]. Most available case reports involve children with multisystem disease who also received radiation to other areas, such as lytic lesions in the pelvis and long bones. Patients generally tolerate the treatment well, experiencing symptomatic relief in chest pain, shortness of breath, and bone pain for at least a year post-radiotherapy [15]. Dosing strategies for pulmonary lymphangiomatosis typically recommend 18–20 Gy, while higher doses are advised for abdominal and skeletal lesions. Lower doses are used when targeting the lung to reduce the risk of radiation pneumonitis and fibrosis of nearby tissue [15]. Interestingly, radiation therapy may be effective in DPL by inducing inflammatory changes and fibrosis within abnormal lymphatic channels, making them nonfunctional [15, 16]. Lung transplantation for end-stage disease has been documented in one case [11].

For recurrent pleural effusions, options such as repeated drainage, pleurodesis, parietal pleurectomy, thoracic duct ligation, and pleuroperitoneal shunt placement can be considered [1, 10, 12, 15]. Standard treatment for chylothorax of any cause includes dietary modifications, specifically adopting a low medium-chain triglyceride/high protein diet to decrease chyle production and restore protein levels [1, 2, 33]. Additionally, octreotide or somatostatin has been used to slow the formation of chylothorax [3, 12].

Prognosis

Diffuse pulmonary lymphangiomatosis is a progressive disease with a generally poor prognosis. The short-term outlook is relatively favorable for patients with minimal or localized disease, which can be managed through observation or surgical removal [13]. Disease symptoms tend to be less severe in adults compared to children [2, 8]. Younger patients up to 16 years old face a mortality rate of up to 40%, whereas adults have nearly a 0% mortality rate [11, 15, 33]. In newborns, the disease is aggressive and almost always fatal [12]. Respiratory failure caused by chylous fluid buildup and infections is the leading cause of death in patients with DPL [18, 19, 33].

References

1. Faul JL, Berry GJ, Colby TV, et al. Thoracic Lymphangiomas, lymphangiectasis, Lymphangiomatosis, and lymphatic dysplasia syndrome. 1999. Am J Respir Crit Care Med, 161(3), pp. 1037–1046.
2. Feng YX, Wang TS, Zhang S, Xu WQ, Liu M, Mao YM, Nong Y. Clinical characteristics and genetic analysis of a patient with diffuse pulmonary lymphangiomatosis: a case report and literature review. BMC Pulm Med. 2025;25(1):72. https://doi.org/10.1186/s12890-025-03544-w. PMID: 39934754; PMCID: PMC11817988.
3. Zhang S, Zhong D, Zhao L, et al. Diffuse pulmonary lymphangiomatosis involving lungs and mediastinal soft tissue. American J Med Sci. 2022;364(1):118–23.
4. Stanley G. R. laboratory models for the investigation of lymphangiomatosis. Microvasc Res. 2014;96:64–7.
5. Lin RY, Zou H, Chen TZ, Wu W, Wang JH, Chen XL, Han QX. Abdominal lymphangiomatosis in a 38-year-old female: case report and literature review. World J Gastroenterol. 2014;20(25):8320–4.
6. Han W, Yang H, Liu J, Li H, Xu H, Liu H, Tang X, Zhao S. Lymphatic malformations involving the thorax in children: a retrospective cohort study. BMC Pulm Med. 2025;25(1):241.
7. Onyeforo E, Barnett A, Zagami D, Deller D, Feather I. Diffuse pulmonary lymphangiomatosis treated with bevacizumab. Respirol Case Rep. 2018;7(1):e00384.
8. Tazelaar HD, Kerr D, Yousem SA, et al. Diffuse pulmonary Lymphangiomatosis. Hum Pathol. 1993;24(10):1313–22.
9. Zhao J, Wu R, Gu Y. Pathology analysis of a rare case of diffuse pulmonary lymphangiomatosis. Ann Transl Med. 2016;4(6):114.
10. Kadakia KC, Patel SM, Yi ES, et al. Diffuse pulmonary lymphangiomatosis. Can Respir J. 2013;20(1):52–4.
11. Luisi F, Torre O, Harari S. Thoracic involvement in generalised lymphatic anomaly (or lymphangiomatosis). Eur Respir Rev. 2016;25:101–3.
12. Riazuddin M, Farouk N, Ali S, Butt M, Arabi T, Sabbah B, Ali M, Alkattan K. Pleural effusion due to lymphangiomatosis and the role of sirolimus: a case report. Ann. Med. Surg. 2023;85(12):6178–81.
13. Yu W, Mi L, Cong J, Cheng W, Chen Y, Gong H. Diffuse pulmonary lymphangiomatosis. Medicine. 2019;98(43):e17349.
14. Zheng G, Tang H, Su R, Liang Y, He Z, Zhang J, Deng J, Bai J, Zhong X. A gene missense mutation in diffuse pulmonary lymphangiomatosis with thrombocytopenia. Medicine (Baltimore). 2020;99(39):e21941. https://doi.org/10.1097/MD.0000000000021941.
15. Purkayastha A, Sharma N, Roy S, Agarwal C. Upfront radiotherapy for diffuse lymphangiomatosis in a child. Int J Adv Med Health Res. 2016;3(2):97–100. https://doi.org/10.4103/2349-4220.195938.

16. Fang X, Huang Z, Zeng Y, Zhu X, Wang S, Yu X, Li X, Wu C, Yi X. Lymphangiomatosis involving the pulmonary and extrapulmonary lymph nodes and surrounding soft tissue. Medicine (Baltimore). 2017;96(49):e9032. https://doi.org/10.1097/MD.0000000000009032.
17. Putta T, Irodi A, Thangakunam B, Oliver A, Gunasingam R. Young patient with generalized lymphangiomatosis. Indian J Radiold Imag. 2016;26(3):411–5. https://doi.org/10.4103/0971-3026.190416.
18. Biscotto I, Rodrigues RS, Forny DN, Barreto MM, Marchiori E. Diffuse pulmonary lymphangiomatosis. J Bras Pneumol. 2019;45(5):e20180412. https://doi.org/10.1590/1806-3713/e20180412. PMID: 31531617; PMCID: PMC7247761.
19. Ernotte C, Médart L, Collignon L. Diffuse pulmonary Lymphangiomatosis. J Belge Radiol. 2018;102(1):64. https://doi.org/10.5334/jbsr.1603.
20. Salcedo Miranda D, Galvis JR, Téllez Rodríguez LJ, Garzón Ramírez JC, Ariza Traslaviña J. Diffuse pulmonary lymphangiomatosis as a differential diagnosis of anterior mediastinal mass. J Surg Case Rep. 2024;2024(9):rjae577. https://doi.org/10.1093/jscr/rjae577. PMID: 39280023; PMCID: PMC11393567.
21. Gurskytė V, Zeleckienė I, Maskoliūnaitė V, Mickys U, Šileikienė V. Successful treatment of diffuse pulmonary lymphangiomatosis with sirolimus. Respir Med Case Rep. 2020;29:101014. https://doi.org/10.1016/j.rmcr.2020.101014. PMID: 32071853; PMCID: PMC7013175.
22. Ito K, Kuse N, Misumi A, Takashi M, Chin H, Ito Y, Miyazaki S, Sakamoto K, Awano N, Inomata M, Kobayashi Y, Kumasaka T, Bae Y, Izumo T. Lymphangiomatosis diagnosed using transbronchial lung cryobiopsy: a case report. Respir Med Case Rep. 2025;56:102239. https://doi.org/10.1016/j.rmcr.2025.102239. PMID: 40502211; PMCID: PMC12152360.
23. Polke M, Polke N, Piel S, Brunnemer E, Wälscher J, Buschulte K, Warth A, Heussel CP, Eichinger M, Frankenstein L, Eichhorn M, Miliauskas S, Herth FJF, Kreuter M. Pulmonary lymphangiomatosis: insights into an ultra-rare disease. Respir Res. 2024;25(1):416. https://doi.org/10.1186/s12931-024-03040-5. PMID: 39593123; PMCID: PMC11600747.
24. Dimiene I, Bieksiene K, Zaveckiene J, Andrulis M, Optazaite DE, Vaguliene N, Zemaitis M, Miliauskas S. Effective initial treatment of diffuse pulmonary Lymphangiomatosis with Sirolimus and propranolol: a case report. Medicina (Kaunas). 2021;57(12):1308. https://doi.org/10.3390/medicina57121308. PMID: 34946253; PMCID: PMC8706407.
25. Aman J, Thunnissen E, Paul MA, van Nieuw Amerongen GP, Vonk-Noordegraaf A. Successful treatment of diffuse pulmonary lymphangiomatosis with bevacizumab. Ann Intern Med. 2012;156(11):839–40. https://doi.org/10.7326/0003-4819-156-11-201206050-00016. PMID: 22665821.
26. Nagano N, Izumi S, Katsuno T, Iikura M, Miyazaki H, Igari T, Okafuji T, Sekihara K, Nagasaka S, Hojo M. A case of diffuse pulmonary lymphangiomatosis with a venous anomaly presenting with acute respiratory failure and hemoptysis. Respir Med Case Rep. 2020;31:101243. https://doi.org/10.1016/j.rmcr.2020.101243. PMID: 33088708; PMCID: PMC7567044.
27. Boscolo E, Pastura P, Glaser K, Goines J, Hammill AM, Adams DM, Dickie P, Hsi Dickie B, Le Cras TD. Signaling pathways and inhibitors of cells from patients with kaposiform lymphangiomatosis. Pediatr Blood Cancer. 2019;66(8):e27790. https://doi.org/10.1002/pbc.27790. Epub 2019 May 2. PMID: 31045327; PMCID: PMC6588438.
28. Maurac A, Debray MP, Crestani B, Taillé C. Thoracic involvement of diffuse lymphangiomatosis successfully treated with sildenafil. BMJ Case Rep 2019 Apr 23;12(4):e228523. doi: https://doi.org/10.1136/bcr-2018-228523. PMID: 31015245; PMCID: PMC6510121.
29. Guo Y, Chen J, Xu B, Zheng Y, Shen K. Causes and manifestations of chylothorax in children in China: experience from a children's medical center, 2007–2017. Pediatr Investig. 2018;2(1):8–14. https://doi.org/10.1002/ped4.12019. PMID: 32851223; PMCID: PMC7331315.
30. Zhang J, Jin H, Wang Y, Bai C, Han Y. A case of diffuse pulmonary lymphangiomatosis with unilateral lung invasion. Oxf Med Case Rep. 2015;2015(10):346–8. https://doi.org/10.1093/omcr/omv059. PMID: 26512334; PMCID: PMC4622182.
31. Lim HJ, Han J, Kim HK, Kim TS. A rare case of diffuse pulmonary lymphangiomatosis in a middle-aged woman. Korean J Radiol. 2014;15(2):295–9. https://doi.org/10.3348/kjr.2014.15.2.295. Epub 2014 Mar 7. PMID: 24642766; PMCID: PMC3955798.
32. Kadakia KC, Patel SM, Yi ES, Limper AH. Diffuse pulmonary lymphangiomatosis. Can Respir J. 2013;20(1):52–4. https://doi.org/10.1155/2013/971350. PMID: 23457676; PMCID: PMC3628648.
33. Satria MN, Pacheco-Rodriguez G, Moss J. Pulmonary lymphangiomatosis. Lymphat Res Biol. 2011;9(4):191–3. https://doi.org/10.1089/lrb.2011.0023. PMID: 22196284; PMCID: PMC3246407.
34. Takahashi K, Takahashi H, Maeda K, Homma S, Uekusa T, Dambara T, Kira S. An adult case of lymphangiomatosis of the mediastinum, pulmonary interstitium and retroperitoneum complicated by chronic disseminated intravascular coagulation. Eur Respir J. 1995;8(10):1799–802. https://doi.org/10.1183/09031936.95.08101799. PMID: 8586141.

35. El Hajj L, Mazieres J, Rouquette I, Boulduc JP, Didier A, Dahan M, Joffre F, Chabbert VC. Diagnostic value of bronchoscopy, CT and transbronchial biopsies in diffuse pulmonary lymphangiomatosis: case report and review of literature. Clin Radiol. 2005;60(8):921–5. https://doi.org/10.1016/j.crad.2005.03.006. PMID: 16039928.

Part III

Rare Causes of Pleural Effusions

6 Chylothorax

Michael Nicholson and Danish Ahmad

Introduction

Chylothorax is a rare pleural effusion that occurs due to the buildup of chyle, a lipid-rich lymphatic fluid, within the pleural cavity [1]. This condition arises from damage or obstruction of the thoracic duct or its tributaries, resulting in lymphatic fluid leakage and subsequently leading to pleural effusion. Representing approximately 2–3% of all pleural effusions, chylothorax may result in considerable morbidity owing to respiratory compromise, nutritional deficiencies, and immune dysfunction [2, 3]. In one review, patients who did not undergo any lymphatic duct intervention exhibited a one-year mortality rate of 47% [4].

Reportedly, the first description of chylothorax is attributed to Bartolet in 1633, several years following the initial characterization of the lymphatic system [5]. In 1685, Diemerbroeck also documented a case resulting from trauma, and in 1875, H. Quincke reported a case that occurred after a fall from a wagon; however, these instances are not thoroughly documented or readily accessible within medical literature [5]. Over the subsequent decades, case reports and case series, primarily concerning traumatic chylothorax, further delineated this condition [6, 7]. In 1946, Lampson described the first successful treatment for traumatic chylothorax, namely, thoracic duct ligation [8]. Since that period, progress in imaging modalities, anatomical knowledge, and molecular analysis has led to a broad spectrum of nontraumatic causes, including malignancies, congenital anomalies, infections, and systemic inflammatory diseases. This ongoing expansion of knowledge regarding the diverse pathophysiology has led to the development of increasingly targeted and efficacious therapeutic approaches [9, 10].

This chapter provides a comprehensive overview of anatomy, pathophysiology, clinical features, diagnostic strategies, and management options for chylothorax.

M. Nicholson
Department of Pulmonary and Critical Care Medicine, Robert Wood Johnson Barnabas Health, East Brunswick, NJ, USA
e-mail: Michael.Nicholson@rwjbh.org

D. Ahmad (✉)
Interventional Pulmonology, Department of Medicine, Fox Chase Cancer Center, Philadelphia, PA, USA
e-mail: Danish.Ahmad@fccc.edu

Anatomy and Physiology

Chyle Formation

The term "chyle" derives from the Greek word "chylos," meaning "juice" [11]. Chyle is a bodily fluid composed of lymphocytes, proteins, electrolytes, free fatty acids, and emulsified fats absorbed from the small intestine during digestion. Approximately 2.4 liters of chyle are transported daily from the intestines to the systemic

F. Ido (ed.), *Rare Pleural Diseases*, https://doi.org/10.1007/978-3-032-14873-5_6

circulation [12]. Dietary triglycerides are a major constituent in the formation of chyle. In the small intestine, triglycerides undergo hydrolysis into free fatty acids and monoglycerides, facilitated by pancreatic lipase and bile salts [13]. These lipids are absorbed by jejunal enterocytes, where they are reconstituted into triglycerides. Since triglycerides and cholesterol esters are insoluble in plasma, they are packaged into lipoprotein particles, known as chylomicrons, to enable systemic transport [14]. Chylomicrons, the principal lipid transporters, are classified as ultralow-density lipoproteins responsible for the translocation of lipids from the gastrointestinal tract to various tissues within the body. They are formed through the assembly of triglycerides with phospholipids, cholesterol, and cholesterol esters. Structurally, a chylomicron comprises a core of triglycerides and cholesterol esters enveloped by a surface layer composed of phospholipids, cholesterol, and specific proteins [15, 16]. These chylomicrons are rich in triglycerides, constituting approximately 90% of their composition. This elevated triglyceride concentration imparts upon chyle its distinctive white or "milky" appearance, a defining characteristic of the fluid [15].

Chyle Transport

Following the digestion of triglycerides into monosaccharides and fatty acids, these substances are transported across the basolateral surface of the small intestinal enterocytes, which are located at the base of the microvilli. These small molecules are then taken up by the small lymphatic vessels located within the microvilli, known as jejunal lacteals. The jejunal lacteals play a vital role in transporting chyle from the small intestine into the lymphatic circulation [12]. Lacteals converge into progressively larger lymphatic vessels, which ultimately merge into a lymphatic reservoir known as the cisterna chyli [17].

The cisterna chyli is a retroperitoneal lymphatic sac situated within the retrocrural space, anterior to the first or second lumbar vertebrae and posterolateral to the abdominal aorta. It receives drainage from two lumbar trunks and one intestinal trunk, functioning as a central reservoir for lymphatic fluid and serving as the origin of the thoracic duct [18]. However, approximately half of all individuals lack a defined cisterna chyli. In these cases, lymphatic trunks directly feed into the thoracic duct, sometimes presenting as focal dilatations of the trunks rather than a single reservoir [18, 19].

The thoracic duct, first described by French anatomist Jean Pecquet in 1651, constitutes the largest lymphatic vessel within the human anatomy. It is responsible for transporting approximately 60–70% of ingested fats, including fat-soluble vitamins [20, 21]. The thoracic duct originates at the cisterna chyli and terminates at the venous angle, where the left subclavian vein and internal jugular vein converge [17]. The total length of the duct approximately measures 35 to 46 centimeters. It extends from the abdomen into the thorax through the aortic hiatus of the diaphragm. The duct proceeds superiorly posterior to the esophagus, positioned between the thoracic aorta to its left and the azygos vein to its right. At the fifth thoracic vertebra (T5) level, the thoracic duct crosses the midline from right to left [21]. This anatomical feature is clinically significant in identifying the side of a pleural effusion attributable to pathology of the thoracic duct. Insults occurring below T5 generally result in right-sided chylothorax, whereas injuries above T5 typically cause left-sided chylothorax [22]. Approximately 50% of all chylous effusions are unilateral on the right side owing to the duct's extended course below T5 [23]. While the course described represents the most frequently observed anatomical pathway, notable variations exist in its course, midline crossing point, and termination of the thoracic duct. These variations may complicate the identification and management of thoracic duct pathologies but underscore the importance of understanding its typical course within clinical practice [19] .

Etiology

Nontraumatic Causes

Malignancy

Malignancy constitutes the most prevalent cause of nontraumatic chylothorax, with lymphoma representing the majority of cases [14, 24]. Non-Hodgkin lymphoma is implicated in approximately 70% of malignant chylothorax cases, whereas Hodgkin lymphoma accounts for around 18% [10, 23, 25]. Other malignancies, including lung, esophageal, and breast cancers, as well as distant metastatic diseases, are less common causes [26].

Malignancy can cause chylothorax mainly through three mechanisms. One is direct infiltration, where tumor cells invade the thoracic duct or lymph nodes, disrupting chyle flow and raising hydrostatic pressure, which then leads to chyle leakage [17, 27]. Another mechanism, lymphatic obstruction, occurs when the thoracic duct is compressed externally by enlarged intrathoracic lymph nodes, which may result from lymphoma, metastatic cancer, or inflammatory conditions. Finally, transdiaphragmatic translocation occurs when malignant lymphatic obstruction within the abdomen results in chyle leakage into the peritoneal cavity. During inspiration, negative thoracic pressure facilitates the migration of chyle into the thoracic cavity via diaphragmatic defects [28–30].

Congenital Abnormalities

Congenital abnormalities, although infrequent, may lead to structural or functional impairments within the lymphatic system, including the thoracic duct. Conditions such as hypoplasia, duplication, and atresia of the thoracic duct can result in abnormal chyle flow, frequently presenting as chylothorax in neonates [31].

Lymphangiomas, also referred to as lymphatic malformations, are benign, multicystic proliferations of lymphatic tissue that may obstruct the flow of the thoracic duct. They can develop in the subcutaneous tissue, mediastinum, lung parenchyma, or chest wall, and are believed to originate from abnormal sequestration of lymphatic vessels during embryonic development. Although their occurrence is rare, constituting approximately 4% of all vascular tumors in pediatric patients, these lesions are typically present at birth, with 90% being identified by the age of two [31, 32].

Other primary lymphatic conditions, such as pulmonary lymphangiectasia, generalized lymphatic anomaly, and central conducting lymphatic anomaly, also disrupt lymphatic flow and may cause chylothorax [32].

Several genetic syndromes are associated with impaired lymphatic drainage, which can lead to the subsequent development of chylothorax. Predominant conditions include Down syndrome, Turner syndrome, and Noonan syndrome. These conditions lead to lymphatic hypoplasia, obstruction, or compromised chyle transport, with severity contingent upon the degree of dysfunction [11, 31, 33].

A rare syndrome associated with chylothorax is Gorham-Stout syndrome, characterized by extensive osteolysis, vascular malformations, and abnormal proliferation of lymphatic channels within bone [34, 35]. These abnormalities impede the thoracic duct, resulting in chylothorax in approximately 17% of cases [36].

Infections

Infections can influence the lymphatic system via multiple mechanisms [11, 26]. Granulomas or abscesses resulting from resolved or active infections may exert external pressure on lymphatic vessels, thereby disrupting the flow of chyle. Additionally, specific pathogens, including *Wuchereria bancrofti*, *Yersinia pestis*, and particular *Salmonella* species, have the capacity to invade lymphatic vessels, leading to impaired lymphatic circulation [11]. Tuberculous and nontuberculous mycobacteria have been observed in conjunction with chylothorax, even in the absence of lymphadenopathy, thereby highlighting multiple mechanisms [26, 37–39].

Miscellaneous

Various systemic diseases and syndromes can cause chylothorax. Lymphangioleiomyomatosis (LAM) involves the abnormal proliferation of smooth muscle-like cells, primarily affecting the lungs. It is most frequently observed in women of reproductive age and can manifest with cystic lung disease [38, 39]. Involvement of the thoracic duct may occur, leading to lymphatic obstruction and chylothorax [40, 41]. Approximately 20–40% of patients with LAM will develop chylothorax during their lifetime [12].

Yellow nail syndrome is a condition characterized by yellow nails, lymphedema, and various respiratory manifestations, including chronic cough and bronchiectasis. Its etiology remains unclear [42]. Pleural effusions are observed in approximately 46% of cases, with 20% of these being chylous and generally bilateral [43]. The underlying mechanism likely involves impaired chyle movement within the lymphatic system. It is suspected to be linked to abnormalities in the lymphatic vessels, although the exact mechanism is not well understood [44].

Sarcoidosis is a systemic inflammatory disorder characterized by the formation of noncaseating granulomas. Although rare, chylous pleural effusions have been documented, frequently attributed to the occlusion of the thoracic duct by enlarged lymphadenopathy. Other potential mechanisms include granulomatous inflammation of the pleura or direct inflammation of lymphatic channels leading to chyle leakage [45].

Rarely, chylothorax can manifest in patients presenting with transudative effusions. This phenomenon is observed in conditions such as chronic heart failure, liver cirrhosis, or nephrotic syndrome. In such instances, elevated hydrostatic pressure within the thoracic duct, resultant from venous hypervolemia, compromises lymphatic flow, thereby resulting in chyle leakage into the pleural cavity [29, 46].

An additional mechanism may occur in liver cirrhosis whereby chylous ascites can develop due to elevated pressure in abdominal lymphatics. Through diaphragmatic fenestrations, chyle can migrate into the thoracic cavity, resulting in chylous pleural effusions. This process mirrors the physiology of hepatic hydrothorax [46].

Approximately 9% of nontraumatic chylothorax cases lack a discernible cause and are categorized as idiopathic. These instances frequently pose challenges in diagnosis and management [47].

Traumatic Causes

Iatrogenic Injury

Traumatic etiologies exhibit the highest prevalence of chylothorax, with iatrogenic injury identified as the primary causative factor [23]. Iatrogenic injuries account for 80% of traumatic chylothorax cases [37]. The most frequent cause of iatrogenic chylothorax is thoracic surgery, with the incidence varying according to the type of procedure [48]. Approximately 0.5–1% of all thoracic surgeries are reportedly complicated by chylothorax [26]. Although this percentage is relatively small, it is estimated that over 530,000 thoracic surgeries are performed annually in the United States alone [49]. Esophagectomy, in particular, carries a significant risk, with an estimated 4% of cases developing chylothorax due to the proximity of the thoracic duct to the aorto-esophageal groove [19, 23, 50]. Other thoracic surgical procedures, such as lung resection, cardiothoracic surgery, and mediastinal lymph node dissection, may also lead to iatrogenic chylothorax, often attributable to the variability in thoracic duct anatomy [19, 51]. Cardiothoracic surgeries report incidences of chylothorax ranging from 2% to 5%, with pediatric surgery for congenital heart defects exhibiting a higher incidence compared to adults [48]. In lung resections, more extensive procedures, such as pneumonectomy, present a higher risk, especially on the right side, owing to more comprehensive mediastinal lymph node dissections [51, 52] .

Thyroid surgeries, although infrequent, also carry a risk of thoracic duct injury. The occurrence is higher when a neck dissection or sternotomy is performed, typically in cases of advanced thyroid carcinoma. A cervical neck dissection may result in chylothorax in 2% of cases, whereas a sternotomy can lead to chylous effusion in up to 7% of cases. The most common site of injury during thyroid surgery is located near the venous angle, where the thoracic duct terminates [53].

Nonsurgical procedures may also result in chylothorax. Central venous catheterization, including procedures such as Swan-Ganz catheter insertion and pacemaker implantation, entails a minor risk. Mechanisms of injury encompass thrombosis, causing external compression or direct trauma to the thoracic duct during subclavian vein catheterization. The overall risk of chylothorax associated with these procedures remains low, with an incidence rate below 0.5% [54].

Trauma

The two most common mechanisms of traumatic injury to the thoracic duct are blunt and penetrating trauma. Gunshot or stab wounds have the potential to lacerate the thoracic duct in the abdomen, thorax, or neck; however, this occurs in only approximately 1% of penetrating traumas [21]. Blunt trauma can cause injury to the thoracic duct through various mechanisms. Rib fractures resulting from blunt chest trauma may shear the duct, leading to chyle leakage. Acute hyperextension of the vertebral column may also stretch and tear the duct. Additionally, the right diaphragmatic crus can transect the thoracic duct in instances of acute blunt trauma [1]. Despite these potential injury mechanisms, the incidence of chylothorax is observed in only 0.2–3% of cases involving blunt trauma cases [55, 56].

Other less common traumatic causes, which are infrequently associated with chylothorax, include acceleration-deceleration incidents such as motor vehicle collisions. These are presumably attributable to the stretching and tearing of the thoracic duct, resulting from sudden changes in velocity [57]. Additionally, maneuvers that elevate intra-abdominal pressure, such as excessive stretching, childbirth, forceful sneezing, coughing, or vomiting, are believed to shear the thoracic duct near the diaphragmatic aperture [58–60]. Although these events are documented in the literature, they are not common causes of chylothorax.

Clinical Presentation

Symptoms

Chylothorax manifests with varying symptoms depending on the underlying etiology, severity, and duration of lymphatic obstruction [14]. Numerous cases initially present without symptoms; the most frequent signs are dyspnea and cough, which are nonspecific and commonly observed in most pleural effusions [23]. A key distinction between chylous effusions and other types is the absence of chest pain and fever. Chyle does not irritate the pleural surface; therefore, it does not trigger an inflammatory response, leading to these symptoms [4, 17].

A rare symptom characteristic of chylothorax is chyloptysis, defined as the expectoration of chylous fluid within sputum. This phenomenon arises from the reflux of chyle from the pleural cavity into the bronchial tree, leading to the production of "milky" sputum [61]. Another uncommon symptom is uncontrolled atrial fibrillation in patients previously stable on amiodarone or digoxin. Generally, these medications are transported via chyle into the venous system; however, in the presence of a chylothorax, they accumulate in the pleural space, resulting in decreased serum levels [62, 63].

The onset and severity of respiratory symptoms depend on the rate of chyle accumulation. Insidious dyspnea is more prevalent with slow accumulation, often observed in nontraumatic etiologies involving smaller obstructions and gradual leaks. Postsurgical chylous effusions generally manifest within 2–10 days following surgical procedures; however, some cases may be identified through routine imaging prior to the emergence of clinical symptoms. Conversely, rapid accumulation of chyle results in more acute symptoms, commonly observed after blunt or penetrating trauma, wherein significant damage to the thoracic duct precipitates large-volume effusions within a brief period [14, 17, 23].

A rare yet life-threatening presentation is tension chylothorax, wherein a considerable volume of chyle exerts compressive force on the mediastinum, resulting in swift hemodynamic and respiratory compromise. The underlying physiology bears resemblance to that of tension pneumothorax. This condition is especially concerning following a pneumonectomy, as lung function may decline precipitously due to mechanical compression of the remaining lung [64].

Symptoms can also vary depending on the underlying cause. Malignant cases may present with constitutional symptoms such as night sweats, weight loss, and fatigue. Infectious causes often present with fever and chills. Additionally, complications such as nutritional deficiencies and immunodeficiencies can arise [23].

Physical Examination

Physical examination findings are nonspecific to chylothorax and reflect the findings of pleural effusions in general. Auscultation will reveal decreased breath sounds and shifting dullness on the side of the effusion. Specific physical examination findings related to the underlying cause can be identified, such as the characteristic yellow nails seen in yellow nail syndrome [17, 43].

Diagnosis

Diagnostic Thoracic Imaging

The initial step in diagnosing a chylothorax involves the identification of a pleural effusion. Various thoracic imaging techniques are instrumental in characterizing pleural effusions and can assist in identifying underlying causes such as malignancy, abscesses, and lymphadenopathy. Specific imaging modalities also permit direct visualization of the lymphatic system, thereby facilitating the assessment of the chyle leak's location and the detection of potential underlying abnormalities contributing to chylothorax formation.

Chest Radiography

Pleural effusions are frequently identified on chest radiographs. The ability to detect pleural effusions through imaging largely depends on their size and the radiographic technique used. A posteroanterior view can detect effusions containing at least 200 mL of pleural fluid, whereas lateral views are more sensitive, capable of identifying effusions as small as 50 mL [65, 66]. While chest radiography serves as a valuable tool for the rapid detection of pleural effusions, it cannot differentiate a chylothorax from other types of pleural effusions. Nonetheless, it can expose underlying etiologies such as pulmonary masses or lymphadenopathy. Alternative imaging techniques are more effective for diagnosing these etiologies [47].

Computed Tomography

Computed tomography (CT) of the chest provides detailed images of pleural effusions, allowing better characterization of their size, complexity, and other fluid attributes compared to chest radiography [47]. CT is also more effective in identifying malignancies, lymphadenopathy, and other thoracic pathologies that can cause chylothorax. In rare cases, the site of lymphatic injury may be visible on CT, but this is uncommon. Dedicated lymphatic imaging is usually needed for precise localization. CT, however, is unable to differentiate chylothorax from other categories of pleural effusions [26].

Thoracic Ultrasonography

A thoracic ultrasound is a rapid, portable, and effective method for assessing pleural effusions. It has demonstrated nearly 100% specificity, sensitivity, and diagnostic accuracy in detecting effusions [67]. Ultrasound can also reveal effusion characteristics such as septations, heterogeneity, and echogenicity. Additionally, it is an invaluable tool for guiding thoracentesis safely and effectively [68]. Nevertheless, thoracic ultrasound is incapable of diagnosing chylothorax.

Lymphatic-Specific Imaging

Computed Tomography Lymphangiography

CT lymphangiography is an invasive procedure wherein water-soluble contrast media is directly administered into the cisterna chyli under CT guidance [69]. This technique highlights central lymphatic structures, such as the thoracic duct, which are not distinctly visible on standard CT imaging. Contrast extravasation aids in identifying the site of chyle leakage [70, 71]. CT lymphangiography enables immediate CT-guided interventions and provides rapid image acquisition, eliminating the interference caused by metal implants—a limitation of magnetic resonance imaging lymphangiography.

Magnetic Resonance Lymphangiography

Magnetic resonance (MR) lymphangiography may be conducted either with or without the use of contrast enhancement. Non-contrast MR lymphangiography is a noninvasive procedure that offers detailed visualization of lymphatic anatomy [72]. However, it is not effective for localizing chyle leaks due to the lack of contrast. Dynamic contrast-enhanced MR lymphangiography, a procedure that involves the invasive intranodal administration of contrast (such as gadolinium) under ultrasound guidance, offers enhanced visualization of chyle leaks and provides exceptional detail of lymphatic structures [73, 74]. This method is valuable due to its high spatial resolution and 3D imaging capabilities [2, 69]. However, its use is limited by factors such as the presence of metal implants, cost, and availability at certain medical centers.

Lymphangioscintigraphy and Single-Photon Emission Computed Tomography

Lymphangioscintigraphy is a minimally invasive nuclear medicine technique that involves the subcutaneous injection of a radiotracer into the lymphatic system [75–77]. Recently, it has been combined with single-photon emission computed tomography (SPECT)) to enhance image quality. While lymphangioscintigraphy alone has limited spatial resolution and lacks clear anatomical landmarks, the addition of SPECT improves anatomical localization of the radiotracer, making the images more practical. This combined approach enables functional assessment of lymphatic flow and the precise localization of chyle leakage [69].

Invasive Lymphangiography

Invasive lymphangiography is regarded as the gold standard for imaging both the central and peripheral lymphatic systems [78]. Initially, pedal lymphangiography was the predominant method, involving the injection of poppy seed-based oil into the interdigital web spaces of the foot, enabling absorption by the lymphatic capillaries and consequently visualizing the entire lymphatic network [69]. This technique has evolved to target more effective sites, such as the inguinal lymph nodes [79]. Once the oil is injected, lymphatic flow is observed using fluoroscopy, enabling real-time identification of lymphatic abnormalities and chyle leakage. Invasive lymphangiography detects leakage in 64–78% of cases and permits therapeutic intervention during imaging, if necessary. Notably, the procedure itself is therapeutic in 30–70% of instances, likely attributable to inflammation induced by the poppy seed-based oil, which occludes the leak [26, 80]. Potential complications encompass oil embolization, lipoid pneumonia, and injection site urticaria [17]. To minimize risks, contrast injections should be restricted to 14 mL. Although highly effective, this procedure is invasive and necessitates qualified operators, thereby limiting its accessibility [69].

Pleural Fluid Analysis

Pleural fluid analysis is essential for diagnosing chylothorax and involves both a macroscopic description of the fluid and several laboratory studies.

The characteristic appearance of chylothorax fluid is "milky" white, attributable to a high lipid concentration. However, this visual characteristic is observed in only 22–44% of cases, rendering it neither sensitive nor specific for the diagnosis of chylothorax [24, 81]. In certain instances, such as with decreased lipid intake or traumatic injury, the fluid may not exhibit a milky appearance [17]. In cases of trauma, the fluid may be blood-tinged or serosanguinous as a result of contamination with blood [9]. Similarly, other effusions, such as pseudochylothorax and empyema, may also present with a whitish appearance due to elevated cholesterol levels or the presence of pus, respectively. Consequently, a milky appearance alone should not serve as the sole diagnostic criterion [23].

Pleural fluid analysis relies on detecting elevated levels of triglycerides and cholesterol. A triglyceride level exceeding 110 mg/dL combined with a cholesterol level below 200 mg/dL is highly sensitive for diagnosing chylothorax [9]. Triglyceride levels greater than 110 mg/dL are found to be non-chylous in only 1% of instances [23]. However, triglyceride levels can be lower in 14% of chylothorax cases, often due to nutritional deficiencies. When triglyceride levels are less than 50 mg/dL, the likelihood of a chylous effusion is very low. For triglyceride levels between 50–110 mg/dL, additional tests, such as pleural fluid-to-serum triglyceride and cholesterol ratios, may be helpful [3]. A pleural fluid-to-serum triglyceride ratio exceeding 1 and a cholesterol ratio below 1 are indicative of chylothorax [14, 24]. The gold standard for diagnosing chylothorax, particularly when pleural fluid triglyceride levels are equivocal, is the detection of chylomicrons through lipoprotein electrophoresis [25].

Additional pleural fluid tests, although nondiagnostic, may aid in supporting the diagnosis. Despite the low protein content of chyle, total protein levels are typically elevated due to the high rate of solute reabsorption into the intravascular space [82]. Lactate dehydrogenase (LDH) levels are generally low in chylous effusions, given that LDH is a large molecule that does not readily traverse into the pleural space unless there is an alteration in the pleural-capillary membrane. An elevation in LDH suggests the presence of concomitant pleural pathology [81]. The discrepancy between total protein and LDH classifies chylous effusions as protein-discordant exudates, wherein they meet the exudative criteria by either total protein or LDH, but not both. Rarely, chylous effusions may present as transudates, usually in hypervolemic states such as liver cirrhosis, heart failure, or nephrotic syndrome [24, 46].

The quantitative cellular composition and cytology of pleural fluid help narrow the differential diagnosis and exclude effusions that may resemble chylothoraces, which can be caused by infection and malignancy. Chylous effusions usually exhibit lymphocyte predominance, typically comprising greater than 70% of the pleural fluid cellular composition. Although this is often observed with malignant effusions, microscopic analysis of pleural fluid cytology by a pathologist can differentiate the two by identifying neoplastic cells. A predominantly neutrophilic effusion is rare and should warrant consideration of an alternative diagnosis, such as infection [26, 81].

Differential Diagnoses

A recognized differential diagnosis for chylothorax is pseudochylothorax, also referred to as chyliform effusions, which is frequently mistaken for chylothorax due to its similar milky appearance [21]. However, there are significant distinctions between the two entities. Pseudochylothorax is characterized as a cholesterol-rich pleural effusion that develops from prolonged pleural effusions. Chronic, exudative effusions result in cellular breakdown, releasing cholesterol and lipid particles into the pleural cavity. Although the appearances may resemble each other, pseudochylothorax is distinguished by its cholesterol composition rather than chyle and does not involve the thoracic duct or lymphatic abnormalities [83].

The diagnosis of pseudochylothorax is supported by a pleural fluid triglyceride level below 50 mg/dL, a cholesterol level exceeding 200 mg/dL, and a pleural fluid-to-serum cholesterol ratio greater than 1, accompanied by a triglyceride ratio less than 1 [83, 84]. Common causes of pseudochylothorax include tuberculous effusions, rheumatoid effusions, chronic hemothorax, and inadequately drained empyema [83].

Other significant differential diagnoses encompass parapneumonic effusions and empyema, which can be distinguished by the presence of notable neutrophils and bacteria in pleural fluid analysis [9]. Hemothorax and malignant effusions may also resemble chylous effusions; however, pleural fluid analysis can distinguish these diagnoses [85].

Management

Currently, no consensus guidelines exist for the management of chylothoraxes, and robust evidence, such as randomized controlled trials, on the treatment of chylothorax remains lacking. Therapeutic strategies, therefore, vary considerably and should be individualized according to the patient's clinical condition, the underlying etiology of the effusion, its respiratory and hemodynamic consequences, the volume and rate of chyle leakage, and the expertise available within the treating center [86]. Chyle leakage is typically categorized according to daily output, with volumes <500 mL/day considered low output and those >1000 mL/day classified as high output [87]. This distinction is clinically relevant, as the severity of leakage often guides therapeutic decision-making. Management options span a continuum, beginning with conservative measures such as dietary modification (e.g., a medium-chain triglyceride diet or total parenteral nutrition) and pharmacological therapy, progressing to interventional procedures (e.g., thoracic duct embolization), and, when necessary, definitive surgical approaches, including thoracic duct ligation [14, 88, 89]. Effective management requires a multidisciplinary team approach, bringing together pulmonologists, thoracic surgeons, interventional radiologists, dietitians, and pharmacists to tailor therapy to the individual patient [9].

Conservative Management

Conservative interventions are typically implemented after the initial effusion has been drained. A combination of multiple conservative measures is frequently employed to maximize efficacy. The primary objective of conservative therapy is to diminish flow through the thoracic duct and facilitate the healing of the leakage site, thereby obviating the necessity for more invasive procedures. Although conservative management is generally more effective in cases of low-output chylothorax, it may still be considered as a trial in high-output cases [12] .

Dietary Modifications

Dietary modifications are frequently considered the initial approach to treatment, given their ease of implementation and prompt application. The emphasis is placed on a no-fat, high-protein diet. Eliminating fat decreases the lipid content within caloric intake, as long-chain triglycerides (the core component of chylomicrons) are removed [90, 91]. Medium-chain triglycerides, however, remain suitable for ingestion as they are directly absorbed into the portal circulation, thus bypassing the lymphatic system [87]. Consuming a high-protein diet helps decrease fat absorption in the intestines. The integration of these strategies results in a reduction of circulating chyle volume [92]. If a modified enteral diet fails to decrease chyle leakage adequately, a strict nothing-by-mouth (NPO) approach combined with total parenteral nutrition (TPN) may be trialed [88]. However, TPN involves risks, including infections, thrombosis, and cholestasis [17]. The efficacy of dietary modifications is unpredictable and exhibits variability among patients. Furthermore, potential risks encompass deficiencies in fat-soluble vitamins and essential fatty acids, which may result in malnutrition and various other complications [91]. This consideration is particularly significant in patients with malignancy-induced chylothorax, who may already be malnourished and frail [12]. Furthermore, most patients perceive the diet as considerably restrictive, leading to low adherence [87].

Pharmacologic Therapy

Somatostatin and its analogs, such as octreotide, have been utilized as pharmacological therapies for chylothorax [93]. They diminish lymph production and lymphatic flow via multiple mechanisms, including the reduction of gastric, biliary, and pancreatic secretions, constriction of smooth muscle within the splanchnic and lymphatic vessels, and augmentation of fecal fat secretion [94, 95]. There is no consensus regarding the dosage, timing, or route of administration, with various regimens employed in clinical practice. For optimal efficacy, these medications should be supplemented with dietary modifications [93, 96].

Alpha-1-adrenergic agonists, such as midodrine and etilefrine, have demonstrated some efficacy in the treatment of chylothorax, although the precise mechanism remains unclear. It is hypothesized to be associated with splanchnic vasoconstriction [97, 98]. Due to limited data, these medications are not routinely recommended for the treatment of chylous effusions.

The primary treatment for a chylothorax is centered on addressing the underlying etiology, as this frequently results in the resolution of the pleural effusion. Accordingly, specific treatment strategies may be employed depending on the causative factor. For instance, sirolimus can be utilized in cases attributable to lymphangioleiomyomatosis [38]. In instances of chylothorax associated with sarcoidosis, corticosteroids are advised [99]. Malignant effusions may resolve with appropriate radiation and chemotherapy. Chylothorax due to hypervolemia can be managed with diuretics and guideline-directed medical therapy [87].

Interventional Procedures

Pleural Drainage

The primary goal of pleural drainage is to relieve respiratory symptoms associated with the effusion; however, it does not usually correct the underlying chylothorax. Drainage provides symptomatic palliation, particularly for dyspnea, while definitive treatment of the underlying cause is pursued. The two most frequently employed drainage techniques are thoracentesis and tube thoracostomy. Selection of the appropriate method should be based on the etiology of the effusion and the rate at which it accumulates [17].

Thoracentesis is commonly chosen as the initial intervention, especially when the nature of the effusion and its likelihood of recurrence are not yet established [66]. Its utility in recurrent chylous effusions is limited, with a reported success rate of only 24% in achieving resolution [100]. In addition, repeated thoracenteses can lead to significant nutritional and immunologic depletion through the ongoing loss of proteins, electrolytes, immunoglobulins, and lymphocytes. For this reason, thoracentesis is generally reserved for patients with slowly accumulating chylous effusions who require only occasional drainage [87].

Tube thoracostomy is often preferred because it permits continuous monitoring of fluid output, enabling clinicians to quantify the degree of chyle loss and detect changes promptly. This information is valuable in determining the need for earlier and more aggressive therapies in cases of high-output chylothorax. Tube thoracostomy also reduces the frequency of repeat pleural procedures, which are themselves associated with risks such as infection, bleeding, and pneumothorax [89, 101]. In postoperative patients, chest tubes are often already in place, and studies demonstrate that small-bore catheters (14 French or smaller) are just as effective as larger-bore tubes for draining chylous effusions [87]. Despite these advantages, prolonged chest tube drainage carries risks similar to repeated thoracentesis, including nutritional and immunologic compromise. Furthermore, chest tubes can serve as a route for chemical pleurodesis when conservative measures or other interventions fail. The effectiveness of pleurodesis is highly dependent on the underlying etiology: success rates as high as 80% have been reported for postoperative, refractory chylous effusions [102, 103], while series involving lymphoma or congenital chylothorax describe success rates of 50–80% [104, 105]. For other causes, outcomes are less certain, as most data are limited to isolated case reports.

A newer strategy for fluid control is the use of indwelling pleural catheters (IPCs). These tunneled catheters allow patients to perform drainage in the outpatient setting, reducing the need for repeated hospital-based procedures [106]. IPCs offer benefits similar to tube thoracostomy, including the ability to monitor ongoing effusion accumulation, while also providing the convenience of at-home management. Additionally, IPCs may facilitate spontaneous pleurodesis and eventual resolution of chylous effusions, although supporting data remain limited [107, 108]. Like other drainage modalities, repeated use of IPCs is associated with nutritional and immunologic losses due to the persistent removal of lymphatic fluid [106].

Thoracic Duct Embolization

Thoracic duct embolization is a percutaneous interventional radiology procedure performed in conjunction with lymphangiography. The technique involves identifying the site of chyle leakage using invasive lymphangiography, followed by sealing the leak through the injection of a foreign material, such as glue or coils. The overall success rate is approximately 60%, with outcomes generally more favorable in nontraumatic chylous effusions, where success rates approach 74% [79, 109]. In some cases, the chyle leak may not be visualized or may be technically challenging to access. The use of inguinal lymph node cannulation, rather than traditional pedal access, has helped overcome some of these limitations [69, 79].

The procedure is contraindicated in patients with severe coagulopathy or an abdominal aortic aneurysm [110]. Acute complications, including fat embolism, biliary leak, and aspiration, occur in approximately 2% of cases [109]. Chronic complications, such as leg swelling, abdominal swelling, and diarrhea, are reported in nearly 14% of patients [111].

Surgical Procedures

Surgical procedures are typically reserved for specific scenarios. While there are no definitive guidelines, surgery is often considered for patients with significantly high-output chylous effusions, those whose high-output effusions do not respond quickly to conservative measures, and patients with low-output effusions who do not improve with conservative management over time. While thresholds may vary, indications for surgery commonly include output greater than 1500 mL in 24 hours, more than 1000 mL/day for five days, greater than 2000 mL over two days, or ongoing chest tube drainage after two weeks of conservative management [88, 112]. A rapidly declining nutritional status may also be an indication to proceed with early surgery [113]. Surgical intervention is often considered earlier for traumatic chylothorax, as these cases tend to respond poorly to conservative treatment [89, 114]. A multidisciplinary approach is essential in determining whether surgery or less-invasive interventional procedures are appropriate.

Thoracic Duct Ligation

Thoracic duct ligation is a surgical procedure that involves suturing the thoracic duct proximal to the site of leakage, thereby preventing the flow of lymphatic fluid through it. The procedure is most commonly performed using video-assisted thoracoscopic surgery (VATS) , although a thoracotomy may be deemed necessary [87, 102]. The surgical approach is typically guided by the suspected location of the chyle leak, which is typically identified via lymphangiography in cases of nontraumatic chylothorax or based on the location of trauma or previous surgical interventions in iatrogenic instances [102]. To assist in the intraoperative identification of the leak, patients may be administered a lipid-rich beverage or lipophilic dye [114]. Surgical thoracic duct ligation is successful in approximately 90% of cases of traumatic chylothorax [89, 113]. Success rates in nontraumatic cases are less clear and are generally considered to be lower [100]. Historically, complications occurred in up to 38% of cases, with a mortality rate of 25%. However, with the advent of VATS and improved preoperative diagnostic techniques, these rates have decreased significantly, and current procedural mortality is estimated at 3% [21, 113].

Pleuroperitoneal Shunt Placement

A pleuroperitoneal shunt is a palliative procedure used to alleviate dyspnea in instances of refractory chylous effusions. Although it is not curative, the procedure entails the implantation of a pump that enables unidirectional flow of chyle from the pleural cavity into the peritoneal cavity, where it can subsequently be reabsorbed [87]. This procedure helps alleviate respiratory symptoms and prevents nutritional deficiencies caused by significant chyle loss. However, it is rarely performed due to common serious complications such as shunt migration, obstruction, infection, and pneumoperitoneum. It is contraindicated in patients with chylous ascites to prevent additional disruption of abdominal lymphatics [115].

Complications

The complications of chylothorax stem from the loss of lymphatic fluid, which contains lipids, proteins, electrolytes, and immune cells [91, 116]. Chyle is abundant in fat-soluble vitamins A, D, E, and K. The leakage of chyle hinders the transportation of these vital vitamins into the bloodstream, thereby resulting in nutritional deficiencies. Albumin, the primary protein found in chyle, exists at concentrations exceeding 4 g/dL. A daily loss of 1 liter of chyle can cause an approximate loss of 30 grams of albumin, which may lead to hypoalbuminemia, hypoproteinemia, and malnutrition [96]. The electrolyte composition of chyle closely mirrors that of plasma; consequently, ongoing loss results in the depletion of essential electrolytes, including sodium, potassium, magnesium, phosphate, chloride, and bicarbonate [23]. Lymphocytes, particularly B cells, are abundantly present in chyle, and their depletion results in immunodeficiency due to both lymphopenia and a deficiency in immunoglobulins [117]. Consequently, persistent chylothorax may render patients more susceptible to opportunistic infections owing to their compromised immune system [116].

Prognosis

The mortality rate of chylothorax was initially reported as 50% in 1948 [23]. However, as our knowledge of the underlying pathology and treatments has advanced, the mortality rate has been gradually declining [100]. The prognosis of chylothorax varies significantly depending on the underlying cause, time to diagnosis, and capacity to intervene effectively [17]. The longer a chylothorax persists, the greater the likelihood of complications such as nutritional and immunodeficiencies [82, 114].

Chylous effusions resulting from benign conditions with a detectable leak typically have a good prognosis, especially if the leak can be definitively managed. Traumatic causes, including iatrogenic injuries, also tend to have a favorable prognosis if promptly diagnosed and treated. However, postoperative chylothorax can considerably raise the 30-day mortality rate [88, 101, 118]. Nontraumatic causes generally tend to have poorer long-term outcomes and a lower resolution rate when compared to traumatic causes [100]. Malignant chylothorax, chronic chylothorax, and bilateral chylous effusions are linked to a worse prognosis and increased risk of both short-term and long-term mortality [119].

References

1. Seitelman E, Arellano JJ, Takabe K, Barrett L, Faust G, Angus LDG. Chylothorax after blunt trauma. J Thorac Dis. 2012;4(3):327–30.
2. Cholet C, Delalandre C, Monnier-Cholley L, Le Pimpec-Barthes F, El Mouhadi S, Arrivé L. Nontraumatic Chylothorax: nonenhanced MR Lymphography. Radiographics. 2020;40(6):1554–73.
3. de Beer HG, Mol MJ, Janssen JP. Chylothorax. Neth J Med. 2000;56(1):25–31.
4. Porcel JM, Bielsa S, Civit C, Aujayeb A, Janssen J, Bodtger U, et al. Clinical characteristics of chylothorax: results from the international collaborative effusion database. ERJ Open Res. 2023;9(5):00091–2023.
5. Olsen AMWG. Chylothorax. J Thoracic Sur. 1944;13(1):53–62.
6. Jahsman W. Chylothorax; Brief review of literature; report of three non-traumatic cases. Ann Intern Med. 1944;21(4)
7. Bauersfeld EH. Traumatic chylothorax from ruptured thoracic duct. JAMA J Am Med Assoc. 1937;109(1):16.
8. Lampson RS. Traumatic chylothorax: a review of the literature and report of a case treated by medi-

astinal ligation of the thoracic duct. J Thorac Surg. 1948;17(6):778–91.
9. Rahman NM, Chapman SJ, Davies RJO. Pleural effusion: a structured approach to care. Br Med Bull. 2004;72:31–47.
10. McWilliams A, Gabbay E. Chylothorax occurring 23 years post-irradiation: literature review and management strategies. Respirology. 2000;5(3):301–3.
11. Rudrappa M, Paul M. Chylothorax. 2024.
12. Rehman K, Sivakumar P. Non-traumatic chylothorax: diagnostic and therapeutic strategies. Breathe. 2022;18(2):210163.
13. Haithcock BE, Lewis MI, McKenna RJ, Feins RH. Pleural effusions and complications. In: Medical Management of the Thoracic Surgery Patient. Elsevier; 2010. p. 420–31.
14. Nair SK, Petko M, Hayward MP. Aetiology and management of chylothorax in adults. Eur J Cardiothorac Surg. 2007 Aug;32(2):362–9.
15. Rahmany S, Jialal I. Biochemistry, Chylomicron. 2024.
16. Zilversmit DB. The composition and structure of lymph chylomicrons in dog, rat, and man. J Clin Invest. 1965;44(10):1610–22.
17. Bhatnagar M, Fisher A, Ramsaroop S, Carter A, Pippard B. Chylothorax: pathophysiology, diagnosis, and management—a comprehensive review. J Thorac Dis. 2024;16(2):1645–61.
18. Moazzam S, O'Hagan LA, Clarke AR, Itkin M, Phillips ARJ, Windsor JA, et al. The cisterna chyli: a systematic review of definition, prevalence, and anatomy. Am J Physiol Heart Circ Physiol. 2022;323(5):H1010–8.
19. Phang K, Bowman M, Phillips A, Windsor J. Review of thoracic duct anatomical variations and clinical implications. Clin Anat. 2014;27(4):637–44.
20. Macfarlane JR, Holman CW. Chylothorax. Am Rev Respir Dis. 1972;105(2):287–91.
21. Pillay TG, Singh B. A review of traumatic chylothorax. Injury. 2016;47(3):545–50.
22. Ray A. Pathogenesis of bilateral chylothorax after injury of the thoracic duct during central venous catheterization. Lung India. 2015;32(6):673–5.
23. McGrath EE, Blades Z, Anderson PB. Chylothorax: Aetiology, diagnosis and therapeutic options. Respir Med. 2010;104(1):1–8.
24. Maldonado F, Hawkins FJ, Daniels CE, Doerr CH, Decker PA, Ryu JH. Pleural fluid characteristics of chylothorax. Mayo Clin Proc. 2009;84(2):129–33.
25. Huggins JT. Chylothorax and cholesterol pleural effusion. Semin Respir Crit Care Med. 2010;31(6):743–50.
26. Riley LE, Ataya A. Clinical approach and review of causes of a chylothorax. Respir Med. 2019;157:7–13.
27. O'Callaghan AM, Mead GM. Chylothorax in lymphoma: mechanisms and management. Ann Oncol. 1995;6(6):603–7.
28. Nadolski G. Nontraumatic Chylothorax: diagnostic algorithm and treatment options. Tech Vasc Interv Radiol. 2016;19(4):286–90.
29. Villena V, de Pablo A, Martín-Escribano P. Chylothorax and chylous ascites due to heart failure. Eur Respir J. 1995;8(7):1235–6.
30. Duletzke NT, Kiraly LN, Martindale RG. Chylothorax and chylous ascites: overview, management, and nutrition. Nutr Clin Pract. 2023;38(3):557–63.
31. Resch B, Sever Yildiz G, Reiterer F. Congenital Chylothorax of the newborn: a systematic analysis of published cases between 1990 and 2018. Respiration. 2022;101(1):84–96.
32. Faul JL, Berry GJ, Colby TV, Ruoss SJ, Walter MB, Rosen GD, et al. Thoracic lymphangiomas, lymphangiectasis, lymphangiomatosis, and lymphatic dysplasia syndrome. Am J Respir Crit Care Med. 2000;161(3 Pt 1):1037–46.
33. Pham KT, Balaguru D, Tammisetti VS, Guevara CJ, Rasmussen JC, Zvavanjanja RC, et al. Multimodality lymphatic imaging of postoperative chylothorax in an infant with Noonan syndrome: a case report. Eur J Med Res. 2020;25(1):55.
34. Radhakrishnan K, Rockson SG. Gorham's disease. Ann N Y Acad Sci. 2008;1131(1):203–5.
35. Nikolaou VS, Chytas D, Korres D, Efstathopoulos N. Vanishing bone disease (Gorham-stout syndrome): a review of a rare entity. World J Orthop. 2014;5(5):694–8.
36. Tie MLH, Poland GA, Rosenow EC. Chylothorax in Gorham's syndrome. Chest. 1994;105(1):208–13.
37. Doerr CH, Allen MS, Nichols FC, Ryu JH. Etiology of Chylothorax in 203 patients. Mayo Clin Proc. 2005;80(7):867–70.
38. Johnson SR, Cordier JF, Lazor R, Cottin V, Costabel U, Harari S, et al. European Respiratory Society guidelines for the diagnosis and management of lymphangioleiomyomatosis. Eur Respir J. 2010;35(1):14–26.
39. Taveira-DaSilva AM, Moss J. Epidemiology, pathogenesis and diagnosis of lymphangioleiomyomatosis. Expert Opin Orphan Drugs. 2016;4(4):369–78.
40. Ryu JH, Doerr CH, Fisher SD, Olson EJ, Sahn SA. Chylothorax in lymphangioleiomyomatosis. Chest. 2003;123(2):623–7.
41. Almoosa KF, McCormack FX, Sahn SA. Pleural disease in lymphangioleiomyomatosis. Clin Chest Med. 2006;27(2):355–68.
42. Maldonado F, Tazelaar HD, Wang CW, Ryu JH. Yellow nail syndrome: analysis of 41 consecutive patients. Chest. 2008;134(2):375–81.
43. Valdés L, Huggins JT, Gude F, Ferreiro L, Alvarez-Dobaño JM, Golpe A, et al. Characteristics of patients with yellow nail syndrome and pleural effusion. Respirology. 2014;19(7):985–92.
44. Hoque SR, Mansour S, Mortimer PS. Yellow nail syndrome: not a genetic disorder? Eleven new cases and a review of the literature. Br J Dermatol. 2007;156(6):1230–4.
45. Israeli-Shani L, King D, Epstein Shochet G, Shitrit D, Wand O. Chylothorax associated with sarcoid-

osis: a review of the literature. Sarcoidosis Vasc Diffuse Lung Dis. 2022;39(4):e2022039.
46. Romero S, Martín C, Hernandez L, Verdu J, Trigo C, Perez-Mateo M, et al. Chylothorax in cirrhosis of the liver: analysis of its frequency and clinical characteristics. Chest. 1998;114(1):154–9.
47. Majdalany BS, Murrey DA, Kapoor BS, Cain TR, Ganguli S, Kent MS, et al. ACR appropriateness criteria ® Chylothorax treatment planning. J Am Coll Radiol. 2017;14(5):S118–26.
48. Kahraman D, Keskin G, Khalil E, Dogan OF. Ten-year clinical experience on Chylothorax after cardiovascular surgery. Heart Surg Forum. 2020;23(1):E081–7.
49. Byrd CT, Williams KM, Backhus LM. A brief overview of thoracic surgery in the United States. J Thorac Dis. 2022;14(1):218–26.
50. Shah RD, Luketich JD, Schuchert MJ, Christie NA, Pennathur A, Landreneau RJ, et al. Postesophagectomy chylothorax: incidence, risk factors, and outcomes. Ann Thorac Surg. 2012;93(3):897–903; discussion 903–4.
51. Chen C, Wang Z, Hao J, Hao X, Zhou J, Chen N, et al. Chylothorax after lung cancer surgery: a key factor influencing prognosis and quality of life. Ann Thorac Cardiovasc Surg. 2020;26(6):303–10.
52. Bryant AS, Minnich DJ, Wei B, Cerfolio RJ. The incidence and management of postoperative chylothorax after pulmonary resection and thoracic mediastinal lymph node dissection. Ann Thorac Surg. 2014;98(1):232–5; discussion 235–7.
53. Merki V, Pichler J, Giger R, Mantokoudis G. Chylothorax in thyroid surgery: a very rare case and systematic review of the literature. J Otolaryngol Head Neck Surg. 2016;45(1):52.
54. Kurekci E, Kaye R, Koehler M. Chylothorax and chylopericardium: a complication of a central venous catheter. J Pediatr. 1998;132(6):1064–6.
55. Kakamad FH, Salih RQM, Mohammed SH, HamaSaeed AG, Mohammed DA, Jwamer VI, et al. Chylothorax caused by blunt chest trauma: a review of literature. Indian J Thorac Cardiovasc Surg. 2020;36(6):619–24.
56. Harvey C, Shin H, Martin S, Perea L. Traumatic chylothorax following blunt thoracic trauma. Trauma Case Rep. 2024;54:101101.
57. Agrawal V, Doelken P, Sahn SA. Seat Belt-induced Chylothorax. Chest. 2007;132(2):690–2.
58. Cammarata SK, Brush RE, Hyzy RC. Chylothorax after childbirth. Chest. 1991;99(6):1539–40.
59. Yekeler E, Ulutas H. Bilateral chylothorax after severe vomiting in a child. Ann Thorac Surg. 2012;94(1):e21–3.
60. Reilly KM. Bilateral Chylothorax. JAMA. 1975;233(6):536.
61. Lim KG, Rosenow EC, Staats B, Couture C, Morgenthaler TI. Chyloptysis in adults: presentation, recognition, and differential diagnosis. Chest. 2004;125(1):336–40.
62. Strange C, Nicolau DP, Dryzer SR. Chylous transport of amiodarone. Chest. 1992;101(2):573–4.
63. Taylor MD, Kim SS, Vaias LJ. Therapeutic digoxin level in chylous drainage with no detectable plasma digoxin level. Chest. 1998;114(5):1482–4.
64. Ammori JB, Pickens A, Chang AC, Orringer MB. Tension chylothorax. Ann Thorac Surg. 2006;82(2):729–30.
65. Hooper C, Lee YCG, Maskell N, BTS Pleural Guideline Group. Investigation of a unilateral pleural effusion in adults: British Thoracic Society pleural disease guideline 2010. Thorax 2010 65 Suppl 2:ii4–i17.
66. Nicholson MJ, Manley C, Ahmad D. Thoracentesis for the diagnosis and Management of Pleural Effusions: the current state of a centuries-old procedure. Journal of Respiration. 2023;3(4):208–22.
67. Xirouchaki N, Magkanas E, Vaporidi K, Kondili E, Plataki M, Patrianakos A, et al. Lung ultrasound in critically ill patients: comparison with bedside chest radiography. Intensive Care Med. 2011;37(9):1488.
68. Prina E, Torres A, Carvalho CRR. Lung ultrasound in the evaluation of pleural effusion. J Bras Pneumol. 2014;40(1):1–5.
69. Schwartz FR, James O, Kuo PH, Witte MH, Koweek LM, Pabon-Ramos WM. Lymphatic imaging: current noninvasive and invasive techniques. Semin Intervent Radiol. 2020;37(3):237–49.
70. Patel S, Hur S, Khaddash T, Simpson S, Itkin M. Intranodal CT lymphangiography with water-soluble iodinated contrast medium for imaging of the central lymphatic system. Radiology. 2022;302(1):228–33.
71. Zhang C, Chen X, Wen T, Zhang Q, Huo M, Dong J, et al. Computed tomography lymphangiography findings in 27 cases of lymphangioleiomyomatosis. Acta Radiol. 2017;58(11):1342–8.
72. Yu DX, Ma XX, Wang Q, Zhang Y, Li CF. Morphological changes of the thoracic duct and accessory lymphatic channels in patients with chylothorax: detection with unenhanced magnetic resonance imaging. Eur Radiol. 2013;23(3):702–11.
73. Chavhan GB, Lam CZ, Greer MLC, Temple M, Amaral J, Grosse-Wortmann L. Magnetic resonance lymphangiography. Radiol Clin North Am. 2020;58(4):693–706.
74. Kim EY, Hwang HS, Lee HY, Cho JH, Kim HK, Lee KS, et al. Anatomic and functional evaluation of central lymphatics with noninvasive magnetic resonance lymphangiography. Medicine (Baltimore). 2016;95(12):e3109.
75. Witte CL, Witte MH, Unger EC, Williams WH, Bernas MJ, McNeill GC, et al. Advances in imaging of lymph flow disorders. Radiographics. 2000;20(6):1697–719.
76. Yoshida RY, Kariya S, Ha-Kawa S, Tanigawa N. Lymphoscintigraphy for imaging of the lymphatic flow disorders. Tech Vasc Interv Radiol. 2016;19(4):273–6.

77. Suga K, Kume N, Hara A, Miura G, Matsunaga N, Sugi K, et al. Abnormal lymphatic flow demonstrated by lymphoscintigraphy in chylothorax correlation with lymphography. Clin Nucl Med. 1999;24(9):716–7.
78. Guermazi A, Brice P, Hennequin C, Sarfati E. Lymphography: an old technique retains its usefulness. Radiographics. 2003;23(6):1541–58; discussion 1559–60.
79. Nadolski GJ, Itkin M. Feasibility of ultrasound-guided intranodal lymphangiogram for thoracic duct embolization. J Vasc Interv Radiol. 2012;23(5):613–6.
80. Alejandre-Lafont E, Krompiec C, Rau WS, Krombach GA. Effectiveness of therapeutic lymphography on lymphatic leakage. Acta Radiol. 2011;52(3):305–11.
81. Agrawal V, Doelken P, Sahn SA. Pleural fluid analysis in chylous pleural effusion. Chest. 2008;133(6):1436–41.
82. Merrigan BA, Winter DC, O'Sullivan GC. Chylothorax. Br J Surg. 1997;84(1):15–20.
83. Lama A, Ferreiro L, Toubes ME, Golpe A, Gude F, Álvarez-Dobaño JM, et al. Characteristics of patients with pseudochylothorax-a systematic review. J Thorac Dis. 2016;8(8):2093–101.
84. Skouras V, Kalomenidis I. Chylothorax: diagnostic approach. Curr Opin Pulm Med. 2010;16(4):387–93.
85. Mercer RM, Corcoran JP, Porcel JM, Rahman NM, Psallidas I. Interpreting pleural fluid results. Clin Med (Lond). 2019;19(3):213–7.
86. Bender B, Murthy V, Chamberlain RS. The changing management of chylothorax in the modern era. Eur J Cardiothorac Surg. 2016;49(1):18–24.
87. Agrawal A, Chaddha U, Kaul V, Desai A, Gillaspie E, Maldonado F. Multidisciplinary management of chylothorax. Chest. 2022;162(6):1402–12.
88. Martucci N, Tracey M, Rocco G. Postoperative Chylothorax. Thorac Surg Clin. 2015;25(4):523–8.
89. Marts BC, Naunheim KS, Fiore AC, Pennington DG. Conservative versus surgical management of chylothorax. Am J Surg. 1992;164(5):532–4; discussion 534–5.
90. Takuwa T, Yoshida J, Ono S, Hishida T, Nishimura M, Aokage K, et al. Low-fat diet management strategy for chylothorax after pulmonary resection and lymph node dissection for primary lung cancer. J Thorac Cardiovasc Surg. 2013;146(3):571–4.
91. Steven BR, Carey S. Nutritional management in patients with chyle leakage: a systematic review. Eur J Clin Nutr. 2015;69(7):776–80.
92. Sriram K, Meguid RA, Meguid MM. Nutritional support in adults with chyle leaks. Nutrition. 2016;32(2):281–6.
93. Kalomenidis I. Octreotide and chylothorax. Curr Opin Pulm Med. 2006;12(4):264–7.
94. Rosti L, Bini RM, Chessa M, Butera G, Drago M, Carminati M. The effectiveness of octreotide in the treatment of post-operative chylothorax. Eur J Pediatr. 2002 Mar;161(3):149–50.
95. Al-Zubairy SA, Al-Jazairi AS. Octreotide as a therapeutic option for management of chylothorax. Ann Pharmacother. 2003;37(5):679–82.
96. Mincher L, Evans J, Jenner MW, Varney VA. The successful treatment of chylous effusions in malignant disease with octreotide. Clin Oncol (R Coll Radiol). 2005;17(2):118–21.
97. Sivakumar P, Ahmed L. Use of an Alpha-1 Adrenoreceptor agonist in the Management of Recurrent Refractory Idiopathic Chylothorax. Chest. 2018;154(1):e1–4.
98. Guillem P, Papachristos I, Peillon C, Triboulet JP. Etilefrine use in the management of post-operative chyle leaks in thoracic surgery. Interact Cardiovasc Thorac Surg. 2004;3(1):156–60.
99. Jarman PR, Whyte MK, Sabroe I, Hughes JM. Sarcoidosis presenting with chylothorax. Thorax. 1995;50(12):1324–5.
100. Maldonado F, Cartin-Ceba R, Hawkins FJ, Ryu JH. Medical and surgical management of chylothorax and associated outcomes. Am J Med Sci. 2010;339(4):314–8.
101. Power R, Smyth P, Donlon NE, Nugent T, Donohoe CL, Reynolds JV. Management of chyle leaks following esophageal resection: a systematic review. Dis Esophagus. 2021;34(11).
102. Paul S, Altorki NK, Port JL, Stiles BM, Lee PC. Surgical management of chylothorax. Thorac Cardiovasc Surg. 2009;57(4):226–8.
103. Lai Y, Zheng X, Yuan Y, Xie TP, Zhao YF, Zhu ZJ, et al. A modified pleurodesis in treating postoperative chylothorax. Ann Transl Med. 2019;7(20):549.
104. Mares DC, Mathur PN. Medical thoracoscopic talc pleurodesis for chylothorax due to lymphoma: a case series. Chest. 1998;114(3):731–5.
105. Nahlovsky J, Matejek T. Chemical Pleurodesis with povidone-iodine in congenital Chylothorax. Indian J Pediatr. 2023;90(6):634.
106. DePew ZS, Iqbal S, Mullon JJ, Nichols FC, Maldonado F. The role for tunneled indwelling pleural catheters in patients with persistent benign chylothorax. Am J Med Sci. 2013;346(5):349–52.
107. Mohamed M, Tan J, Kalpurath KK. Non-Hodgkin lymphoma manifesting as massive malignant chylothorax: successful management with chemotherapy and ambulatory drainages using indwelling pleural catheter. Intern Med J. 2015;45(9):980–3.
108. Jimenez CA, Mhatre AD, Martinez CH, Eapen GA, Onn A, Morice RC. Use of an indwelling pleural catheter for the management of recurrent chylothorax in patients with cancer. Chest. 2007;132(5):1584–90.
109. Kim PH, Tsauo J, Shin JH. Lymphatic interventions for Chylothorax: a systematic review and meta-analysis. J Vasc Interv Radiol. 2018;29(2):194–202.e4.
110. Stecker MS, Fan CM. Lymphangiography for thoracic duct interventions. Tech Vasc Interv Radiol. 2016;19(4):277–85.

111. Laslett D, Trerotola SO, Itkin M. Delayed complications following technically successful thoracic duct embolization. J Vasc Interv Radiol. 2012;23(1):76–9.
112. Selle JG, Snyder WH, Schreiber JT. Chylothorax: indications for surgery. Ann Surg. 1973;177(2):245–9.
113. Schild HH, Strassburg CP, Welz A, Kalff J. Treatment options in patients with chylothorax. Dtsch Arztebl Int. 2013;110(48):819–26.
114. Misthos P, Kanakis MA, Lioulias AG. Chylothorax complicating thoracic surgery: conservative or early surgical management? Updat Surg. 2012;64(1):5–11.
115. Romero S. Nontraumatic chylothorax. Curr Opin Pulm Med. 2000;6(4):287–91.
116. Liao S, von der Weid PY. Lymphatic system: an active pathway for immune protection. Semin Cell Dev Biol. 2015;38:83–9.
117. Wasmuth-Pietzuch A, Hansmann M, Bartmann P, Heep A. Congenital chylothorax: lymphopenia and high risk of neonatal infections. Acta Paediatr. 2004;93(2):220–4.
118. Al-Sahaf M. Postoperative chylothorax. Shanghai Chest. 2021;5:28.
119. Milsom JW, Kron IL, Rheuban KS, Rodgers BM. Chylothorax: an assessment of current surgical management. J Thorac Cardiovasc Surg. 1985;89(2):221–7.

Urinothorax

7

Truong-An Andrew Ho and Samantha Pettigrew

Introduction

Urinothorax, defined by the presence of urine in the pleural space, is an extremely rare cause of a pleural effusion. In the 1800s, the presence of fetal or neonatal ascites was attributed to Syphilis until Fordyce collected many cases and disproved this notion. His review mentioned the presence of urinary tract abnormalities in several cases. However, ascites was not yet linked to urinary obstruction [1]. Cases of fetal ascites were continually documented for several decades. In 1953, Josephine Lord described two cases in addition to reviewing prior literature, concluding that several appeared directly linked to urinary obstruction as the underlying etiology. Pleural effusions were not yet observed in this setting; however, autopsies did note atelectasis of the lungs [2]. A year later, the presence of significant lung collapse associated with ascites observed during postmortem analysis was further reported by France and Beck in 1954 [3, 4]. Over a decade later, in 1968, Corriere et al. described two cases in which right-sided effusions and hydronephrosis co-occurred. Interestingly, the effusions resolved after relieving the urinary obstruction [5]. He attempted to reproduce this relationship between hydronephrosis and pleural effusion using a canine model by ligating the right ureter and lymphatic ducts in varying combinations. The results demonstrated the accumulation of perirenal tissue edema; however, they were unsuccessful at producing a pleural effusion. The lower position of the kidneys in relationship to the diaphragm in dogs was cited as a potential cause for the failure to produce a pleural effusion [5]. In 1970, H. C. Stoerk et al. demonstrated the development of ascites and hydrothorax in rats and guinea pigs following bilateral ureteral ligation [6]. In the subsequent year, 1971, Gerald W. Friedland and colleagues introduced the term "urinothorax" following their observation of a left pleural effusion containing substantial urea levels in a neonate with posterior urethral abnormalities valves [7]. Currently, urinothorax is considered a rare cause of pleural effusion, with fewer than 100 cases documented since its initial identification. With up to 20% of pleural effusions lacking a definitive diagnosis, urinothorax may be underreported due to a lack of recognition [8].

T.-A. A. Ho · S. Pettigrew (✉)
Department of Thoracic Medicine and Surgery, Temple University, Philadelphia, PA, USA
e-mail: truong-an.ho@tuhs.temple.edu; Samantha.Pettigrew@tuhs.temple.edu

F. Ido (ed.), *Rare Pleural Diseases*, https://doi.org/10.1007/978-3-032-14873-5_7

Epidemiology and Risk Factors

Epidemiologic data concerning urinothorax are limited to case reviews. In 2017, the most recent and comprehensive systematic literature review identified a total of 88 cases. The median age at presentation was 45 years, with a range from 0 to 84 years, suggesting that urinothorax can manifest across all age groups. The condition was marginally more prevalent in males (61.4%), with a reported male-to-female ratio of 1.6 [3].

Urinothorax is predominantly unilateral (87%) rather than bilateral (12.9%). In cases of unilateral presentation, the right side was affected in 58.1% of instances, while the left side was involved in 41.9% of cases. The pleural effusion encompassed more than two-thirds of the hemithorax in 64.4% of cases, between one-third and two-thirds in 23.3%, and less than one-third in 12.3%. Typically, the effusions occur ipsilaterally to the obstructed side in approximately two-thirds of cases; however, contralateral occurrences are also observed [3]. The development of a urinothorax following the inciting event most frequently occurs within 2 days; however, it has been documented to range from several hours to as long as 2 months [9].

The etiologies of urinothorax can be classified into two categories: obstructive and traumatic [9–11]. Traumatic etiologies constitute 75% of all cases of urinothorax, with iatrogenic surgical injuries being the most frequently reported, occurring in 24% of cases [3]. Surgical causes have been evidenced, for instance, after a total abdominal hysterectomy with inadvertent bladder perforation, ovarian tumor resection with ureteral ligation, and following adrenalectomy [12–18]. Other causes associated with renal, ureteral, and bladder injury include acute obstruction due to renal calculi (18%), blunt trauma (13%), percutaneous nephrostomy (12%), lithotomy (12%), extracorporeal shock wave lithotripsy (ESWL) (7.5%), and renal transplantation (7.5%) [3, 19, 20]. Very rarely, urinothorax has been reported in association with percutaneous renal cryoablation, and ureteroscopy [21]. Recognition of iatrogenic causes can be identified within hours following a renal biopsy or up to several weeks following renal transplantation, occurring at the ureteroneocystostomy site [22].

Blunt trauma is the most commonly reported non-iatrogenic cause of urinothorax, typically resulting from motor vehicle or motorcycle accidents. This results in direct injury to the kidneys, ureter, or bladder, in addition to reported injuries to the diaphragm [23–27]. Penetrating trauma has also been reported to cause a urinothorax, such as that occurring following gunshot wounds [28, 29]. In nearly all trauma-related cases, the injury results in urine leaking into the peritoneal or retroperitoneal space, followed by extravasation into the pleural cavity. The diagnosis of the urinothorax in such instances can be delayed for several days as the patient undergoes treatment for multisystemic injuries [23–29].

Obstructive etiologies account for nearly 25% of cases, with prostate disease, bladder cancer, and urethral valves representing approximately 77% of cases [3]. Reported prostate causes include both prostate adenocarcinoma and benign prostate hypertrophy [30, 31]. Other non-urothelial malignant causes reported include renal cancer causing direct obstructive hydronephrosis, as well as metastasis to the bladder and ureters from colorectal carcinoma, lymphoma, and vaginal cancer [22, 32–34]. Non-neoplastic etiologies include a large renal cyst accompanied by renal pelvis obstruction, intraoperative rupture of a renal cyst, pyelonephritis, retroperitoneal fibrosis secondary to metastatic cancer (i.e., metastatic neuroectodermal sarcoma), and a gravid uterus at 35 weeks of gestation, causing bilateral ureteral obstruction [3, 5, 22, 35–37].

Pathophysiology

Urinothorax formation requires either an obstruction to the urinary tract or trauma to the kidneys, ureters, or bladder. In the absence of trauma, either bilateral obstruction or unilateral obstruction with an abnormally functioning contralateral kidney is necessary for the development of a urinothorax [3, 9–11]. In instances of isolated unilateral obstruction with a normal functioning contralateral kidney, trauma is generally presumed, even if not evidently visible [3, 11]. Two main theoretical mechanisms have been identified that explain how urine enters the pleural space, involving a direct and an indirect pathway [3, 9]. Following obstruction or injury to the kidneys or urinary tract, urine may extravasate into the perirenal or retroperitoneal region [3, 9–11]. The extravasated urine in the retroperitoneum may also form into an encapsulated collection, termed a urinoma [11, 38]. The direct pathway occurs when urine enters the pleural space through diaphragmatic defects, fenestrations, or fistulas [9, 10, 39]. The indirect path refers to the uptake of extravasated urine into the subdiaphragmatic retroperitoneal lymphatic vessels, which drain into the pleural lymphatics [3, 9, 10]. In either pathway, the formation of a urinothorax is only possible when the fluid accumulation rate surpasses the pleural lymphatics' removal rate [5, 9, 40]. These pathways generally result in the development of an ipsilateral urinothorax; however, contralateral and bilateral urinothoraces have been described [3, 9, 16, 20, 33, 41, 42].

Clinical Features

The signs and symptoms of urinothorax vary significantly, depending on the underlying etiology. The initial clinical presentation can range from anuria or oliguria and shortness of breath in patients with urinary obstruction to multisystem failure with septic or hemorrhagic shock following infection or trauma, respectively [9, 43, 44]. The most significant clinical indicator of urinothorax is the combination of a new pleural effusion with urinary abnormalities. Urinary symptoms may include suprapubic or flank pain, an inability to void, and hematuria [3, 43, 45]. The severity of pulmonary symptoms depends on the size of the pleural effusion, the rate of accumulation, baseline pulmonary function, and the presence of comorbidities. It ranges from an asymptomatic presentation to severe shortness of breath, dyspnea, and cough [13, 43, 44, 46, 47]. The signs may include suprapubic or costodiaphragmatic angle tenderness, decreased urine output, diminished thoracic breath sounds, and dullness to percussion. In cases of sepsis or traumatic etiologies, presenting signs may be more extreme and include septic or hemorrhagic shock, ascites, and multisystemic failure [20, 43, 48–52].

Diagnosis

Several key features in pleural fluid analysis strongly indicate the presence of a urinothorax. The appearance and odor of the pleural fluid may also serve as diagnostic indicators, as the fluid may resemble and emit an odor similar to urine. However, such observations are infrequently documented, reported in fewer than 10% of cases [3, 10, 14, 23, 30, 46, 53–55]. Pleural fluid analyses in cases of urinothorax are predominantly transudative, comprising 50–70% of such instances [3, 9]. Pleural fluid lactate dehydrogenase (LDH) levels can exhibit substantial variation, ranging from 25 to 3475 IU/L, depending on the etiology [3, 10, 46, 56]. Pleural fluid total protein levels are generally low, with a reported median of 0.93 g/dl. Additionally, only 15.9% of cases of urinothorax exhibited pleural fluid total protein levels exceeding 3 g/dL [9, 11, 40]. The pH level is also notably low, with a median reported pH of 7.24 (range: 6.8–8.4), and 61% of cases exhibited a pH value of less than 7.30 [3]. A transudative effusion with low pH significantly narrows the differential diagnosis of an effusion [53]. Urinothorax has previously been documented as the only cause of an acidic transudative effusion. However, it may also be observed in cases of inadvertent infusion of normal saline, such as in scenarios involving an extravascular central venous catheter [13, 46, 57]. The pH range reflects the urine content and may be influenced by urine alkalization and specific bacterial infections, such as those caused by Proteus and Klebsiella species [9, 12, 57, 58].

Pleural fluid creatine levels are not routinely measured for all analyzed pleural effusions; however, they should be assessed when urinothorax is suspected. The pleural fluid-to-serum creatine (PFSC) ratio should be calculated, and traditionally, a cutoff value exceeding one is considered highly indicative of the diagnosis [10, 54]. This cutoff value is highly sensitive, with 97.9% of confirmed cases demonstrating a ratio greater than 1 [3]. The mean PFSC has ranged from 2.9 to 9.15 [3, 56]. Values for PFSC in patients with urinothorax have been documented as low as 1.17 and reaching a peak of 19.8 [46]. The specificity of PFSC is somewhat limited, as a study demonstrated that nearly 12% of patients with non-urinothorax pleural effusions exhibited a PFSC greater than 1. However, the mean value was 1.17, with a maximum observed value of 1.64 [46].

Imaging

Suspected urinothoraces, based on clinical context and pleural fluid studies, require imaging confirmation. A chest X-ray frequently reveals a pleural effusion depending on the volume of fluid accumulation; however, when utilized in isolation, it is insufficient to diagnose a urinothorax. Urinothoraces are predominantly unilateral effusions; nonetheless, bilateral effusions have been documented [3, 9, 44, 59].

Thoracic ultrasound offers the advantage of increased sensitivity in identifying smaller pleural effusions and may additionally offer valuable insights into renal abnormalities, including hydronephrosis, ascites, or the formation of a urinoma [19, 21, 57, 60].

Thoracic non-contrast computed tomography (CT) can reveal pleural effusions, hydronephrosis, and perinephric fluid collections; however, it lacks sensitivity for detecting urine extravasation. Contrast-enhanced CT of the chest, especially when combined with CT urography, can detect urine leakage from the kidneys and/or ureters and demonstrate the presence of a urinoma or nephropleural fistula (Fig. 7.1a, b) [61–65].

When CT is unavailable, an intravenous urography (IVU) or pyelogram (IVP), in which iodinated contrast is intravascularly infused with subsequent X-rays obtained during the excretory phase, can be utilized to detect leaks from the urinary system. A pyelogram can also be performed retrograde by instilling the contrast agent into the bladder during a cystoscopy [19, 48, 66–68].

In instances where CT findings are inconclusive, a nuclear medicine scan known as dynamic renal scintigraphy, using radioactive tracers such as 99mTC diethylenetriaminepentaacetic acid, 99mTC ethylene dicysteine, or 99mTC mercaptoacetyltriglycine, allows for visualization of radiotracer translocation of urine from the peritoneal or retroperitoneal space into the pleural cavity (Fig. 7.1c) [9, 10, 44, 52, 69, 70].

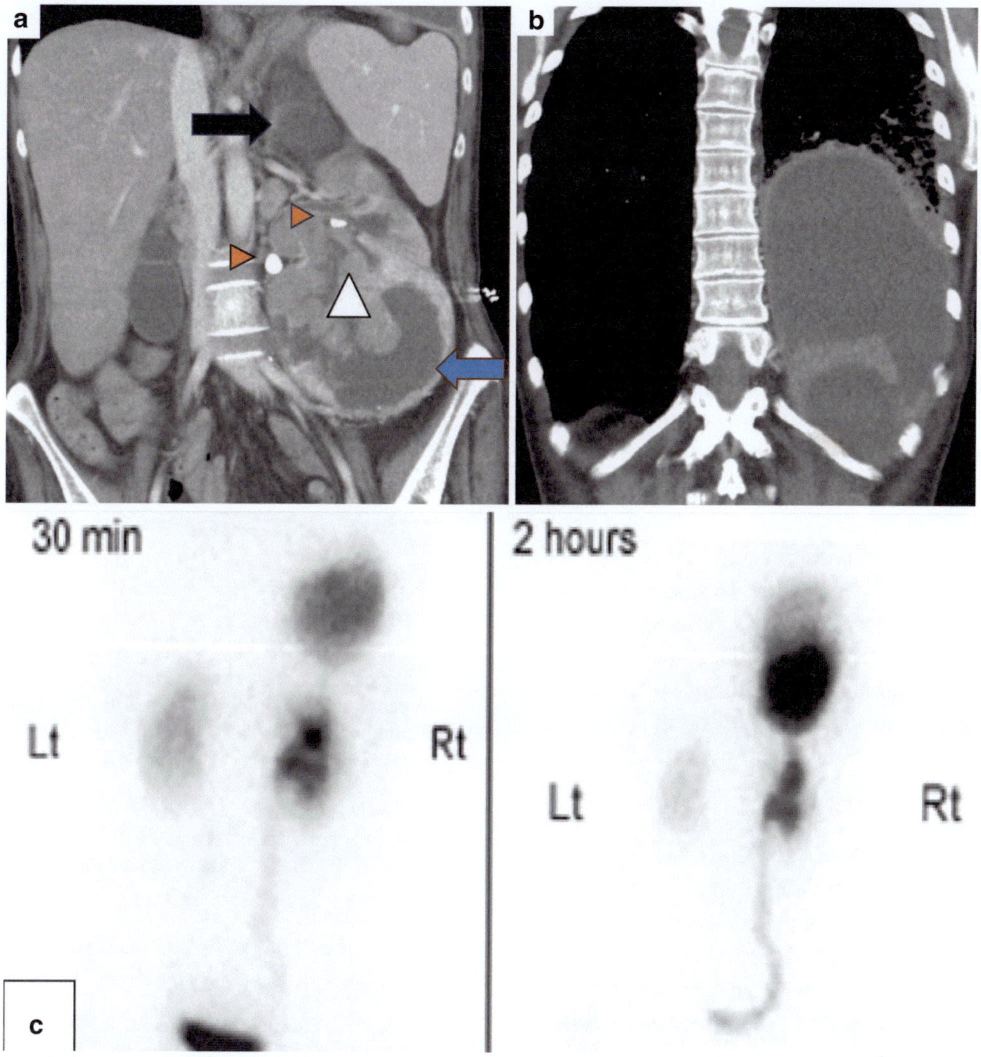

Fig. 7.1 (**a**) Contrast-enhanced coronal computed tomography (CT) of the abdomen demonstrating a large left renal pelvic mass (white triangle). A urinoma is visible superior to the left kidney (black arrow), accompanied by dilated left renal calyces (blue arrow) and multiple renal calculi (orange arrowheads). (**b**) Contrast-enhanced coronal CT of the chest showing continuity between the abdominal urinoma and the left pleural space through a diaphragmatic defect, resulting in a large left pleural effusion consistent with urinothorax. (**c**) Renal scintigraphy performed with technetium-99 m ethylene dicysteine (^{99m}Tc-EC) obtained from a different patient. Static planar images obtained at 30 min and 2 h after tracer injection demonstrate radiotracer accumulation within the renal collecting system as well as abnormal tracer activity within the thoracic cavity, consistent with urinary leakage into the pleural space (urinothorax)

Treatment

The primary treatment for urinothorax focuses on addressing the underlying urinary issue to prevent further leakage of urine into the pleural cavity. This method has shown a high success rate, even without pleural drainage [3, 9, 13]. In contrast, thoracentesis alone has a low likelihood of fully resolving the pleural effusion unless it is combined with urological intervention. Chest tube drainage has been performed on multiple occasions; however, pleural fluid output persisted until targeted treatment addressing the source of urine leakage was undertaken [48, 55, 62, 71, 72]. More invasive procedures, including surgical drainage, pleurodesis, and decortication, have all been performed with varying results, depending on the clinical context [3]. In one case of urinothorax resulting from penetrating trauma, a video-assisted thoracoscopic surgery with conversion to an open thoracotomy failed to resolve the pleural effusion until a ureteral stent to mitigate the source of urine extravasation was subsequently performed [29]. Thoracic surgical interventions, although uncommon, have been performed, such as diaphragmatic repairs in cases of defects or fistulas that facilitate the translocation of fluid from the peritoneum to the pleural cavity [27, 28, 73]. Interventions targeting urinary pathology vary based on etiology and include nephrostomy, nephrectomy, double-J stents, and sclerotherapy of a nephron-pleural fistula using 0.1% povidone-iodine instillation [3, 36, 39, 74, 75]. Ultimately, the treatment depends on the mechanism of injury, and each case requires an individualized approach. Due to the rarity of urinothorax, collaboration among pulmonology, urology, and radiology is recommended.

Conclusion

Urinothorax demands a high index of suspicion and should be considered in all patients presenting with pleural effusion, especially when urinary obstruction or injury is suspected. Performing a pleural fluid analysis is highly recommended and can support diagnosis through the pleural fluid-to-serum creatinine ratio. The variability in fluid analysis results may depend on the underlying cause of the urinothorax. As more cases are reported and data expand, cutoff values may be refined. Routine imaging includes chest X-ray and ultrasound, which can demonstrate pleural effusions. CT chest in combination with CT urography, pyelogram, and renal scintigraphy can confirm urine extravasation from the renal system. Addressing and correcting the root cause typically results in the rapid resolution of symptoms and effusions. Increased awareness and case reporting are crucial for better understanding urinothorax and improving diagnostic accuracy.

References

1. Fordyce W. Intra-uterine ascites: its obstetrical significance and pathology. Edinburgh: The University of Edinburgh; 1893.
2. Lord JM. Foetal Ascites. Arch Dis Child. 1953;28:398–403.
3. Toubes ME, Lama A, Ferreiro L, et al. Urinothorax: a systematic review. J Thorac Dis. 2017;9:1209–18.
4. France NE, Back EH. Neonatal ascites associated with urethral obstruction. Arch Dis Child. 1954;29:565–8.
5. Corriere JN, Miller WT, Murphy JJ. Hydronephrosis as a cause of pleural effusion. Radiology. 1968;90:69–84.
6. Stoerk HC, Laragh JH, Aceto RM, Budzilovich T. Edema and ascites following the ligation of both ureters in rats. Am J Pathol. 1970;58:51–67.
7. Friedland GW, Axman MM, Love T. Neonatal "urinothorax" associated with posterior urethral valves. Br J Radiol. 1971;44:471–4.
8. Ansari T, Idell S. Management of undiagnosed persistent pleural effusions. Clin Chest Med. 1998;19:407–17.
9. Austin A, Jogani SN, Brasher PB, Argula RG, Huggins JT, Chopra A. The Urinothorax: a comprehensive review with case series. Am J Med Sci. 2017;354:44–53.
10. Bramley K, Puchalski JT. Defying Gravity. Clin Chest Med. 2013;34:39–46.
11. Garcia-Pachon E, Romero S. Urinothorax: a new approach. Curr Opin Pulm Med. 2006;12:259–63.
12. Kinasewitz G. Transudative effusions. Eur Respir J. 1997;10:714–8.
13. Judson MA, Sahn SA. The pleural space and organ transplantation. Am J Respir Crit Care Med. 1996;153:1153–65.

14. Ryu JH, Tomassetti S, Maldonado F. Update on uncommon pleural effusions. Respirology. 2011;16:238–43.
15. Amro O, Webb-Smith F, Sunderji S. A rare complication of Total abdominal hysterectomy. Obstet Gynecol. 2009;114:482–4.
16. Dimitriadis G, Tahmatzopoulos A, Kampantais S, Ioannidis S, Radopoulos D, Katsikas V. Unilateral urinothorax can occur contralateral to the affected kidney. Scand. J. Urol. 2013;47:242–3.
17. Mikhail E, Seri A, Ralston K, Valvani A, Kalynych Z. Urinothorax and pseudo-azotemia following total abdominal hysterectomy: a case report. AME Case Rep. 2024;8:25.
18. Puthenveedu DKA. Urinothorax: a rare postoperative complication of Adrenalectomy. J Clin Diagn Reasoning. 2016;10:11–2.
19. Kelley M, Spieler B, Rouse C, Karl B, Marshall R, Carbonella G. Urinothorax: a rare complication of percutaneous nephrostomy. Radiol Case Rep. 2019;14:729–33.
20. Oguzulgen İK, Oguzulgen Aİ, Sınık Z, Köktürk O, Ekim N, Karaoglan Ü. An unusual cause of urinothorax. Respiration. 2002;69:273–4.
21. Ng H, Wang K, Cartledge J, et al. Urinothorax following percutaneous image-guided renal cryoablation. Radiol Case Rep. 2020;15:2348–52.
22. Salcedo JR. Urinothorax: report of 4 cases and review of the literature. J Urol. 1986;135:805–8.
23. Chawla A, Chaudhary G, Chawla M, Chawla R, Chawla P. Case of urinothorax—a rare presentation. Lung India. 2020;37:53–6.
24. Lahiry SK, Alkhafaji AH, Brown AL. Urinothorax following blunt trauma to the kidney. J Trauma. 1978;18:608–610.
25. Parvathy U, Saldanha R, Balakrishnan KR. Blunt abdominal trauma resulting in urinothorax from a missed uretero-pelvic junction avulsion: case report. J Trauma. 2003;54:187–9.
26. Hase T, Kodama M, Domasu S, Nakamura K, Morita K, Traumi T, Nakagama K, Nakamura K. A case of urothorax that manifested as posttraumatic pleural effusion after a motorcycle crash. J Trauma. 1999;56:967–9.
27. Capellier G, Gaussorgues P, Boyer F, Claud B. Diagnostic d'un panchement pleural posttraumatique. Ann Fr Anesth Reanim. 1989;8:131–2.
28. Gandhi R, Dhandapani B, Barvadheesh R. Combination injuries of diaphragm and urinary bladder resulting urinothorax. J Minimal Access Surg. 2015;11:149–50.
29. Connors C, Faizi Z, Ratnasekera A. A rare case of urinothorax as a result of penetrating trauma. Am Surg. 2023;89:2813–5.
30. Battah A, Farouji A, DaCosta T, Ahmad A, Kazmi R, DaCosta T Jr, Miller R, Farouji I. Urinothorax, a rare complication of rupture renal calyx. Radiol Case Rep. 2023;18:2335–8.
31. Belis A, Franklin D. Pleural effusion secondary to ureteral obstruction. Urology. 1979;14:27–9.
32. Tal Y, Weinberg I, Ben-Yehuda A, Duvdevani M. Unilateral obstructive urinothorax secondary to colorectal carcinoma. Isr Med Assoc J. 2015;17:321–2.
33. Karkoulias K, Sampsonas F, Kaparianos A, Tsiamita M, Tsoukalas G, Spiropoulos K. Urinothorax: an unexpected cause of pleural effusion in a patient with non-Hodgkin lymphoma. Eur Rev Med Pharmacol Sci. 2007;11:373–4.
34. Glozman T, Kooner S, Kostowniak C, Pacheco R, Zhang Y, Dumas CL, Chopra A. A rare case of infected urinothorax. Respir Med Case Rep. 2024;47:101989.
35. Gulec H, Degerli S, Ozayar E, Bercin F, Sahin S. Pleural effusion due to intraoperative rupture of an infected renal cyst. Korean J Anesthesiol. 2012;62:497–8.
36. Abusnina W, Bukamur H, Koc Z, Najar F, Munn N, Zeid F. Urinothorax caused by xanthogranulomatous pyelonephritis. Case Rep Pulmonol. 2018;2018:1–3.
37. Weiss Z, Shalev E, Zuckerman H, Shental J, Barzilay E. Obstructive renal failure and pleural effusion caused by the gravid uterus. Acta Obstet Gynecol Scand. 1986;65:187–9.
38. Anjum T, Ikram M, Abdulhameed R, Khan A, Mirza ZR. Urinoma: a rare but potential differential of acute abdomen. Cureus. 2024;16:e67368.
39. Aeron R, Goel S, Goel A, Kumar V. Spontaneous nonobstructive nephropleural fistula with an autoimmune disorder causing massive urinothorax: a rare association. BMJ Case Rep bcr-2017-221601. 2017.
40. Ferreiro L, Toubes ME, Suárez-Antelo J, Rodríguez-Núñez N, Valdés L. Clinical overview of the physiology and pathophysiology of pleural fluid movement: a narrative review. ERJ Open Res. 2024;10:00050–2024.
41. Muzhrachi A, Prasad KV. Bilateral urinothorax following spontaneous extravasation from the kidney-speculation of an anatomical pathway for the transport of the extravasated urine to the pleural cavities: a case report and review of the literature. Qatar Med J. 2008;17:71–4.
42. Gupta R, Singh P. Urinothorax - a rare cause of pleural effusion. JK Sci. 2014;16:86–8.
43. Agrawal S, Chipde S, Dosi R, Ranjan V. Urinothorax: a path, less travelled: case report and review of literature. J Nat Sci Biol Med. 2015;6:213.
44. Ralston MD, Wilkinson RH. Bilateral urinothorax identified by technetium-99m DPTA renal imaging. J Nucl Med. 1986;27:56–9.
45. Sullivan A, Lanham T, Bohra N, Ellis B, Kahn D. Urine in the lung: an uncommon cause of transudative pleural effusion. Respir Med Case Rep. 2020;31:101220.
46. Garcia-Pachon E, Padilla-Navas I. Urinothorax: case report and review of the literature with emphasis on biochemical diagnosis. Respiration. 2004;71:533–6.
47. Thomas R, Jenkins S, Eastwood PR, Lee YCG, Singh B. Physiology of breathlessness associ-

ated with pleural effusions. Curr Opin Pulm Med. 2015;21:338–45.
48. Dregoesc D, Kelley R, Lick D. An unusual case of urinothorax after percutaneous nephrostolithotomy. J Family Med Prim Care. 2019;8:2155–7.
49. Izzo L, Caputo M, De Toma G, Izzo P, Bolognese A, Basso L. Urinoma and urinothorax: report of a case. Am Surg. 2008;74:62–3.
50. Powers RE, Estrada-Y-Martin RM, Cherian SV. Urinothorax: an under-reported cause of pleural effusions. QJM. 2022;115:862–3.
51. McLean A, Bartman MT, Winton EB. Case report: acute dyspnea secondary to urinothorax following ureteroscopy. Urol Case Rep. 2023;51:102565.
52. Bhattacharya A, Venkataramarao SH, Kumar S, Mittal BR. Urinothorax demonstrated on 99mTc ethylene dicysteine renal scintigraphy. Nephrol Dial Transplant. 2007;22:1782–3.
53. Light RW. Pleural diseases. 5th ed. Baltimore: Lippincott Williams & Wilkins; 2007.
54. Pierson DJ. Respiratory considerations in the patient with renal failure. Respir Care. 2006;51:413–22.
55. Chandra A, Pathak A, Kapur A, Russia N, Bhasin N. Urinothorax: a rare cause of severe respiratory distress. Indian J Crit Care Med. 2014;18:320–2.
56. Stark DD, Shanes JG, Baron RL. Biochemical features of urinothorax. Arch Intern Med. 1982;142:1509–11.
57. Miller KS, Wooten S, Sahn S. Urinothorax: a cause of low pH transudative pleural effusions. Am J Med. 1988;85:448–9.
58. Bichler K-H, Eipper E, Naber K, Braun V, Zimmermann R, Lahme S. Urinary infection stones. Int J Antimicrob Agents. 2002;19:488–98.
59. Laskaridis L, Kampantais S, Toutziaris C, Chachopoulos B, Perdikis I, Tahmatzopoulos A, Dimitriadis G. Urinothorax—an underdiagnosed cause of acute dyspnea: report of a bilateral and of an ipsilateral urinothorax case. Case Rep Emerg Med. 2012;2012:1–3.
60. Buyukcelik M, Satar N, Celik U, Yildizdas D, Dursun H, Soran M, Anarat A. An unusual cause of pleural effusion, urinothorax in a child with urinary stone disease. Pediatr Nephrol. 2005;20:1487–9.
61. González-Montaos A, Rodríguez-Otero I, Chávarri-Ibáñez E. Urinothorax secondary to bilateral rupture of the ureters: an unusual case of pleural exudate. Arch Bronconeumol. 2023;59:389–90.
62. Batura D, Haylock-Vize P, Naji Y, Tennant R, Fawcett K. Management of iatrogenic urinothorax following ultrasound guided percutaneous nephrostomy. Radiol Case. 2014;8:34–40.
63. Abdel-Rahman AM. Urinothorax: a rare finding after urinary intervention. Clin Respir J. 2017;11:529–31.
64. Ahmad Para S, Ansari FM, Ahmad Dar Y, Wani MS, Bhat AH, Latief Lone A. Slowly developing urinothorax in a child due to intrapleural migration of DJ stent-a rare complication of percutaneous nephrolithotomy. Radiol Case Rep. 2022;17:3877–81.
65. Artiles Medina A, Laso García I, Duque Ruiz G, Hevia Palacios M, Arias Funez F, Burgos Revilla FJ. Spontaneous urinoma debuting as retroperitoneal abscess: report of 2 cases and literature review. Transl Androl Urol. 2021;10:963–8.
66. Baugh AD, Youssef E, Hasan SS, Siddiqui NS, Elsamoloty H, Shahrour K, Javaid T. Nephropleural fistula effectively managed with serial thoracentesis: a case report. J Endourol Case Rep. 2016;2:212–4.
67. Casallas A, Castaneda-Cardona C, Rosselli D. Urinothorax: case report and systematic review of the literature. Urol Ann. 2016;8:91.
68. Dyer RB, Chen MYM, Zagoria RJ. Intravenous urography: technique and interpretation. Radiographics. 2001;21:799–824.
69. Lee TW, Jang HN, Cho HS, Choi SM, Choi B-H, Bae E, Chang S-H, Park DJ. Urinothorax after ultrasonography-guided renal biopsy: a case report. BMC Nephrol. 2018;19:104.
70. Jelic S, Sampogna RV. Detection of unrecognized urinothorax with renal scintigraphy. Kidney Int. 2009;76:353–4.
71. Hendriks J, Michielsen D, Van Schil P, Wyndaele J-J. Urinothorax: a rare pleural effusion. Acta Chir Belg. 2002;102:274–5.
72. Wei B, Takayama H, Bacchetta MD. Urinothorax: an uncommon cause of pleural effusion. Respir Med CME. 2009;2:179–80.
73. Vallianou N, Gennimata V, Constantinou F, Karamanolakis D, Grigorakis A. Synchronous urinothorax and uroperitoneum. Am J Emerg Med. 2018;36:1922.e1–2.
74. Bahjat AS, Sadeeq KJ, Tahir AMS, Mohammed AA. Urinothorax causing massive left side pleural effusion in a young lady; case report and literature review. Urol Case Rep. 2019;26:100957.
75. Andreia Freitas, Telmo Coelho, Sara Beça, Tiago Gregório. Pleural effusion secondary to obstructive uropathy: a case of urinothorax. Eur J Case Rep Intern Med. 2020;7:001865.

Duropleural Fistula

8

Timothy Daly, Firas Ido, and Thomas Zanders

Introduction

A duropleural fistula (DPF), also known as a subarachnoid–pleural fistula (SAPF), is an abnormal communication of iatrogenic, genetic, or idiopathic origin between the subarachnoid space and the pleural cavity, resulting in the accumulation of cerebrospinal fluid (CSF) within the pleural space. Because the fluid originates outside the pleural vasculature, this condition is classified as a pleural effusion of extravascular origin (PEEVO) [1–8].

The first documented case of a DPF was reported in 1959. The patient, a 19-year-old male with paraplegia following a gunshot wound, initially showed no evidence of pleural effusion for several years. After receiving a paraspinal alcohol injection to manage spastic paralysis, he developed a right-sided pleural effusion 6 weeks later. Upon recurrence after thoracentesis, thoracotomy revealed a direct communication between the subarachnoid and pleural spaces, confirming the presence of a DPF [9]. Since that time, additional case reports have emerged, though DPF remains an exceptionally rare clinical entity. Diagnostic accuracy has improved significantly with the advent of advanced spinal imaging and the identification of beta-2 transferrin, a CSF-specific protein, within pleural fluid. The use of beta-2 transferrin in diagnosis was first described by Meurman et al. in 1979 [10]. Prior to this discovery, detection of CSF in pleural fluid relied on albumin and prealbumin ratios determined by protein electrophoresis [11].

DPF can be broadly classified as traumatic or nontraumatic. Primary risk factors include blunt thoracic trauma and surgical procedures involving thoracotomy or spinal access (e.g., discectomy) [9–11]. Penetrating injuries such as gunshot wounds account for only a small subset of cases. Primary intrathoracic malignancies, such as primary spinal tumors, metastatic lesions, and paraspinal malignant mesothelioma, have also been implicated [12]. The increased use of anterior approach discectomy since the 1990s has heightened the risk of pleural injury due to the close proximity of the dural sac [13].

Rarely, Gorham–Stout syndrome (GSS), a condition characterized by lymphangiomatous proliferation leading to massive osteolysis and Chiari malformations (CMs), has been associated with DPF formation [6, 14]. Additionally, iatrogenic CSF–pleural communications may be intentionally created in the form of ventriculopleural shunts (VPLS), used for the management of normal pressure hydrocephalus (NPH) when

T. Daly · F. Ido · T. Zanders (✉)
Department of Pulmonary and Critical Care Medicine, St. Luke's University Health Network, Bethlehem, PA, USA
e-mail: timothy.daly@sluhn.org; firas.ido@sluhn.org; Thomas.zanders@sluhn.org

F. Ido (ed.), *Rare Pleural Diseases*, https://doi.org/10.1007/978-3-032-14873-5_8

the peritoneal cavity is unsuitable for drainage (e.g., due to infection, malignancy, or bowel obstruction) [15–18]. When CSF production exceeds pleural absorption, a pleural effusion ensues [19, 20]. To date, fewer than 100 cases of DPF have been reported in the literature. The following sections detail the pathophysiology, clinical presentation, diagnostic approach, and therapeutic management of duropleural fistulas.

Pathophysiology

The timeline for the development of a duropleural fistula varies significantly according to the underlying etiology and mechanism of injury. Depending on the site and nature of the insult, fistula formation may occur within hours or may take several months to manifest. For instance, one case documented the development of a DPF 4 months after a transthoracic discectomy, while another described a patient who developed a fistula 2 years following extensive lumbar disk surgery [7, 13]. Similarly, a traumatic subarachnoid–pleural fistula was reported 1.5 years after blunt thoracic trauma [21]. Conversely, other cases have demonstrated early-onset fistula formation within hours to days of the initial injury [8].

The risk of DPF formation is particularly elevated in patients with impaired wound healing, such as those with diabetes mellitus, immunocompromised states, or those undergoing chemotherapy [22]. Moreover, the combined use of chemotherapy and radiotherapy further heightens susceptibility due to their cytotoxic and necrotizing effects on surrounding pulmonary and pleural tissues [23]. Following the initial insult, a localized inflammatory response is triggered, characterized by the release of cytokines such as tumor necrosis factor-alpha (TNF-α) and interleukin-13 (IL-13) from activated cells in the affected region. These mediators recruit T and B lymphocytes, initiating an acute inflammatory cascade. As the process transitions to the chronic phase, fibroblasts proliferate and deposit collagen and extracellular matrix fibers, promoting tissue repair. In the context of a DPF, this reparative process inadvertently leads to the formation of a tract between the subarachnoid and pleural compartments [24, 25]. In postoperative cases, the proximity of two suture lines, one dural and one pleural, within inflamed tissue may predispose to fistula formation during healing. Once established, the fistulous tract remains patent due to the hydrostatic pressure gradient between the central nervous system (CNS) and the thoracic cavity [24]. The negative intrapleural pressure, especially during inspiration, further facilitates unidirectional flow of CSF into the pleural space. Because the parietal pleura is more vascularized and lymphatic than the visceral pleura, it plays a predominant role in fluid dynamics within the pleural space. When CSF influx exceeds compensatory drainage, an effusion develops [26–30].

Certain congenital disorders are recognized as predisposing factors for the development of a duropleural fistula, most notably Gorham–Stout syndrome and Chiari malformation type II. Gorham–Stout syndrome is a rare condition characterized by idiopathic intraosseous angiomatous proliferation, leading to progressive osteolysis and resorption of bone [31, 32]. When spontaneous osteolysis involves the thoracic spine, structural weakening can result in microtears of the adjacent parietal pleura and dural sac, thereby facilitating the formation of a pathologic communication between the subarachnoid and pleural spaces [33, 34]. In Chiari malformation type II, there is a strong association with DPF development due to congenital alterations in the neural tube and spinal anatomy. The frequent coexistence of myelomeningocele allows for direct communication between the subarachnoid space and extrathecal compartments, predisposing to persistent cerebrospinal fluid leakage. Furthermore, surgical repair of these congenital malformations can further compromise dural integrity, substantially increasing the risk of subsequent duropleural fistula formation [35–39].

Clinical Features

The clinical presentation of a duropleural fistula is highly variable and depends mainly on the underlying etiology. Symptoms attributable to the pleural effusion component are generally nonspecific, commonly including dyspnea, orthopnea, and exertional shortness of breath. Less frequently, patients may report fever, chills, tachypnea, malaise, nonproductive cough, diaphragmatic spasm, or decreased appetite. A hallmark clinical clue suggestive of a DPF is the development of a new pleural effusion in conjunction with neurologic symptoms, particularly when these manifestations occur soon after spinal or pleural injury or intervention [40, 41].

The most frequent neurological manifestation is headache, typically severe in nature and often exacerbated following thoracentesis [42, 43]. The headache classically worsens in the upright position and improves when supine, a pattern characteristic of spontaneous intracranial hypotension (SIH) [12, 44]. This postural component results from the migration of cerebrospinal fluid from the central nervous system, where the hydrostatic pressure is higher, into the pleural space, creating a relative CSF deficit intracranially [45, 46]. Other neurological symptoms may include neck pain or stiffness, generalized weakness, vomiting, and paresthesias affecting the extremities or trunk, all reflecting disturbances in CSF pressure dynamics or direct neural involvement [47, 48].

Diagnosis

The diagnosis of a duropleural fistula is primarily established through pleural fluid analysis, typically obtained via thoracentesis. Lumbar puncture is typically unnecessary for diagnostic confirmation. The pleural effusion may be transudative or exudative, depending on the underlying etiology, although it is most often transudative in nature [49]. In addition to standard pleural fluid studies, beta-2 transferrin testing should be specifically requested in the evaluation of any unexplained pleural effusion suspected to originate from a CSF source [69]. This protein is exclusively synthesized in the cochlea of the inner ear, and its presence in pleural fluid is pathognomonic for a cerebrospinal fluid leak. The sensitivity and specificity of beta-2 transferrin for detecting CSF fistulas range from 94–100% and 98–100%, respectively [64, 65]. Beta-2 transferrin is a monomeric glycoprotein detectable by gel electrophoresis and immunofixation, with very high analytical sensitivity, requiring as little as 3 μL of fluid for detection [10, 70, 71–74]. In addition to beta-2 transferrin, beta-trace protein (BTP) has emerged as a novel biomarker for identifying CSF leaks, including dural fistulae [75]. Discovered in the late twentieth century, BTP is a low-molecular-weight enzyme involved in prostaglandin metabolism and constitutes a major protein component of CSF [76]. Secreted predominantly by the leptomeninges, its detection in pleural fluid is highly specific for DPF. Although no standardized pleural reference range exists, one study reported mean pleural BTP levels of 2.16 mg/L in patients without DPF and serum levels of 0.38–0.86 mg/L. In contrast, patients with confirmed DPF demonstrated markedly elevated levels, averaging 14 mg/L [13].

The gross appearance of the pleural fluid is typically clear and watery, with very low protein levels (usually <1 g/dL), a pH near 7.55, a glucose concentration around 100 mg/dL, and low lactate dehydrogenase (LDH) levels (Fig. 8.1b). Cellular analysis often reveals a macrophage-predominant differential [6, 7, 66, 67]. These effusions characteristically reaccumulate rapidly, often within days of thoracentesis, unless the fistulous tract is definitively repaired [13, 68].

Depending on presenting symptoms, initial radiologic evaluation may include chest radiography, computed tomography (CT), or magnetic resonance imaging (MRI) of the thorax and spine. While these modalities provide useful anatomic information, specialized imaging is required to directly visualize a DPF [50–57]. Pleural effusions associated with DPF are typically large, unilateral, and simple-appearing (Fig. 8.1a) [13, 42, 53]. Once a DPF is suspected, the imaging modalities of choice for localizing the fistulous tract are magnetic resonance (MR) cisternography and computed tomography cisternography. MR cisternography demonstrates superior sensitivity compared to CT (90% vs. 86%) and is particularly effective for detecting small or slow CSF leaks [58, 59]. CT dynamic

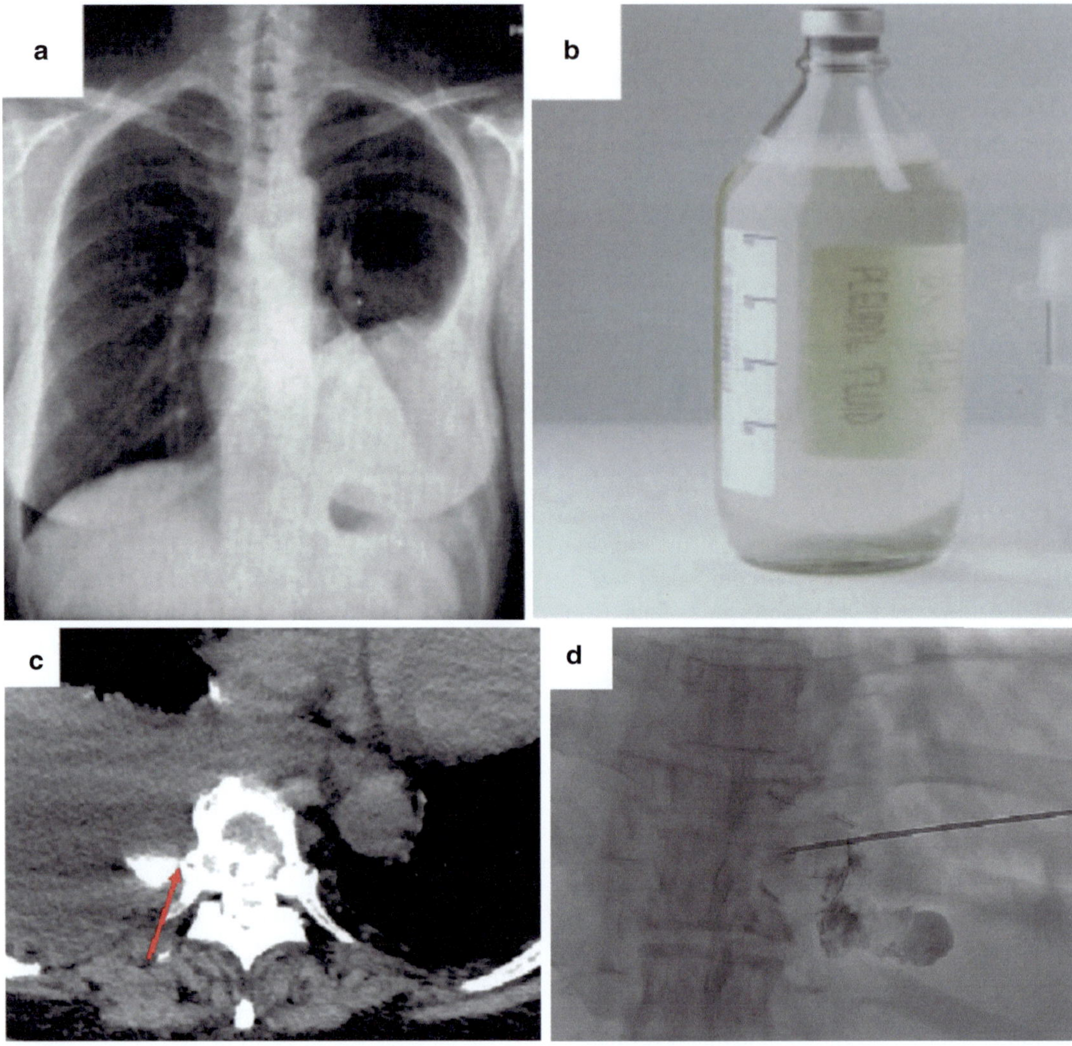

Fig. 8.1 Features of a duropleural fistula
(**a**) Chest radiograph showing a large left pleural effusion.
(**b**) Pleural fluid obtained by thoracentesis from a patient with a duropleural fistula, demonstrating a clear, water-like appearance consistent with a transudative, low-protein effusion.
(**c**) Computed tomographic myelography from a different case reveals a right pleural effusion with contrast extravasation between the subarachnoid and pleural spaces, confirming the presence of a duropleural fistula.
(**d**) Using stereotactic fluoroscopy guidance, the duropleural fistula is sealed with injection of acrylic glue.

Attribution: Panels A–B reprinted from *CHEST*, Vol 114(6), Monla-Hassan J., Eichenhorn M., Spickler E., Talati S., Nockels R., Hyzy R., "Duropleural Fistula Manifested as a Large Pleural Transudate: An Unusual Complication of Transthoracic Diskectomy," pp. 1786–1789, Copyright © 1998. American College of Chest Physicians. Published by Elsevier Inc. Reproduced by permission of Elsevier through RightsLink License No. 6130610906479 for *Rare Pleural Disease* (Springer Nature, 2026).

Panels C–D reprinted from *Respiratory Medicine and Research*, Vol 80, Moncomble E., Al Kahf S., Clerc S., Ikka L., Lonjon G., Planquette B., "Subarachnoid-pleural fistula: To drain or not to drain," Article 100,786, Copyright © 2021 Elsevier Masson SAS. Reproduced by permission of Elsevier through RightsLink License No. 6130610563328 for *Rare Pleural Disease* (Springer Nature, 2026).

myelography serves as a valuable alternative, permitting positional adjustments to enhance visualization of pressure-dependent leaks during inspiration, standing, or contrast timing, based on the suspected location of the defect (Fig. 8.1c) [60–62]. An additional, though less frequently utilized, modality is radionuclide myelography, which involves the injection of a radiotracer into the subarachnoid space and the subsequent tracking of tracer migration into the pleural cavity. While relatively invasive, this technique remains a diagnostic option when other imaging studies are inconclusive [63].

Treatment and Prognosis

The treatment of a duropleural fistula typically requires active intervention, as spontaneous closure is exceedingly rare. Conservative management alone is generally unsuccessful due to the persistent pressure gradient between the subarachnoid and pleural spaces [3, 25]. Noninvasive positive pressure ventilation (NPPV), used in combination with chest tube drainage or lumbar CSF diversion, has been reported to facilitate fistula closure by counteracting the negative intrathoracic pressure that perpetuates CSF leakage. Successful closure has been documented within 5–14 days of therapy [77, 78]. Even low ventilatory pressures, such as 6 cm H_2O inspiratory and 4 cm H_2O expiratory pressure, have been sufficient to promote resolution in select cases [57]. Despite these reports, surgical repair remains the definitive treatment for most patients. Surgical techniques include direct closure of the dural or pleural defect using graft materials, such as cadaveric dural–pleural grafts, muscle flaps, or omental flaps [25, 79]. In some cases, duroplasty with vascularized tissue grafts is performed to enhance durability and reduce recurrence risk [42, 80, 81]. When primary suturing is not feasible due to defect size or location, onyx embolization—an endovascular technique employing a liquid embolic agent—has been successfully used in select case reports. Acrylic glue injection of the fistula under fluoroscopic guidance has also been performed (Fig. 8.1d) [82].

For cases in which the DPF arises in association with a ventriculopleural shunt, management focuses on reducing CSF flow into the pleural space and preventing reaccumulation of fluid. Options include repeated thoracentesis, externalization of the shunt, relocation of the shunt to the contralateral hemithorax or peritoneal cavity, and, in refractory cases, placement of a tunneled pleural catheter to avoid repeated invasive procedures. However, the latter approach is rarely employed due to the significant infection risk, including the potential for ascending infection into the central nervous system, making it an undesirable long-term solution [83, 84]. In patients with DPF secondary to Gorham–Stout syndrome, adjunctive therapies such as radiation therapy, vitamin D supplementation, anti-osteoclastic medications, and alpha-2b interferon have been reported to achieve favorable outcomes [6].

Following intervention, close clinical and radiologic monitoring is essential to detect complications. One of the most common is rebound intracranial hypertension, resulting from rapid restoration of normal CSF volume and pressure after repair. This typically manifests as a frontal or periorbital headache, occasionally accompanied by nausea and vomiting [85, 86]. Chronic, unresolved DPF-associated effusions may lead to fibrothorax, characterized by pleural fibrosis and restrictive ventilatory impairment. In such cases, surgical decortication combined with correction or revision of the CSF shunt is often required to alleviate dyspnea and restore pulmonary function [87, 88].

References

1. Saini P, Callejas L, Gudi M, Grosu HB. Recurrent pleural effusion due to duropleural fistula. J Bronchology Interv Pulmonol. 2014;21(3):265–6.
2. Jahn K, Winkler K, Tiling R, Brandt T. Intracranial hypotension syndrome due to duropleural fistula after thoracic diskectomy. J Neurol (Germany). 2001;248:1101–3.
3. Maskin LP, Raimondi A, Hlavnicka A, Díaz MF, Roura N, Wainsztein N. Duropleural fistula revealed by neurological manifestations: an unusual cause of pleural effusion. Anaesth Intensive Care. 2010;38(1):201–3.

4. Maeda D, Kosuda S, Kusano S, Fujikawa Y. Pleural cerebrospinal fluid input and output kinetics dynamically demonstrated by In-111 DTPA myelography in a patient with pleural cerebrospinal fluid fistulae. Clin Nucl Med. 2004;29(12):836–7.
5. Rosen PR, Chaudhuri TK. Radioisotope myelography in the detection of pleural-dural communication as a source of recurrent meningitis. Clin Nucl Med. 1983;8(1):28–30.
6. Agrawal R, Mohammed I, Reilly PG. Duropleural fistula as a consequence of Gorham-stout syndrome: a combination of 2 rare conditions. J Thorac Cardiovasc Surg. 2006;131(5):1205–6.
7. Huggins JT, Sahn SA. Duro-pleural fistula diagnosed by beta2-transferrin. Respiration. 2003;70(4):423–5.
8. Sarwal V, Suri RK, Sharma OP, Baruah A, Singhi P, Gill S, et al. Traumatic subarachnoid-pleural fistula. Ann Thorac Surg. 1996;62(6):1622–6.
9. Milloy FJ, Correll NO, Langston HT. Persistent subarachnoid-pleural space fistula; report of a case. J Am Med Assoc. 1959;169(13):1467.
10. Meurman OH, Irjala K, Suonpää J, Laurent B. A new method for the identification of cerebrospinal fluid leakage. Acta Otolaryngol. 1979;87(3–4):366–9.
11. Reisinger PW, Lempart K, Hochstrasser K. [New methods of diagnosing cerebrospinal fluid fistulas using beta 2-transferrin or prealbumin--principles and methodology]. Laryngol Rhinol Otol (Stuttg). 1987; 66(5):255–259.
12. Heyer CM, Theile A, Weisser H, Reichert J, Horch C, Mueller K-M, et al. Subarachnoid-pleural fistula as a complication of malignant pleural mesothelioma. Respirology. 2006;11(4):502–5.
13. Monla-Hassan J, Eichenhorn M, Spickler E, Talati S, Nockels R, Hyzy R. Duropleural fistula manifested as a large pleural transudate: an unusual complication of transthoracic diskectomy. Chest. 1998;114(6):1786–9.
14. Patel DV. Gorham's disease or massive osteolysis. Clin Med Res. 2005;3(2):65–74.
15. Torres Lanzas J, Ríos Zambudio A, Martínez Lage JF, Roca Calvo MJ, Poza M, Parrilla PP. Ventriculopleural shunt to treat hydrocephalus. Arch Bronconeumol. 2002;38(11):511–4.
16. Hoffman HJ, Hendrick EB, Humphreys RP. Experience with ventriculo-pleural shunts. Childs Brain. 1983;10(6):404–13.
17. Martínez-Lage JF, Torres J, Campillo H, Sanchez-del-Rincón I, Bueno F, Zambudio G, et al. Ventriculopleural shunting with new technology valves. Childs Nerv Syst. 2000;16(12):867–71.
18. Alam S, Manjunath NM. Severe respiratory failure following ventriculopleural shunt. Indian J Crit Care Med. 2015;19:690–2.
19. Henningfeld J, Loomba RS, Encalada S, Magner K, Pfister J, Matthews A, et al. Pleural effusion in a child with a ventriculoperitoneal shunt and congenital heart disease. Springerplus. 2016;5:90.
20. Fowler JB, De Jesus O, Mesfin FB. Ventriculoperitoneal Shunt. In Treasure Island (FL); 2024.
21. Jimenez MF, Roca R, Alvarez C, Loinaz C, Toledo J. Persistent pleural effusion and post-traumatic subarachnoidal-pleural fistula. Eur. J. Cardiothorac. Surg. 1991;5(10):554–6.
22. Moncomble E, Al Kahf S, Clerc S, Ikka L, Lonjon G, Planquette B. Subarachnoid-pleural fistula: to drain or not to drain. Respir Med Res. 2021;80:100786.
23. Kapoor H, Gulati V, Gulati A, Donuru A, Parekh M. Comprehensive imaging review of pleural fistulas from diagnosis to management. Radiographics. 2022;42(7):1940–55.
24. Hentschel SJ, Rhines LD, Wong FC, Gokaslan ZL, McCutcheon IE. Subarachnoid-pleural fistula after resection of thoracic tumors. J Neurosurg. 2004;100(4 Suppl Spine):332–6.
25. Eli I, Guan J, Karsy M, Mazur MD, Dailey A. A case of ventral spinal cord herniation from a chronic Dural-pleural fistula resulting in thoracic myelopathy. Cureus. 2019;11:e6123.
26. Shen-Wagner J, Gamble C, MacGilvray P. Pleural effusion: diagnostic approach in adults. Am Fam Physician. 2023;108(5):464–75.
27. Miserocchi G. Mechanisms controlling the volume of pleural fluid and extravascular lung water. Eur Respir Rev. 2009;18(114):244–52.
28. Felekis VA. The suction mechanism as a factor in intrathoracic oedema, connective tissue, or pleural effusion. Med Hypotheses. 2002;59(4):462–7.
29. Yalcin NG, Choong CKC, Eizenberg N. Anatomy and pathophysiology of the pleura and pleural space. Thorac Surg Clin. 2013;23(1):1–10. v
30. Heller JG, Kim HS, Carlson GW. Subarachnoid--pleural fistulae--management with a transdiaphragmatic pedicled greater omental flap: report of two cases. Spine (Phila, Pa 1976). 2001;26(16):1809–13.
31. Schneider KN, Gosheger G, Andreou D. Gorham-Stout Syndrome. Dtsch Arztebl Int. 2019;116(29–30):507.
32. Yildiz TS, Kus A, Solak M, Toker K. The Gorham-stout syndrome: one lung ventilation with a bronchial blocker. A case of Gorham's disease with chylothorax. Paediatr Anaesth. 2009;19:190–1.
33. Itkin M, McCormack FX. Nonmalignant adult thoracic lymphatic disorders. Clin Chest Med. 2016;37(3):409–20.
34. Takahashi A, Ogawa C, Kanazawa T, Watanabe H, Suzuki M, Suzuki N, et al. Remission induced by interferon alfa in a patient with massive osteolysis and extension of lymph-hemangiomatosis: a severe case of Gorham-stout syndrome. J Pediatr Surg. 2005;40(3):E47–50.
35. Somoza-Cano FJ, Al Armashi AR, Hammad F, Patell K, Ravakhah K. Arnold-Chiari malformation and scoliosis: a chronic lung collapse mimicking sepsis. Cureus. 2021;13:e15292.
36. Schmid S, Bevot A, Neunhoeffer F, Michel J, Kumpf MU, Reimold M, et al. Chronic pleural effusion in ventriculoperitoneal shunt due to diaphragmatic CSF fistula: report of a case treated by endoscopic choroid plexus coagulation and literature review. Pediatr Neurosurg. 2023;58:160–7.

37. Porcaro F, Procaccini E, Paglietti MG, Schiavino A, Petreschi F, Cutrera R. Pleural effusion from intrathoracic migration of a ventriculo-peritoneal shunt catheter: pediatric case report and review of the literature. Ital J Pediatr. 2018;44(1):42.
38. Glatstein MM, Roth J, Scolnik D, Haham A, Rimon A, Koren L, et al. Late presentation of massive pleural effusion from intrathoracic migration of a ventriculoperitoneal shunt catheter: case report and review of the literature. Pediatr Emerg Care. 2012;28(2):180–2.
39. Hilmani S, Mesbahi T, Bouaggad A, Lakhdar A. A rare complication of ventriculoperitoneal shunt: pleural effusion without intrathoracic ventriculoperitoneal shunt catheter. Surg Neurol Int. 2020;11:291.
40. Gayen S. Malignant pleural effusion: presentation, diagnosis, and management. Am J Med. 2022;135(10):1188–92.
41. Beaudoin S, Gonzalez AV. Evaluation of the patient with pleural effusion. Can Med Assoc J = J l'Association médicale Can. 2018;190(10):E291–5.
42. D'Souza R, Doshi A, Bhojraj S, Shetty P, Udwadia Z. Massive pleural effusion as the presenting feature of a subarachnoid-pleural fistula. Respiration. 2002;69(1):96–9.
43. Pollack II, Pang D, Hall WA. Subarachnoid-pleural and subarachnoid-mediastinal fistulae. Neurosurgery. 1990;26(3):519–25.
44. Lin S-F, Weng H-Y. Postural headaches due to cerebrospinal fluid leakage through subarachnoid-pleural fistula: a case report. Headache. 2017;57(3):467–71.
45. Dobrocky T, Nicholson P, Häni L, Mordasini P, Krings T, Brinjikji W, et al. Spontaneous intracranial hypotension: searching for the CSF leak. Lancet Neurol. 2022;21(4):369–80.
46. Magnaes B. Body position and cerebrospinal fluid pressure. Part 2: clinical studies on orthostatic pressure and the hydrostatic indifferent point. J Neurosurg. 1976;44(6):698–705.
47. Chen P-H, Li C-R, Gan C-W, Yang T-H, Chang C-S, Chan F-H. Rare combination of traumatic subarachnoid-pleural fistula and intracranial subdural hygromas: a case report. World J Clin Cases. 2023;11:5173–8.
48. Knecht B. [Otoliquorrhrea. Causes and Treatment]. Wien Klin Wochenschr. 1963; 75:588–591.
49. Dalphy A, Burkett A. Pleural cerebrospinal fluid shunting causing trapped lung: a respiratory physician's approach to management and prevention. Respir Med Case Rep. 2018;25:303–5.
50. Kranz PG, Luetmer PH, Diehn FE, Amrhein TJ, Tanpitukpongse TP, Gray L. Myelographic techniques for the detection of spinal CSF leaks in spontaneous intracranial hypotension. AJR Am J Roentgenol. 2016;206(1):8–19.
51. Dobrocky T, Grunder L, Breiding PS, Branca M, Limacher A, Mosimann PJ, et al. Assessing spinal cerebrospinal fluid leaks in spontaneous intracranial hypotension with a scoring system based on brain magnetic resonance imaging findings. JAMA Neurol. 2019;76(5):580–7.
52. Tay AS-MS, Maya M, Moser FG, Nuño M, Schievink WI. Computed tomography vs heavily T2-weighted magnetic resonance Myelography for the initial evaluation of patients with spontaneous intracranial hypotension. JAMA Neurol. 2021;78(10):1275–6.
53. Ohana N, Benharroch D, Sheinis D. Pleural Dural fistula after anterior excision of thoracic disc hernia: suggested repair procedure. Ann Thorac Surg. 2019;107(3):e191–3.
54. Huang W, Yuan C, Patel KM, Mei A, Avilla K, Zhang X, et al. Transthoracic ultrasound to predict exudative pleural effusion etiology. J Ultrasound Med. 2025;44(8):1343–53.
55. Sorino C, Mondoni M, Lococo F, Marchetti G, Feller-Kopman D. Optimizing the management of complicated pleural effusion: from intrapleural agents to surgery. Respir Med. 2022;191:106706.
56. Broaddus VC, Wiener-Kronish JP, Berthiaume Y, Staub NC. Removal of pleural liquid and protein by lymphatics in awake sheep. J Appl Physiol. 1988;64(1):384–90.
57. Kurata Y, Yoshimoto M, Takebayashi T, Kawaguchi S, Yamashita T. Subarachnoid-pleural fistula treated with noninvasive positive pressure ventilation: a two-case report and literature review. Spine (Phila, Pa 1976). 2010;35(18):E908–11.
58. Eberhardt KE, Hollenbach HP, Deimling M, Tomandl BF, Huk WJ. MR cisternography: a new method for the diagnosis of CSF fistulae. Eur Radiol. 1997;7(9):1485–91.
59. Chazen JL, Talbott JF, Lantos JE, Dillon WP. MR myelography for identification of spinal CSF leak in spontaneous intracranial hypotension. AJNR Am J Neuroradiol. 2014;35(10):2007–12.
60. Luetmer PH, Mokri B. Dynamic CT myelography: a technique for localizing high-flow spinal cerebrospinal fluid leaks. AJNR Am J Neuroradiol. 2003;24(8):1711–4.
61. Amrhein TJ, Gray L, Malinzak MD, Kranz PG. Respiratory phase affects the conspicuity of CSF-venous fistulas in spontaneous intracranial hypotension. AJNR Am J Neuroradiol. 2020;41(9):1754–6.
62. Kranz PG, Amrhein TJ, Gray L. CSF venous fistulas in spontaneous intracranial hypotension: imaging characteristics on dynamic and CT Myelography. AJR Am J Roentgenol. 2017;209(6):1360–6.
63. Hofstetter KR, Bjelland JC, Patton DD, Woolfenden JM, Henry RE. Detection of bronchopleural-subarachnoid fistula by radionuclide myelography: case report. J Nucl Med. 1977;18(10):981–3.
64. Deseyne S, Vanhouteghem K, Hallaert G, Delanghe J, Malfait T. Subarachnoidal-pleural fistula (SAPF) as an unusual cause of persistent pleural effusion. Beta-trace protein as a marker for SAPF. Case report and review of the literature. Acta Clin Belg. 2015;70(1):53–7.
65. Haft GF, Mendoza SA, Weinstein SL, Nyunoya T, Smoker W. Use of beta-2-transferrin to diagnose CSF leakage following spinal surgery: a case report. Iowa Orthop J. 2004;24:115–8.

66. Seehusen DA, Reeves MM, Fomin DA. Cerebrospinal fluid analysis. Am Fam Physician. 2003;68(6):1103–8.
67. Smith JC, Cohen E. Beta-2-transferrin to detect cerebrospinal fluid pleural effusion: a case report. J Med Case Rep. 2009;3:6495.
68. Mohan G, Bhide P, Agrawal A, Kaul V, Chaddha U. A practical approach to pseudoexudative pleural effusions. Respir Med. 2023;214:107279.
69. Bluestone CD. Implications of beta-2 transferrin assay as a marker for perilymphatic versus cerebrospinal fluid labyrinthine fistula. Am J Otol. 1999;20:701.
70. Rauch SD. Transferrin microheterogeneity in human perilymph. Laryngoscope. 2000;110(4):545–52.
71. Fransen P, Sindic CJ, Thauvoy C, Laterre C, Stroobandt G. Highly sensitive detection of beta-2 transferrin in rhinorrhea and otorrhea as a marker for cerebrospinal fluid (C.S.F.) leakage. Acta Neurochir. 1991;109(3–4):98–101.
72. Sloman AJ, Kelly RH. Transferrin allelic variants may cause false positives in the detection of cerebrospinal fluid fistulae. Clin Chem. 1993;39(7):1444–5.
73. Levenson MJ, Desloge RB, Parisier SC. Beta-2 transferrin: limitations of use as a clinical marker for perilymph. Laryngoscope. 1996;106(2 Pt 1):159–61.
74. Seltzer J, Babadjouni A, Wrobel BB, Zada G. Resolution of chronic aspiration pneumonitis following endoscopic Endonasal repair of spontaneous cerebrospinal fluid fistula of the Skull Base. J Neurol Surg Rep. 2016;77:e73–6.
75. Meco C, Oberascher G, Arrer E, Moser G, Albegger K. Beta-trace protein test: new guidelines for the reliable diagnosis of cerebrospinal fluid fistula. Otolaryngol Neck Surg. 2003;129(5):508–17.
76. Bachmann G, Achtelik R, Nekic M, Michel O. [Beta-trace protein in diagnosis of cerebrospinal fluid fistula]. HNO. 2000; 48(7):496–500.
77. Yoshor D, Gentry JB, LeMaire SA, Dickerson J, Saul J, Valadka AB, et al. Subarachnoid-pleural fistula treated with noninvasive positive-pressure ventilation. Case report. J Neurosurg. 2001;94(2 Suppl):319–22.
78. Schlag HR, Muquit S, Hristov TB, Morassi G, Boszczyk BM, Shafafy M. Subarachnoidal pleural fistula after resection of intradural thoracic disc herniation and multimodal treatment with noninvasive positive pressure ventilation (NPPV). Eur Spine J. 2016;25(1):155–9.
79. Brown WH, Stothert JCJ. Traumatic subarachnoid-pleural fistula. J Trauma. 1985;25(11):1105–7.
80. Raffa SJ, Benglis DM, Levi AD. Treatment of a persistent iatrogenic cerebrospinal fluid-pleural fistula with a cadaveric dural-pleural graft. Spine J. 2009;9(4):e25–9.
81. Sahota S, Nassr A, Khan MH, Marsh RW, Moran SL, Arnold PM, et al. Treatment of a thoracic dural-pleural fistula with a vascularized omental flap: a case report. Spine (Phila, Pa 1976). 2012;37(11):E683–5.
82. Madhavan AA, Cutsforth-Gregory JK, Oushy SH, Borg N, Brinjikji W. Combined CSF-venous fistula and middle meningeal artery embolization for treatment of spontaneous intracranial hypotension. Interv Neuroradiol. 2022;31:15910199221109044.
83. Rinaldo L, Lanzino G, Elder BD. Predictors of distal malfunction after ventriculoperitoneal shunting for idiopathic normal pressure hydrocephalus and the effect of general surgery involvement. Clin Neurol Neurosurg. 2018;174:75–9.
84. Willison CD, Kopitnik TA, Gustafson R, Kaufman HH. Ventriculopleural shunting is used as a temporary diversion. Acta Neurochir. 1992;115(1–2):67–8.
85. Kranz PG, Amrhein TJ, Gray L. Rebound intracranial hypertension: a complication of epidural blood patching for intracranial hypotension. AJNR Am J Neuroradiol. 2014;35(6):1237–40.
86. Mamlouk MD, Shen PY, Sedrak MF, Dillon WP. CT-guided fibrin glue occlusion of cerebrospinal fluid-venous fistulas. Radiology. 2021;299(2):409–18.
87. Yellin A, Findler G, Barzilay Z, Simansky DA, Lieberman Y. Fibrothorax associated with a ventriculopleural shunt in a hydrocephalic child. J Pediatr Surg. 1992;27(12):1525–6.
88. Khan TA, Khalil-Marzouk JF. Fibrothorax in adulthood caused by a cerebrospinal fluid shunt in the treatment of hydrocephalus. J Neurosurg. 2008;109(3):478–9.

9 Hemothorax

Joseph Evans and Dustin Manchester

Introduction

A hemothorax is defined as the accumulation of blood within the pleural space, typically characterized by a pleural fluid-to-blood hematocrit ratio greater than 50%. However, hemothoraces that persist for an extended period may become diluted, resulting in a reduction in the pleural fluid hematocrit to 25%–50% [1]. Among all etiologies, blunt and penetrating thoracic or abdominal trauma account for the majority of hemothorax cases [2, 3]. Thoracic injuries are observed in approximately 60% of all polytrauma patients [1, 3]. In the United States, an estimated 300,000 trauma-related hemothoraces occur annually, contributing to 16,000–30,000 fatalities each year [2, 4].

In cases of blunt chest trauma, rib fractures serve as a strong indicator of underlying hemothorax, with an incidence of 6.7% in patients without rib fractures compared to 81.4% in those with more than two rib fractures [5]. Less commonly, hemothoraces may result from iatrogenic or spontaneous causes. Iatrogenic hemothorax is a rare complication of invasive thoracic procedures, including chest tube placement (1–2%), thoracentesis (<0.5%), and central venous catheter insertion (0.4–1%) [6–9].

The most frequent cause of spontaneous hemothorax is pneumothorax. In such cases, shearing forces acting on the pleura and adjacent lung parenchyma may rupture blood vessels, resulting in hemothorax in approximately 5% of patients due to the absence of the tamponade effect [1]. Other spontaneous causes include coagulopathies (e.g., hemophilia and anticoagulant therapy), vascular anomalies (e.g., arteriovenous malformations [AVMs] and aneurysms), connective tissue disorders (e.g., neurofibromatosis type 1 [NF1] and Ehlers–Danlos syndrome [EDS]), pleural neoplasms, thoracic endometriosis, extracorporeal membrane oxygenation (ECMO), pulmonary sequestration, and pulmonary embolism (PE) [1, 10–12]. Hemothorax secondary to PE is exceedingly rare, occurring in less than 1% of cases [11].

The mechanisms underlying hemothorax formation vary depending on the etiology. Thymoma, a tumor arising from the thymic gland in the anterior mediastinum, can occasionally bleed spontaneously into the mediastinum or pleural space [1]. Aortic injury or rupture, particularly involving the descending thoracic aorta, may also result in hemothorax, most commonly on the left side. EDS is a rare connective tissue disorder with a prevalence of approximately 1 in 5000. The vascular subtype, which affects type IV collagen, predisposes patients to arterial rupture and pul-

J. Evans
Department of General Surgery, St. Luke's University Health Network, Bethlehem, PA, USA
e-mail: joseph.evans@sluhn.org

D. Manchester (✉)
Department of Thoracic Surgery, St. Luke's University Health Network, Bethlehem, PA, USA
e-mail: dustin.manchester@sluhn.org

F. Ido (ed.), *Rare Pleural Diseases*, https://doi.org/10.1007/978-3-032-14873-5_9

monary bleb formation, both of which can precipitate hemothorax [1]. Similarly, neurofibromatosis type 1 (NF-1), with a prevalence of 1 in 3000, can lead to spontaneous hemothorax through tumor invasion of vascular walls or hypertrophy and subsequent rupture of fragile vessels [1]. Hereditary hemorrhagic telangiectasia (HHT) is an autosomal dominant vascular disorder associated with arteriovenous malformations (AVMs). While recurrent epistaxis is the most common manifestation, pulmonary AVMs, particularly within the left lower lobe, may rupture at any age, leading to spontaneous hemothorax [1]. Additionally, primary and metastatic tumors, especially those involving the lung and pleura, can erode into adjacent vasculature, resulting in intrapleural bleeding [1]. In all such instances, involvement of large-caliber arteries may result in tension physiology and hemodynamic compromise, which can be fatal if untreated [12].

The overall mortality rate associated with hemothorax is approximately 9.4%, although this varies with clinical and injury-related factors. Adverse prognostic indicators include a low Glasgow Coma Scale (GCS) score on presentation, advanced age, penetrating chest trauma, long bone fractures, fractures involving more than five ribs, and concomitant hepatic or splenic injury [13].

Clinical Features

The clinical presentation of hemothorax depends on its underlying etiology, the rate of bleeding, and the total volume of blood accumulated within the pleural space. Common symptoms include dyspnea, tachypnea, pleuritic chest pain, and hemoptysis. As blood accumulates, compression atelectasis of the ipsilateral lung may occur, resulting in ventilation–perfusion (V/Q) mismatch and subsequent hypoxemia [12].

A massive hemothorax, defined as an intrapleural blood volume exceeding 1500 mL, can cause mediastinal shift toward the contralateral hemithorax [14]. This produces tension physiology, manifesting as severe respiratory distress, hemodynamic instability, use of accessory respiratory muscles, diminished or absent breath sounds, dullness to percussion, chest wall tenderness (in traumatic cases), and jugular venous distension [1, 4, 15].

Initially, intrapleural blood accumulation causes compressive atelectasis of the adjacent lung parenchyma. Over time, chronic hemothorax may lead to the development of a trapped lung, which fails to re-expand even after adequate drainage [2]. These mechanical and physiologic changes ultimately contribute to persistent V/Q mismatching and right-to-left physiologic shunting [16].

Diagnosis

The diagnosis of a hemothorax requires pleural fluid analysis demonstrating a pleural fluid-to-blood hematocrit ratio greater than 50% [1]. Chest radiography (CXR) remains one of the most commonly performed imaging modalities for patients presenting with trauma or respiratory distress. The sensitivity and specificity of CXR for detecting pleural effusion vary with fluid volume and patient positioning [3, 17].

Thoracic ultrasound provides a faster and more sensitive means of detecting pleural fluid than CXR, particularly in hemodynamically unstable patients. It demonstrates a sensitivity of 67% and specificity of 99% for identifying hemothorax [12]. In addition to rapid bedside availability, ultrasound is superior for detecting small effusion volumes and avoids ionizing radiation exposure [18]. However, diagnostic accuracy is operator-dependent [19], and image quality may be reduced in patients with large body habitus [20]. A significant advantage of ultrasound is its ability to simultaneously assess the abdomen and pelvis, providing valuable information about associated visceral injuries and intra-abdominal bleeding sources [20, 22, 23]. While ultrasound is a useful diagnostic tool, CXR provides complementary information, including identification of rib fractures, mediastinal widening or shift, pneumothorax, and evaluation of the entire hemithorax [21].

Several ultrasound signs can help differentiate a simple effusion from hemothorax. The thoracic spine sign, visualization of vertebral bodies above the diaphragm, is suggestive of pleural fluid, with a sensitivity of 74% and specificity of 93% [24]. The high-density sign also indicates pleural fluid and exhibits a sensitivity of 89% and a specificity approaching 100% [25]. The hematocrit sign, characterized by layering densities within the pleural fluid representing gravitational sedimentation of red blood cells, is highly suggestive of hemothorax (Fig. 9.1a) [26]. Another useful indicator, the swirl (or plankton) sign, refers to dynamic, echogenic swirling within the pleural space, indicating active bleeding [27].

Computed tomography (CT) plays a pivotal role in confirming and characterizing hemothorax. Compared to CXR and ultrasound, CT provides additional diagnostic information—including precise fluid density measurements (Hounsfield units), identification of septations, loculations, and associated parenchymal or osseous injury (Fig. 9.1b) [28]. Blood within the pleural cavity typically measures 35–70 HU, whereas simple serous fluid averages 0–20 HU [29]. Coagulated blood generally registers between 50 and 90 HU [30]. Contrast-enhanced CT may reveal active extravasation, while CT angiography can localize the source of bleeding, particularly in aortic or intercostal artery injuries [31].

In the acute setting, magnetic resonance imaging (MRI) has limited utility, particularly for trauma-related hemothorax. MRI is more valuable for characterizing mediastinal and pleural masses, such as mesothelioma, chondrosarcoma, or angiosarcoma, and other rare etiologies [32]. Magnetic resonance angiography (MRA) is rarely used but may serve as an alternative in patients with contrast allergies [33, 63].

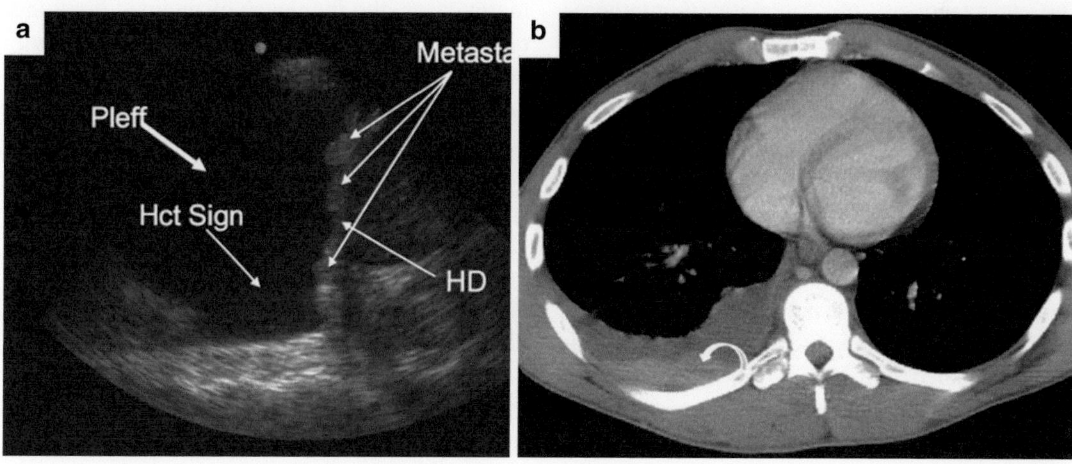

Fig. 9.1 Imaging features of the hematocrit sign. (**a**) Thoracic ultrasonography demonstrating a hypoechoic pleural effusion with a hyperechoic dependent layer, corresponding to sedimented cellular components. Multiple nodular pleural lesions are also visualized along the parietal pleura. *HD* = hemidiaphragm. (**b**) Computed tomography (CT) of the chest showing a right pleural effusion with a dependent layer of increased attenuation (white curved arrow), consistent with blood sedimentation within the effusion ("hematocrit sign")

Attribution: Panel A reprinted from Palas J., Matos A.P., Mascarenhas V., Herédia V., Ramalho M. *Multidetector Computer Tomography: Evaluation of Blunt Chest Trauma in Adults. Radiology Research and Practice.* 2014; Article ID 864369. https://doi.org/10.1155/2014/864369.
Panel B reprinted from *CHEST*, Vol 140(5), Koenig S.J., Narasimhan M., Mayo P.H., "Thoracic Ultrasonography for the Pulmonary Specialist," pp. 1332–1341,

Pleural fluid sampling remains essential for definitive diagnosis and can be obtained by thoracentesis or tube thoracostomy. Standard analysis includes lactate dehydrogenase (LDH), total protein, pH, and cell counts [34]. Virtually all hemothoraces meet Light's criteria for exudative pleural effusions. Measurement of the pleural fluid hematocrit is critical, as a pleural fluid-to-blood hematocrit ratio greater than 50% confirms the diagnosis [35]. The pleural fluid typically appears grossly bloody, with red blood cell counts exceeding 100,000 cells/μL and elevated LDH, though these findings are nonspecific. A low pH and glucose level may suggest a secondary infected hemothorax [17].

Treatment

Traumatic Hemothorax

The management of traumatic hemothorax depends primarily on the volume of pleural blood accumulation and the patient's hemodynamic status. Most cases are treated conservatively, focusing on observation and symptomatic management [36]. Approximately 18% of patients with chest trauma require tube thoracostomy, while only 2% necessitate surgical intervention [13, 37]. Small, unilateral hemothoraces measuring <300 mL in hemodynamically stable patients can be managed with observation alone [38]. This approach has been associated with lower tube thoracostomy rates, shorter hospital and ICU stays, and no increase in pulmonary complications, readmission, or 30-day mortality [38]. Conservative management involves clinical and radiographic monitoring for at least 6 hours, ensuring adequate pain control and repeat imaging to assess for interval progression. For larger hemothoraces, hemopneumothoraces, or those associated with respiratory distress or hemodynamic instability, tube thoracostomy, performed via open or percutaneous technique, is indicated [2, 3, 12, 39, 40]. Although uncommon, spontaneous hemothoraces are also generally managed with tube thoracostomy [1]. According to ATLS guidelines, surgical intervention is recommended when initial chest tube drainage exceeds 1500 mL of blood or when output exceeds 250 mL per hour for three consecutive hours [4]. Additional indications include clotted hemothorax, cardiac tamponade, significant vascular or chest wall injury, diaphragmatic or esophageal disruption, and cardiac trauma [4, 36, 50]. Chest tube size may vary, but 28-Fr tubes have been shown to be as effective as larger 36- to 40-Fr tubes, with comparable rates of pneumonia, empyema, and retained hemothorax (RH). In hemodynamically stable patients, small-bore (14-Fr) percutaneous tubes yield outcomes similar to larger tubes, with equivalent duration, complication, and failure rates [43]. Likewise, no significant differences have been reported in reinsertion rates, image-guided drainage, VATS, or thoracotomy requirements between different tube sizes [41–44].

A retained hemothorax, defined as residual pleural blood following drainage, can lead to pneumonia, fibrothorax, or trapped lung. In traumatic cases, the incidence of retained hemothorax is approximately 29%, often correlated with larger initial pleural volumes [64]. Intrapleural lavage via the existing chest tube is an effective adjunct treatment. Using a three-way stopcock, warm saline can be instilled into the pleural space and then evacuated with suction. Both open and percutaneous tubes can be used for lavage, with studies showing that 14-Fr percutaneous tubes achieve drainage volumes comparable to those of 28-Fr chest tubes [45]. Lavage has been associated with reduced retained hemothorax rates to as low as 5%, shorter tube duration, reduced need for VATS, and decreased hospital length of stay [45, 46]. Early intervention is key—when chest tubes are placed within 24 hours of trauma, lavage reduces retained hemothorax rates from 21% to 10% and lowers the need for secondary procedures (e.g., repeat tube insertion, VATS, thrombolysis, or thoracotomy) by 44% [47]. Once chest tubes are in place, frequent monitoring of drainage volume and character is essential. Traditionally, tubes were removed when drainage decreased below 100–150 mL per day, though recent studies suggest that removal is safe with outputs up to 200 mL per day [48, 49].

Video-assisted thoracoscopic surgery (VATS) provides several advantages over open thoracotomy, including enhanced visualization, less postoperative pain, and lower overall morbidity [51]. VATS is indicated for retained hemothoraces in hemodynamically stable patients capable of single-lung ventilation. Optimal timing is within 48–72 hours post-trauma, which is associated with lower morbidity, reduced mortality, and fewer conversions to thoracotomy [52, 53]. Delayed intervention increases the risk of pleural adhesions and fibrothorax; for example, when VATS is postponed until day 6, the conversion rate to open thoracotomy rises to 15.8% [12]. Despite appropriate intervention, up to 25% of patients require a second operation, and 5% may need a third, with bleeding-related complications occurring in 7% [54].

Intrapleural fibrinolytic therapy has demonstrated promise in reducing the need for surgery. A review of published data revealed that fibrinolytic therapy prevented surgical intervention in over 80% of retained hemothorax cases [55]. However, there are no formal guidelines for its use, and randomized trials are still needed to define its role and standardize protocols [55].

Transcatheter arterial embolization (TAE), though infrequently performed, is a valuable option in traumatic hemothorax secondary to vascular injury, particularly from rib fracture-related intercostal artery damage [56, 57]. Contrast-enhanced CT may reveal active extravasation, guiding embolization. Persistent chest tube output or delayed hemothorax should raise suspicion for intercostal artery injury [58].

Prognosis

The majority of hemothoraces resolve following initial management with either observation or tube thoracostomy. Small hemothoraces can often be treated conservatively, as the intrapleural blood is gradually reabsorbed over several weeks. However, 5–30% of patients may develop a retained hemothorax requiring additional intervention [12, 16]. RH is associated with significant morbidity and mortality, including increased risks of pneumonia, fibrothorax, and trapped lung [12, 54].

Mortality rates vary depending on etiology and severity. Iatrogenic hemothoraces, such as those resulting from malpositioned chest tubes or central line placements, carry a mortality rate of 3–7%. In contrast, traumatic hemothoraces have reported mortality rates ranging from 10–18%, with rates rising to 20–25% in patients presenting with massive hemothorax (>1500 mL) accompanied by hemodynamic instability [59].

Other reported complications associated with hemothorax include infection or empyema (4–25%), fibrothorax (1–5%), recurrent bleeding (<5%), loculated pleural effusion (10–20%), and trapped lung (<5%) [17, 20, 60].

Furthermore, initial management of a hemothorax with tube thoracostomy is not without risk. The overall complication rate associated with this procedure has been reported to be as high as 30% [61]. The most common complication is malposition of the chest tube, which may result in intraparenchymal, intrafissural, extrapleural, or obstructed placement [62].

Following complete drainage of the hemothorax and removal of the chest tube, patients typically undergo follow-up within 1–2 weeks under the supervision of thoracic surgery [49]. Repeat imaging, most commonly chest radiography or, occasionally, computed tomography, is recommended to confirm resolution of the hemothorax. The timing and modality of follow-up imaging may vary based on institutional protocols and surgeon preference [49].

References

1. Patrini D, Panagiotopoulos N, Pararajasingham J, Gvinianidze L, Iqbal Y, Lawrence DR. Etiology and management of spontaneous haemothorax. J Thorac Dis. 2015;7(3):520–6.
2. Boersma WG, Stigt JA, Smit HJ. Treatment of haemothorax. Respir Med. 2010;104(11):1583–7. https://doi.org/10.1016/j.rmed.2010.08.006.
3. Broderick SR. Hemothorax: etiology, diagnosis, and management. Thorac Surg Clin. 2013;23(1):89–96. vi-vii.

4. Mahoozi HR, Volmerig J, Hecker E. Modern management of traumatic hemothorax. J Trauma Treat. 2016;5(3):1000326.
5. Liman ST, Kuzucu A, Tastepe AI, Ulasan GN, Topcu S. Chest injury due to blunt trauma. Eur J Cardiothorac Surg. 2003;23(3):374–8. https://doi.org/10.1016/s1010-7940(02)00813-8.
6. Hernandez MC, El Khatib M, Prokop L, Zielinski MD, Aho JM. Complications in tube thoracostomy: systematic review and meta-analysis. J Trauma Acute Care Surg. 2018;85(2):410–6. https://doi.org/10.1097/TA.0000000000001840. PMID: 29443856; PMCID: PMC6081248.
7. Havelock T, Teoh R, Laws D, Gleeson F, BTS Pleural Disease Guideline Group. Pleural procedures and thoracic ultrasound: British Thoracic Society pleural disease guideline 2010. Thorax. 2010;65(Suppl 2):ii61–76. https://doi.org/10.1136/thx.2010.137026.
8. Sagar AE, Ost DE. The future of interventional pulmonology. Flexible Bronchoscopy. 2020;8:263–70.
9. McGee DC, Gould MK. Preventing complications of central venous catheterization. N Engl J Med. 2003;348(12):1123–33. https://doi.org/10.1056/NEJMra011883.
10. Lee EY, Boiselle PM, Cleveland RH. Multidetector CT evaluation of congenital lung abnormalities. Radiol Clin North Am. 2011;49(1):137–60.
11. Lee DZ, Whittaker M, Al-Mohammad A. An unusual presentation of pulmonary embolism. BMJ Case Rep. 2012;2012:bcr2012006210. https://doi.org/10.1136/bcr-2012-006210. PMID: 22878987; PMCID: PMC4542928.
12. Zeiler J, Idell S, Norwood S, Cook A. Hemothorax: a review of the literature. Clin Pulm Med. 2020;27(1):1–12. https://doi.org/10.1097/CPM.0000000000000343.
13. Kulshrestha P, Munshi I, Wait R. Profile of chest trauma in a level I trauma center. J Trauma. 2004;57(3):576–81.
14. American College of Surgeons. Advanced trauma life support (ATLS) student course manual. 10th ed. Chicago: American College of Surgeons; 2018.
15. Gutierrez G, Reines HD, Wulf-Gutierrez ME. Clinical review: hemorrhagic shock. Crit Care. 2004;8(5):373–81. https://doi.org/10.1186/cc2851. Epub 2004 Apr 2. PMID: 15469601; PMCID: PMC1065003.
16. Scott MF, Khodaverdian RA, Shaheen JL, Ney AL, Nygaard RM. Predictors of retained hemothorax after trauma and impact on patient outcomes. Eur J Trauma Emerg Surg. 2017;43(2):179–84. https://doi.org/10.1007/s00068-015-0604-y. Epub 2015 Nov 30.
17. Light RW. Pleural disease. 6th ed. Philadelphia: Lippincott Williams & Wilkins; 2013.
18. Sisley AC, Rozycki GS, Ballard RB, Namias N, Salomone JP, Feliciano DV. Rapid detection of traumatic effusion using surgeon-performed ultrasonography. J Trauma. 1998;44(2):291–6.; discussion 296–7. https://doi.org/10.1097/00005373-199802000-00009.
19. Staub LJ, Biscaro RRM, Kaszubowski E, Maurici R. Chest ultrasonography for the emergency diagnosis of traumatic pneumothorax and haemothorax: a systematic review and meta-analysis. Injury. 2018;49(3):457–66. https://doi.org/10.1016/j.injury.2018.01.033. Epub 2018 Feb 8.
20. Brooks A, Davies B, Smethhurst M, Connolly J. Emergency ultrasound in the acute assessment of haemothorax. Emerg Med J. 2004;21(1):44–6. https://doi.org/10.1136/emj.2003.005438. PMID: 14734374; PMCID: PMC1756377.
21. McEwan K, Thompson P. Ultrasound to detect haemothorax after chest injury. Emerg Med J. 2007;24(8):581–2. https://doi.org/10.1136/emj.2007.051334. Erratum in: Emerg Med J 2007; 24(12):867. PMID: 17652688; PMCID: PMC2660093.
22. Rozycki GS, Feliciano DV, Schmidt JA, Cushman JG, Sisley AC, Ingram W, Ansley JD. The role of surgeon-performed ultrasound in patients with possible cardiac wounds. Ann Surg. 1996;223(6):737–44; discussion 744–6. https://doi.org/10.1097/00000658-199606000-00012. PMID: 8645047; PMCID: PMC1235223.
23. Kithinji SM, Lule H, Acan M, Kyomukama L, Muhumuza J, Kyamanywa P. Efficacy of extended focused assessment with sonography for trauma using a portable handheld device for detecting hemothorax in a low resource setting; a multicenter longitudinal study. BMC Med Imaging. 2022;22(1):211. https://doi.org/10.1186/s12880-022-00942-y. PMID: 36456990; PMCID: PMC9716853.
24. Dickman E, Terentiev V, Likourezos A, Derman A, Haines L. Extension of the thoracic spine sign: a new sonographic marker of pleural effusion. J Ultrasound Med. 2015;34(9):1555–61. https://doi.org/10.7863/ultra.15.14.06013. Epub 2015 Aug 12.
25. Dietrich CF, Mathis G, Cui XW, Ignee A, Hocke M, Hirche TO. Ultrasound of the pleurae and lungs. Ultrasound Med Biol. 2015;41(2):351–65. https://doi.org/10.1016/j.ultrasmedbio.2014.10.002.
26. Lam J, Montague S. Hematocrit sign elucidates cause of abdominal pain. Pocus J. 2021;6(1):8–9. https://doi.org/10.24908/pocus.v6i1.14751. PMID: 36895502; PMCID: PMC9979907.
27. Impellizzeri P, Levi G, Piamonti D, Locorotondo C, Marchetti GP. The smoke swirl. Chest. 2024;166(2):e47–9. https://doi.org/10.1016/j.chest.2024.02.041.
28. Kaewlai R, Avery LL, Asrani AV, Novelline RA. Multidetector CT of blunt thoracic trauma. Radiographics. 2008;28(6):1555–70. https://doi.org/10.1148/rg.286085510.
29. Del Marmol O, Coulier B. "black" and "white" blood on unenhanced CT. J Belg Soc Radiol. 2019;103(1):16. https://doi.org/10.5334/jbsr.1733. PMID: 30828698; PMCID: PMC6396038.
30. Sangster GP, González-Beicos A, Carbo AI, Heldmann MG, Ibrahim H, Carrascosa P, Nazar M, D'Agostino HB. Blunt traumatic injuries of the lung parenchyma, pleura, thoracic wall, and intrathoracic

airways: multidetector computer tomography imaging findings. Emerg Radiol. 2007;14(5):297–310. https://doi.org/10.1007/s10140-007-0651-8. Epub 2007 Jul 11.
31. Dewhurst C, 'O'Neill S, O'Regan K, Maher M. Demonstration of the course of the posterior intercostal artery on CT angiography: relevance to interventional radiology procedures in the chest. Diagn Interv Radiol. 2012;18(2):221–4. https://doi.org/10.4261/1305-3825.DIR.4366-11.1. Epub 2011 Nov 28.
32. Carter BW, Benveniste MF, Madan R, Godoy MC, Groot PM, Truong MT, Rosado-de-Christenson ML, Marom EM. IASLC/ITMIG staging system and lymph node map for Thymic epithelial neoplasms. Radiographics. 2017;37(3):758–76. https://doi.org/10.1148/rg.2017160096.
33. Ludwig DR, Shetty AS, Broncano J, Bhalla S, Raptis CA. Magnetic resonance angiography of the thoracic vasculature: technique and applications. J Magn Reson Imaging. 2020;52(2):325–47. https://doi.org/10.1002/jmri.27067. Epub 2020 Feb 14.
34. Beaudoin S, Gonzalez AV. Evaluation of the patient with pleural effusion. CMAJ. 2018;190(10):E291–5. https://doi.org/10.1503/cmaj.170420. PMID: 29530870; PMCID: PMC5849448.
35. Azfar Ali H, Lippmann M, Mundathaje U, Khaleeq G. Spontaneous hemothorax: a comprehensive review. Chest. 2008;134(5):1056–65. https://doi.org/10.1378/chest.08-0725.
36. Meyer DM. Hemothorax related to trauma. Thorac Surg Clin. 2007;17(1):47–55. https://doi.org/10.1016/j.thorsurg.2007.02.006.
37. Wells BJ, Roberts DJ, Grondin S, Navsaria PH, Kirkpatrick AW, Dunham MB, Ball CG. To drain or not to drain? Predictors of tube thoracostomy insertion and outcomes associated with drainage of traumatic hemothoraces. Injury. 2015;46(9):1743–8. https://doi.org/10.1016/j.injury.2015.04.032. Epub 2015 May 7.
38. Al Tannir AH, Biesboer EA, Tentis M, Seadler M, Patin BB, Golestani S, et al. Implementation of 300-mL Rule for Management of Traumatic Hemothorax. J Am Coll Surg. 2024 Oct 16;239(5):422–9.
39. Molnar TF. Thoracic trauma: which chest tube when and where? Thorac Surg Clin. 2017;27(1):13–23. https://doi.org/10.1016/j.thorsurg.2016.08.003.
40. Mowery NT, Gunter OL, Collier BR, Diaz JJ, Haut E, Hildreth A, et al. Practice management guidelines for management of hemothorax and occult pneumothorax. J Trauma. 2011;70(2):510–8.
41. Inaba K, Lustenberger T, Recinos G, Georgiou C, Velmahos GC, Brown C, et al. Does size matter? A prospective analysis of 28-32 versus 36-40 French chest tube size in trauma. J Trauma Acute Care Surg. 2012;72(2):422–7.
42. Maezawa T, Yanai M, Huh JY, Ariyoshi K. Effectiveness and safety of small-bore tube thoracostomy (≤20 Fr) for chest trauma patients: A retrospective observational study. Am J Emerg Med. 2020;38(12):2658–60. https://doi.org/10.1016/j.ajem.2020.09.028. Epub 2020 Sep 16. PMID: 33039219.
43. Kulvatunyou N, Joseph B, Friese RS, Green D, Gries L, O'Keeffe T, Tang AL, Wynne JL, Rhee P. 14 French pigtail catheters placed by surgeons to drain blood on trauma patients: is 14-Fr too small? J Trauma Acute Care Surg. 2012;73(6):1423–7. https://doi.org/10.1097/TA.0b013e318271c1c7.
44. Patel NJ, Dultz L, Ladhani HA, Cullinane DC, Klein E, McNickle AG, Bugaev N, Fraser DR, Kartiko S, Dodgion C, Pappas PA, Kim D, Cantrell S, Como JJ, Kasotakis G. Management of simple and retained hemothorax: A practice management guideline from the eastern Association for the Surgery of trauma. Am J Surg. 2021;221(5):873–84. https://doi.org/10.1016/j.amjsurg.2020.11.032. Epub 2020 Nov 17.
45. McLauchlan NR, Igra NM, Fisher LT, Byrne JP, Beyer CA, Geng Z, Schmulevich D, Brinson MM, Dumas RP, Holena DN, Hynes AM, Rosen CB, Shah AN, Vella MA, Cannon JW. Open versus percutaneous tube thoracostomy with and without thoracic lavage for traumatic hemothorax: a novel randomized controlled simulation trial. Trauma Surg Acute Care Open. 2023;8(1):e001050. https://doi.org/10.1136/tsaco-2022-001050. PMID: 36967862; PMCID: PMC10030794.
46. Al Tannir AH, Biesboer EA, Golestani S, Tentis M, Maring M, Gellings J, Peschman JR, Murphy PB, Morris RS, Elegbede A, de Moya MA, Carver TW. Thoracic cavity irrigation prevents retained hemothorax and decreases surgical intervention in trauma patients. J Trauma Acute Care Surg. 2024;97(1):90–5. https://doi.org/10.1097/TA.0000000000004324. Epub 2024 Mar 25.
47. Carver TW, Berndtson AE, McNickle AG, Boyle KA, Haan JM, Campion EM, Biffl WL, Carroll AN, Sise MJ, Berndt KS, Burris JM, Kopelman TR, Blank JJ, Seamon MJ, Peschman JR, Morris RS, Kugler NW, Conrardy RD, Szabo A, de Moya MA. Thoracic irrigation for prevention of secondary intervention after thoracostomy tube drainage for hemothorax: a Western trauma association multicenter study. J Trauma Acute Care Surg. 2024;97(5):724–30. https://doi.org/10.1097/TA.0000000000004364. Epub 2024 May 20.
48. Younes RN, Gross JL, Aguiar S, Haddad FJ, Deheinzelin D. When to remove a chest tube? A randomized study with subsequent prospective consecutive validation. J Am Coll Surg. 2002;195:658–62.
49. Golden P. Follow-up chest radiographs after traumatic pneumothorax or hemothorax in the outpatient setting: a retrospective review. Int J Trauma Nurs. 1999;5:88–94.
50. Cakmak M, Yuksel M, Kandemir MN. Characteristics of the patients undergoing surgical treatment for pneumothorax: a descriptive study. J Pak Med Assoc. 2016;66(5):554–8.

51. Ahmad T, Ahmed S, Hussain N, Sheikh K. Thoracoscopic evacuation of retained post-traumatic hemothorax. J Col Phys Surg Pak. 2013;23:234–6. (Ludwig C, Koryllos A. Management of chest trauma. J Thorac Dis 2017;9:S172–S7)
52. Carrillo EH, Richardson JD. Thoracoscopy in the management of hemothorax and retained blood after trauma. Curr Opin Pulm Med. 1998;4:243–6.
53. Lin HL, Huang WY, Yang C, et al. How early should VATS be performed for retained haemothorax in blunt chest trauma? Injury. 2014;45:1359–64.
54. DuBose J, Inaba K, Demetriades D, Scalea TM, O'Connor J, Menaker J, Morales C, Konstantinidis A, Shiflett A, Copwood B, AAST Retained Hemothorax Study Group. Management of post-traumatic retained hemothorax: a prospective, observational, multi-center AAST study. J Trauma Acute Care Surg. 2012;72(1):11–22.; discussion 22–4; quiz 316. https://doi.org/10.1097/TA.0b013e318242e368.
55. Holsen MR, Tameron AM, Evans DC, Thompson M. Intrapleural tissue plasminogen activator for traumatic retained Hemothorax. Ann Pharmacother. 2019;53(10):1060–6.
56. Hagiwara A, Yanagawa Y, Kaneko N, Takasu A, Hatanaka K, Sakamoto T, Okada Y. Indications for transcatheter arterial embolization in persistent hemothorax caused by blunt trauma. J Trauma. 2008;65(3):589–94. https://doi.org/10.1097/TA.0b013e318181d56a.
57. Lohan R, Leow KS, Ong MW, Goo TT, Punamiya S. Role of intercostal artery embolization in management of traumatic hemothorax. J Emerg Trauma Shock. 2021;14(2):111–6. https://doi.org/10.4103/JETS.JETS_157_20. Epub 2021 Apr 27. PMID: 34321811; PMCID: PMC8312918.
58. Carrillo EH, Heniford BT, Senler SO, Dykes JR, Maniscalco SP, Richardson JD. Embolization therapy as an alternative to thoracotomy in vascular injuries of the chest wall. Am Surg. 1998;64(12):1142–8. PMID: 9843332.
59. Velmahos GC, et al. Srch Surg. 1999;134(5):506–11. (American college of surgeons Trauma committee—ATLS 10th ed. (2018))
60. Navsaria PH, De Bruyn P, Nicol AJ. Penetrating abdominal vena cava injuries. Eur J Vasc Endovasc Surg. 2005;30(5):499–503.
61. Miller KS, Sahn SA. Chest tubes. Indications, technique, management and complications. Chest. 1987;91(2):258–64. https://doi.org/10.1378/chest.91.2.258.
62. Jones CW, Rodriguez RD, Griffin RL, McGwin G, Jansen JO, Kerby JD, Bosarge PL. Complications associated with placement of chest tubes: A trauma system perspective. J Surg Res. 2019;239:98–102. https://doi.org/10.1016/j.jss.2019.01.012. Epub 2019 Feb 27.
63. Dobrilovic N, Sadiq I, Vognar LA, Fingleton JG. Magnetic resonance angiography demonstrating active spontaneous intercostal bleeding. J Emerg Med. 2013;44(1):171–2.
64. Prakash PS, Moore SA, Rezende-Neto JB, Trpcic S, Dunn JA, Smoot B, et al. Predictors of retained hemothorax in trauma: results of an Eastern Association for the Surgery of Trauma multi-institutional trial. J Trauma Acute Care Surg. 2020;89(4):679–85.

Meigs Syndrome

10

Firas Ido

History of the Eponym

Meigs syndrome refers to the triad of a benign solid ovarian tumor, pleural effusion, and ascites, which resolve following resection of the tumor [1]. Prior to the twentieth century, the presence of ascites in conjunction with an intraperitoneal mass was nearly always presumed malignant. Scarce case reports emerged of repeated paracentesis in patients with untreated pelvic tumors monitored for several years, strongly hinting at the benign nature of the tumor, although unconfirmed by pathology [2, 3]. In 1866, Otto Von Spielberg, a professor of obstetrics in Breslau, Poland, described the first case of hydrothorax, ascites, and a roughly 60-lb ovarian fibroma, which was confirmed with histology during autopsy. Since the diagnosis occurred postmortem, documentation regarding the resolution of the pleural effusion and ascites following resection was not possible [4, 5]. In 1887, Albert Demons of Bordeaux, France, described nine cases of permanent resolution of pleural effusions after complete resection of ovarian lesions, which in his cases were cystic [6]. Nearly 15 years later, in 1902, at a Surgical conference in Paris, France, Demons elaborated on the interrelatedness of ascites and pleural effusions in association with fibromas of the ovaries and the broad ligament. Recognizing the rapid resolution of the pleural effusion following resection of the ovarian tumor, Demons stressed the importance of focusing on resecting the tumor rather than performing therapeutic drainage of the pleural effusion unless clinically necessary [7, 8]. Medical reports of the syndrome nearly disappeared for 30 years until Joe Vincent Meigs, a professor of Gynecology at Harvard Medical School, revived awareness of these findings following his description of three cases of the syndrome involving ovarian fibromas in a book titled "Tumors of the Female Pelvic Organs" in 1934 [9, 10]. Additionally, he presented and eventually published several cases at the American Association of Obstetricians, Gynecologists, and Abdominal Surgeons conference in 1936 [11]. The following year, in 1937, Jonathan E. Rhoads and A.W. Terrell at the University of Pennsylvania published a case of this triad, attributing and coining the name Meigs syndrome for the first time [12]. In 1948, in recognition of the contributions of Albert Demons, having presented the first case that included all essential components of the syndrome, Dr. Funck-Brentano advocated adding Demons' name as part of the eponym assigned to the syndrome [13]. Joe Meigs welcomed this idea; however, the eponym "Demons–Meigs" has been inconsistently used to describe both the classic triad, which limits the tumor to a benign ovarian fibroma, and a pseudo-syndrome, which includes all benign tumors of the ovaries,

F. Ido (✉)
Department of Pulmonary and Critical Care Medicine, St. Luke's University Health Network, Bethlehem, PA, USA
e-mail: firas.ido@sluhn.org

F. Ido (ed.), *Rare Pleural Diseases*, https://doi.org/10.1007/978-3-032-14873-5_10

fallopian tubes, and broad ligament [14–16]. By 1954, Meigs had published a review of all reported cases and firmly established the first formal diagnostic criteria, which entailed the presence of a benign ovarian fibroma, ascites, pleural effusion (unilateral or bilateral), and documented resolution of the ascites and pleural effusion after tumor removal [17]. His review of all associated histopathologic descriptions associated with the triad led to an arbitrary expansion of the included tumor types based on the frequency of occurrence. This included fibroma of the ovary, granulosa cell tumors, thecomas, and Brenner tumors. He excluded all other kinds of tumors due to the rarity with which pleural effusions occurred [18]. Since then, several eponym variants have emerged. The term atypical or incomplete Meigs is reserved for pelvic tumors with only a pleural effusion present [19]. Pseudo-Meigs syndrome is further categorized into benign and malignant subtypes, both of which are associated with pleural effusion and ascites. The benign form includes all other benign abdominal or pelvic tumors external to the ovaries, fallopian tubes, and broad ligament. The malignant type refers to malignant ovarian tumors, both primary and metastatic, without evidence of intraperitoneal/intrapleural spread based on negative peritoneal and pleural fluid cytology [20, 21]. Finally, pseudo-pseudo-Meigs (also known as Tjalma syndrome) involves a combination of ascites and pleural effusion associated with systemic lupus erythematosus and elevated cancer antigen-125 (CA-125) in the absence of an ovarian tumor [22, 23]. This chapter reviews the pathophysiology, clinical presentation, diagnosis, and treatment of the classic Meigs syndrome, which is limited to ovarian fibroma and fibroma-like tumors of the ovaries.

Epidemiology

Meigs syndrome is a rare condition, and global epidemiologic data regarding its incidence and prevalence are scarce. Benign ovarian fibromas and fibroma-like tumors account for up to 5% of ovarian tumors [24]. Historically, the reported occurrence of Meigs syndrome was estimated to be only 1% of benign ovarian tumors; however, this may underrepresent the true incidence, as awareness and recognition have increased during the past few decades [25]. A study evaluating a local population noted that Meigs syndrome occurred in 3% of patients with benign ovarian neoplasms [26]. The presence of ascites without a pleural effusion is more common, with an incidence of 10–15% [27]. The lack of Meigs syndrome developing with all benign ovarian tumors highlights the vital role of additional factors influencing the accumulation of fluid within the serous membrane compartments. Tumor size greater than 10 cm and the presence of a myxoid component within the tumor were determined to be potentially necessary components for the formation of peritoneal fluid (Fig. 10.1c) [28].

Meigs syndrome occurs most commonly postmenopause during the fifth and sixth decades, which coincides with the peak age at which the development of benign ovarian fibromas typically occurs. Meigs syndrome prior to the third decade is rare, occurring in approximately 5–6% of all cases [29, 30]. Several documented cases have been encountered during pregnancy [31–33]. Cases involving children and adolescents have also been reported but are rare [34, 35].

Of the different types of benign tumors that define the classic Meigs syndrome, fibromas and fibrothecomas were found to be the cause in 91.4% of cases, benign granulosa cell tumors in about 4.7%, and Brenner tumors in 1.6% of cases [36]. The pleural effusion typically occurs in 70% of cases on the right, 20% bilaterally, and 10% on the left and does not coincide with the location of the tumor [37].

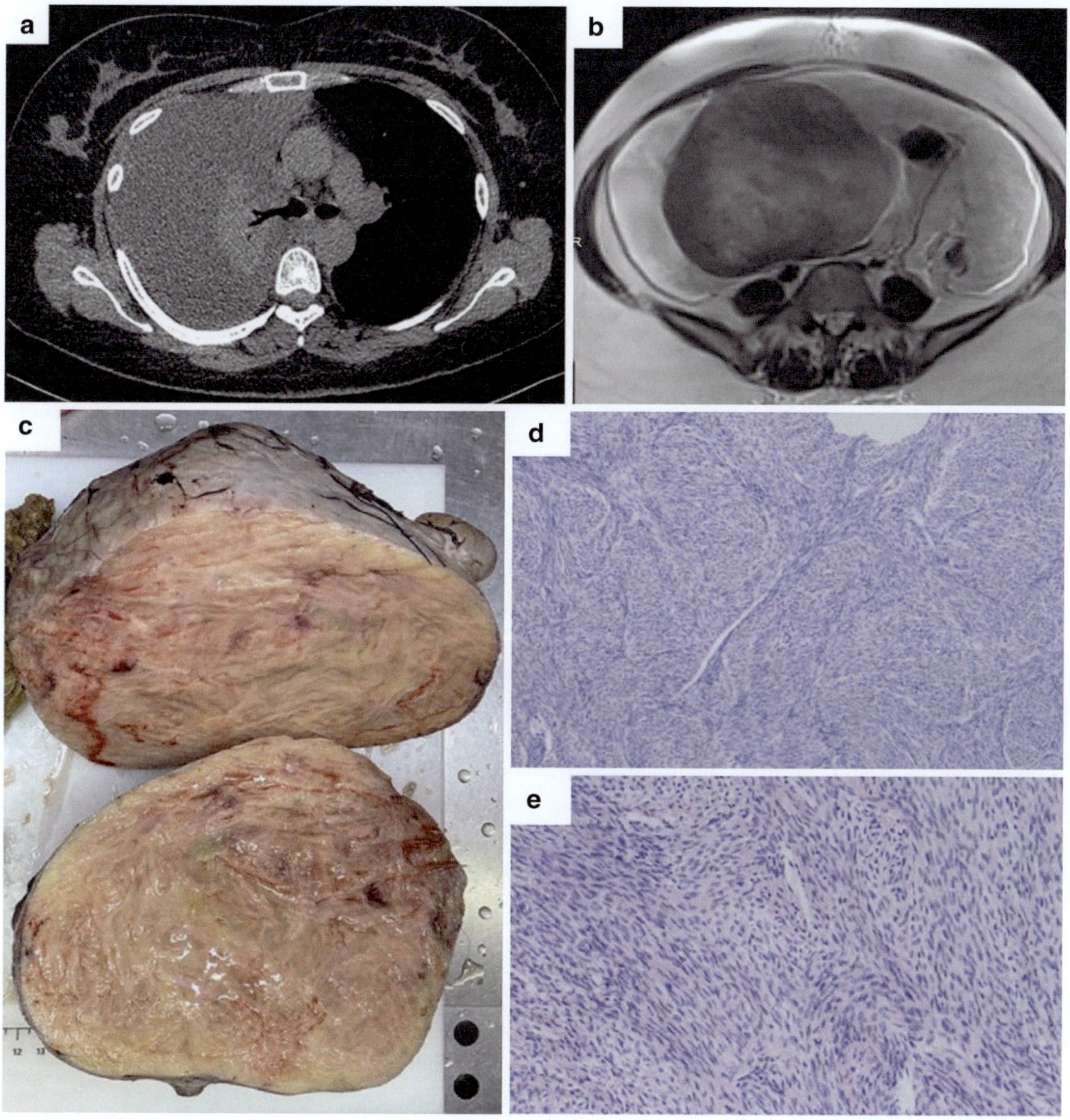

Fig. 10.1 Radiologic and histopathologic features of Meigs syndrome secondary to a right ovarian fibroma
(**a**) Computed tomography (CT) of the thorax demonstrating a large right pleural effusion causing complete collapse of the right lung
(**b**) Magnetic resonance imaging (MRI) of the pelvis showing a large solid ovarian mass measuring 14.5 × 15.5 × 14.3 cm with associated ascites
(**c**) Postoperative cross-section of the resected tumor revealing a solid, densely cellular, firm, yellow-tan mass
(**d**) Hematoxylin and eosin (H&E)–stained histologic section at ×20 magnification showing densely packed spindle cells within a collagenous stroma; (**e**) higher magnification (×40) highlighting uniform spindle cell morphology and stromal composition

Attribution: Reprinted from Seong J., Ravshan A., Narkhodzha S., Saida K., Jamshid A., Bahriddin B., Biloliddin S. *Meigs' syndrome with elevated CA-125 and HE-4: a case report and literature review. Frontiers in Medicine.* 2025; 12:1533388. https://doi.org/10.3389/fmed.2025.1533388. © 2025 Seong et al. This is an open-access article distributed under the terms of the Creative Commons Attribution License (CC BY), which permits use, distribution, and reproduction in any medium, provided the original authors and the publisher are credited and the original publication is cited in accordance with academic standards

Pathophysiology

The mechanism underlying the formation of excess peritoneal and pleural fluid remains poorly understood, with several theories proposed. One hypothesis suggests that edematous tumors actively secrete fluid, which then extravasates through the thin epithelial lining of the lesion into the surrounding cavity. Indeed, resected fibromas placed in dry containers have been observed to produce measurable fluid within hours, further supporting this theory [38]. An alternative theory attributes fluid accumulation to mechanical factors, specifically torsion of the tumor pedicle, which may impair venous and lymphatic drainage, leading to secondary fluid exudation. However, this explanation is considered less robust, as both freely mobile tumors and those firmly adherent to adjacent structures have been shown to develop ascites (18). Recently, elevated levels of vascular endothelial growth factor (VEGF), fibroblast growth factor (FGF), and interleukin-6 (IL-6) were noted in ascitic, pleural fluid, as well as serum. All three declined significantly, weeks following complete resection of the tumor. The presence of these cytokines suggests a potential role in inflammation, resulting in increased peritoneal permeability [39, 40]. Leptin, an adipocyte protein hormone involved in body weight regulation, has been shown to be low in ascites, pleural fluid, and serum in patients with Meigs syndrome. Levels increased significantly following resection, indicating a potential role in the pathophysiology; however, this inverse relationship remains unclear [41].

The accumulation of pleural fluid secondary to ascites is postulated to occur through several potential mechanisms. One theory proposes that ascitic fluid migrates from the peritoneal cavity into the pleural space via the subdiaphragmatic lymphatic channels. This was supported by the fact that India ink, when instilled into the peritoneal cavity, was subsequently detected within the pleural space. The biochemical characteristics of the pleural and peritoneal fluids were found to be remarkably similar [42]. Additionally, Lemons and Higgins, using canines, conducted several experiments that demonstrated the appearance of peritoneal fluid within the dorsal diaphragmatic lymphatics within several minutes. Interestingly, there was a significant delay in observing the peritoneal fluid if the diaphragm was paralyzed. They also postulated that the preference for fluid accumulation within the right pleural space was due to the more pronounced lymphatic plexus on the right side. The flow of peritoneal fluid into the pleural space was considered unidirectional, as injection into the chest cavity did not demonstrate flow in the opposite direction [43]. In contrast, Hodari and Hodgkinson performed a lymphangiogram in a case of Meigs syndrome, which demonstrated the accumulation of the tracer within the right pleural space and without detection within the peritoneal fluid, suggesting an alternative pathway via the pulmonary lymphatics [44]. Peritoneal fluid may also migrate into the chest cavity through small apertures surrounding the diaphragm. The negative intrathoracic pressure during inhalation is thought to potentially play a role in facilitating the movement of peritoneal fluid, resulting from a higher pressure difference [18].

Clinical Features

The signs and symptoms of Meigs syndrome include both pulmonary and abdominal symptoms, reflecting the sites of fluid accumulation. Abdominal distention and dyspnea are the two most commonly reported symptoms, occurring nearly in equal frequency. Shortness of breath, which is essentially always present, can be accompanied by a nonproductive cough or chest pain. Abdominal pain was very infrequently reported and typically occurs in the lower abdomen. Additional signs or symptoms include leg edema, anorexia, and urinary abnormalities such as increased urinary frequency or difficulty voiding. Menorrhagia and metrorrhagia have also been reported, particularly in hormone-secreting ovarian tumors [17, 45, 46].

Diagnosis

The diagnosis of Meigs syndrome requires fulfillment of all criteria, which include the presence of ascites, pleural effusion, and histopathologic confirmation of a benign ovarian tumor, as established by Meigs (fibroma, thecoma, granulosa cell tumor, and Brenner tumor) (Fig. 10.1d–e). Furthermore, diagnostic confirmation necessitates evidence of the resolution of both ascites and pleural effusion following the complete resection of the ovarian tumor [47]. The incidence of pericardial effusion has been infrequently documented; nevertheless, it is not included within the diagnostic criteria and, consequently, is not required [48–51]. Although transvaginal ultrasound offers high-quality imaging than transabdominal ultrasound and is the preferred initial modality for isolated adnexal masses, the presence of ascites requires excluding malignancy [52–55]. Transabdominal and thoracic ultrasound, when readily available, can detect ascites and pleural effusion [56, 57]. With appropriate expertise, ultrasound can frequently distinguish between benign and malignant tumors [58]. If the adnexal mass exhibits indeterminate features, MRI may offer better diagnostic capabilities by providing more detailed information on the tumor's contents (Fig. 10.1b) [59–63]. Contrast-enhanced computed tomography (CT) of the thoracic and abdominopelvic cavities possesses the advantage of effectively identifying pleural effusion, ascites, and adnexal masses (Fig. 10.1a). A benign ovarian tumor mass may present as either homogeneous or heterogeneous, exhibiting contrast enhancement of its solid components [64, 65]. Furthermore, computed tomography provides valuable insights into nodal metastasis in cases of suspected malignancy [66]. Compared to transvaginal ultrasound, CT and MRI provide additional detail regarding surrounding anatomic structures, further enhancing the preoperative evaluation [67, 68]. ^{18}F-FDG PET/CT is solely indicated for the assessment of metastatic lesions. Consequently, it is not necessary for patients diagnosed with Meigs syndrome. PET/CT scan can aid in distinguishing between benign and malignant tumors, with the former exhibiting only minimal FDG uptake, thereby facilitating the acquisition of pertinent preoperative information for diagnosis [69, 70].

The presence of an adnexal mass along with a pleural effusion necessitates excluding malignancy as the underlying cause. Thoracentesis is the most commonly performed procedure for sampling pleural fluid [71–73]. The effusion may extend over two-thirds of the hemithorax in 30% of cases and less than one-third in 36% of cases. Furthermore, the effusion is frequently exudative in nearly 72% of instances. In 20% of cases, the effusion may also be hemorrhagic. Approximately 70% of the time, the effusion occurs on the right side and does not coincide with the location of the adnexal mass. The mean pleural fluid lactate dehydrogenase (LDH) and total protein levels are reported to be 184 IU/L and 4.3 g/dL, respectively [46, 74]. Pleural fluid quantitative cellular analysis typically demonstrates low cellularity, with fewer than 1000 cells/μL [75]. The leukocyte differential is frequently lymphocytic predominant, without evidence of malignant cells [48, 76]. Interestingly, pleural fluid may also contain high amounts of amylase, which is postulated to stem from the fallopian tubes, due to the close proximity of the adnexal mass [77].

Peritoneal fluid sampling may also be necessary, especially if clinically significant, particularly in symptomatic cases [78, 79]. Similar to pleural analysis, the peritoneal fluid is typically exudative in two-thirds of cases and can appear bloody in approximately 17% of cases [46]. The cancer antigen 125 (CA-125), a protein used as a tumor marker for ovarian malignancy, has also been found to be elevated in both peritoneal and pleural fluid in the presence of a benign tumor [80, 81]. The exact mechanism for the elevated tumor marker is unknown; however, immunohistochemical staining for CA-125 has demonstrated increased expression from the reactive mesothelial cells overlying the tumor, rather than the tumor bed [82]. Higher levels of CA-125 were associated with a larger ascitic volume [83]. Since CA-125 can be elevated in pleural fluid, peritoneal fluid, and serum, the detection of this marker cannot be used as an adjunct for diagnosing malignancy. Following complete resection of the adnexal mass, levels return to normal within several weeks [84, 85].

Treatment

Curative treatment of Meigs syndrome requires complete resection of the adnexal mass. This is often performed with an exploratory laparotomy and salpingo-oophorectomy [17, 86]. Given the competing diagnosis of the clinical picture, which mimics an underlying malignancy, a gynecologic surgery referral is warranted [87]. Following resection, the ascites and pleural effusion typically resolve rapidly within days and are thought to occur through reabsorption via the lymphatics, with subsequent excretion [18]. As the role of thoracentesis is primarily diagnostic, in the absence of tumor removal, reaccumulation of fluid will continue to occur. Serial thoracentesis or pleural catheter insertion for continued pleural space drainage may serve as a bridge to surgery [86]. Irradiation of the tumor preoperatively in a patient with a granulosa cell tumor requiring a delay period prior to surgery was reported historically; however, this is no longer performed and is not recommended as the standard of care. The results, however, showed a decrease in the need for repeated thoracentesis and an improvement in symptoms until total resection was performed [88].

Prognosis

The prognosis following resection is favorable with resolution of ascites and the pleural effusion and without recurrence. The fluid within the abdominal and pleural cavity typically resolves within days, and CA-125 levels normalize within weeks. Since Meigs syndrome is curable upon complete surgical resection, lifespan is not impacted and returns to that of the general population [89, 90]. Information regarding the prognosis of inoperable cases is limited, but it likely depends on other factors, such as age, tumor size, and comorbidities.

References

1. Light RW. Pleural diseases. Philadelphia: Lippincott Williams & Wilkins; 2007.
2. Lucas MC, Taylor RR. Joe Vincent Meigs and the evolution of Meigs syndrome. J Pelvic Surg. 2001;7(4):191–5.
3. Griffin JP. Dame Mary Page–the first recorded case of Meigs' syndrome? J R Coll Physicians Lond. 1996;30(5):465.
4. Baskett TF. Spiegelberg, Otto von (1830–1881): Spiegelberg's criteria for ovarian pregnancy. In: Eponyms and names in obstetrics and gynaecology. Cambridge: Cambridge University Press; 2019. p. 403.
5. Spiegelberg O. Fibrom des Eierstockes von enormer Grösse. Monnatschrift Geburtskunde Frauen. 1866;28:415–25.
6. Démons A. Epanchements pleurétiques compliquantles kystes de l'ovaire. Bull Mem Soc Chi Paris. 1887;13:771–6.
7. Demons A. Sur un point de l'évolution clinique des fibromes de l'ovaire et des ligaments larges. In: Alcan Félix, editor. Quinzième Congrès de Chirurgie de Paris; 1902. p. 739–40. Paris.
8. Lurie S. Meigs' syndrome: the history of the eponym. Eur J Obstet Gynecol Reprod Biol. 2000;92(2):199–204.
9. Powell JL. Powell's pearls: joe Vincent Meigs, MD (1892-1963). Obstet Gynecol Surv. 2006;61(12):753–4.
10. Meigs JV. Tumors of the female pelvic organs. 1934.
11. Meigs JV, Cass JW. Fibroma of the ovary with ascites and hydrothorax. Am J Obstet Gynecol. 1937;33(2):249–67.
12. Rhoads JE, Terrell AW. Ovarian fibroma with ascites and hydrothorax (Meigs syndrome): a case. JAMA. 1937;109:1684.
13. Funk Brentano P. Limitation and extension of the Meigs demon syndrome. Med Press. 1949;57(25):341–92.
14. Brun JL. Demons syndrome revisited: a review of the literature. Gynecol Oncol. 2007;105(3):796–800.
15. Guelzim Y, Bennasser A, Marrakchi S, Houssaini AS, Idoubba S, Boujida I, et al. Demons-Meigs syndrome caused by a giant ovarian fibroma: a case report. Radiol Case Rep. 2024;19(7):2585–9.
16. Nohuz E, Alaboud M, El-Drayi B, Tamburro S, Kachkach S, Varga J. Demons-Meigs pseudosyndrome mimicking the symptoms of pregnancy: a case report. J Reprod Infertil. 2014;15(4):229–32. PMID: 25469326; PMCID: PMC4227981.
17. Meigs JV. Fibroma of the ovary with ascites and hydrothorax – Meigs' syndrome. Am J Obstet Gynecol. 1954;67(5):962–87.

18. Meigs JV. Pelvic tumors other than fibromas of the ovary with ascites and hydrothorax. Obstet Gynecol. 1954;3(5):471–86.
19. McNulty TF, Muccino JA. Meigs' syndrome–an incomplete form with severe hydrothorax. Conn Med. 1966;30(4):267–70.
20. Weise M, Westphalen S, Fayyazi A, Emons G, Krauss T. Pseudo-Meigs syndrome: uterine leiomyoma with bladder attachment associated with ascites and hydrothorax – a rare case of a rare syndrome. Oncol Res Treat. 2002;25(5):443–6.
21. Peparini N, Chirletti P. Ovarian malignancies with cytologically negative pleural and peritoneal effusions: demons' or Meigs' pseudo-syndromes? Int J Surg Pathol. 2009;17(5):396–7.
22. Tan Q, Xu LF, Yan T, Huang CH, Tao Y, Huang WH, et al. Deciphering the puzzle: a case report of Tjalma syndrome (pseudo-pseudo Meigs' syndrome) with profoundly elevated CA-125 and pleural effusion. Front Immunol. 2023;14.
23. Tjalma WA. Ascites, pleural effusion, and CA 125 elevation in an SLE patient, either a Tjalma syndrome or, due to the migrated Filshie clips, a pseudo-Meigs syndrome. Gynecol Oncol. 2005;97(1):288–91. https://doi.org/10.1016/j.ygyno.2004.12.022.
24. Chechia A, Attia L, Temime RB, Makhlouf T, Koubaa A. Incidence, clinical analysis, and management of ovarian fibromas and fibrothecomas. Am J Obstet Gynecol. 2008;199(5):473.e1–4.
25. Aziz S, Hanaa L, Noha A, Najia Z, Amina L, Aicha K, et al. Meigs syndrome: about an uncommon case report. Clin J Obstet Gynecol. 2023;6(1).
26. Imran H, Haidar F, Akhatar SS. Prevalence of Meigs syndrome. Pak J Med Health Sci. 2019;13(2):656–9.
27. Saha S, Robertson M. Meigs' and Pseudo-Meigs' syndrome. Australas J Ultrasound Med. 2012;15(1):29–31.
28. Samanth KK, Black WC. Benign ovarian stromal tumors associated with free peritoneal fluid. Am J Obstet Gynecol. 1970;107(4):538–45.
29. Latta RJ, Lee PD. Meigs' syndrome in a young woman. J Adolesc Health Care. 1981;1(4):313–5. https://doi.org/10.1016/s0197-0070(81)80012-5.
30. Parwate NS, Patel SM, Arora R, Gupta M. Ovarian fibroma: a clinico-pathological study of 23 cases with review of literature. J Obstet Gynaecol India. 2016;66(6):460–5. https://doi.org/10.1007/s13224-015-0717-6. Epub 2015 Jul 29. PMID: 27821988; PMCID: PMC5080219.
31. Foster HW. Meigs' syndrome complicated by pregnancy. J Natl Med Assoc. 1971;63(5):372–3. PMID: 5121155; PMCID: PMC2608640.
32. Ziruma A, Hukuimwe M, Nyakura M, Majangara R, Venge M. A rare case of Meigs syndrome in pregnancy. Pan Afr Med J. 2019;33:36. https://doi.org/10.11604/pamj.2019.33.36.18653. PMID: 31384351; PMCID: PMC6658162.
33. Nowak M, Podciechowski L, Krawczyk T, Wilczynski J. Meigs' syndrome and virilizing ovarian fibrothecoma complicating pregnancy. A case report and review of the literature. Neuro Endocrinol Lett. 2009;30(2):192–4.
34. Knaus WE, Campos J, Rose W. Meigs' syndrome; a report of a case in a child. J Pediatr. 1953;43(1):88–91. https://doi.org/10.1016/s0022-3476(53)80093-4.
35. Norris HJ, Jensen RD. Relative frequency of ovarian neoplasms in children and adolescents. Cancer. 1972;30(3):713–9. https://doi.org/10.1002/1097-0142(197209)30:3<713::aid-cncr2820300319>3.0.co;2-g.
36. Nemeth AJ, Patel SK. Meigs syndrome revisited. J Thorac Imaging. 2003;18(2):100–3. https://doi.org/10.1097/00005382-200304000-00009.
37. Corrin B, Nicholson AG. Pathology of the lungs. 3rd ed. Elsevier; 2011.
38. Rubin IC, Novak J, Squire JJ. Ovarian fibromas and theca-cell tumors: report of 78 cases with special reference to production of ascites and hydrothorax (Meigs' syndrome). Am J Obstet Gynecol. 1944;48(5):601–16.
39. Abramov Y, Anteby SO, Fasouliotis SJ, Barak V. Markedly elevated levels of vascular endothelial growth factor, fibroblast growth factor, and interleukin 6 in Meigs syndrome. Am J Obstet Gynecol. 2001;184(3):354–5.
40. Abramov Y. The role of inflammatory cytokines in Meigs' syndrome. Obstet Gynecol. 2002;99(5):917–9.
41. Abramov Y, Anteby SO, Fatum M, Fasouliotis SJ, Barak V. The kinetics of leptin in Meigs' syndrome. Gynecol Oncol. 2001;83(2):316–8.
42. Meigs JV, Armstrong SH, Hamilton HH. A further contribution to the syndrome of fibroma of the ovary with fluid in the abdomen and chest, Meigs' syndrome. Am J Obstet Gynecol. 1943;46(1):19–37.
43. Lemon WS, Higgins GM. Lymphatic absorption of particulate matter through the normal and the paralyzed diaphragm. Am J Med Sci. 1929;178(4):536–47.
44. Hodari AA, Hodgkinson CP. Lymphangiogram of Meigs' syndrome: report of a case. Obstet Gynecol. 1968;32(4):477–81.
45. Calmenson M, Dockerty MB, Bianco JJ. Certain pelvic tumors associated with ascites and hydrothorax. Surg Gynecol Obstet. 1947;84(2):181–91. PMID: 20279451.
46. Krenke R, Maskey-Warzechowska M, Korczynski P, Zielinska-Krawczyk M, Klimiuk J, Chazan R, et al. Pleural effusion in Meigs' syndrome—transudate or exudate? Medicine. 2015;94(49):e2114.
47. Majzlin G, Stevens FL. Meigs' syndrome. Case report and review of literature. J Int Coll Surg. 1964;42:625–30.
48. Okuda K, Noguchi S, Narumoto O, Ikemura M, Yamauchi Y, Tanaka G, et al. A case of Meigs' syndrome with preceding pericardial effusion in advance of pleural effusion. BMC Pulm Med. 2016;16(1).
49. Qaisar S, Osman F, Pitt M. Resolution of pericardial effusion after removal of ovarian fibroma–a Meigs'-like syndrome. J R Soc Med. 2005;98(7):313–4. https://doi.org/10.1177/014107680509800706. PMID: 15994592; PMCID: PMC1168915.

50. Patanè S, Marte F, Di Bella G, Davi' M. Pericardial effusion with elevated serum carbohydrate antigen 125 levels and ovarian tumor mass. Int J Cardiol. 2008;127(3):e105–7. https://doi.org/10.1016/j.ijcard.2007.01.094. Epub 2007 Apr 19.
51. Arnáiz-García ME, González-Santos JM, López-Rodriguez J, Dalmau-Sorli MJ, Bueno-Codoñer ME, Arnáiz J. Meigs-like syndrome presenting as cardiac tamponade. Rev Port Cardiol. 2013;32(6):547–8. https://doi.org/10.1016/j.repc.2012.12.016. Epub 2013 Jun 27.
52. American College of Obstetricians and Gynecologists' Committee on Practice Bulletins – Gynecology. Practice bulletin no. 174: evaluation and management of adnexal masses. Obstet Gynecol. 2016;128(5):e210–26. https://doi.org/10.1097/AOG.0000000000001768.
53. Shen-Gunther J, Mannel RS. Ascites as a predictor of ovarian malignancy. Gynecol Oncol. 2002;87(1):77–83. https://doi.org/10.1006/gyno.2002.6800.
54. Leibman AJ, Kruse B, McSweeney MB. Transvaginal sonography: comparison with transabdominal sonography in the diagnosis of pelvic masses. AJR Am J Roentgenol. 1988;151(1):89–92. https://doi.org/10.2214/ajr.151.1.89.
55. Mendelson EB, Bohm-Velez M, Joseph N, Neiman HL. Gynecologic imaging: comparison of transabdominal and transvaginal sonography. Radiology. 1988;166(2):321–4. https://doi.org/10.1148/radiology.166.2.3275976.
56. Rudralingam V, Footitt C, Layton B. Ascites matters. Ultrasound. 2017;25(2):69–79. https://doi.org/10.1177/1742271X16680653. Epub 2016 Dec 1. PMID: 28567101; PMCID: PMC5438051.
57. Soni NJ, Franco R, Velez MI, Schnobrich D, Dancel R, Restrepo MI, Mayo PH. Ultrasound in the diagnosis and management of pleural effusions. J Hosp Med. 2015;10(12):811–6. https://doi.org/10.1002/jhm.2434. Epub 2015 Jul 28. PMID: 26218493; PMCID: PMC4715558.
58. Roseland ME, Maturen KE, Shampain KL, Wasnik AP, Stein EB. Adnexal mass imaging: contemporary guidelines for clinical practice. Radiol Clin North Am. 2023;61(4):671–85. https://doi.org/10.1016/j.rcl.2023.02.002.
59. Mitchell S, Gleeson J, Tiwari M, et al. Accuracy of ultrasound, magnetic resonance imaging and intra-operative frozen section in the diagnosis of ovarian tumours: data from a London tertiary Centre. BJC Rep. 2024;2:50. https://doi.org/10.1038/s44276-024-00068-4.
60. Bazot M, Daraï E, Nassar-Slaba J, Lafont C, Thomassin-Naggara I. Value of magnetic resonance imaging for the diagnosis of ovarian tumors: a review. J Comput Assist Tomogr. 2008;32(5):712–23. https://doi.org/10.1097/RCT.0b013e31815881ef.
61. Grab D, Flock F, Stohr I, Nussle K, Rieber A, Fenchel S, et al. Classification of asymptomatic adnexal masses by ultrasound, magnetic resonance imaging, and positron emission tomography. Gynecol Oncol. 2000;77:454–9.
62. Sohaib SA, et al. The role of magnetic resonance imaging and ultrasound in patients with adnexal masses. Clin Radiol. 2005;60:340–8.
63. Valentini AL, Gui B, Miccò M, Mingote MC, De Gaetano AM, Ninivaggi V, Bonomo L. Benign and suspicious ovarian masses-MR imaging criteria for characterization: pictorial review. J Oncol. 2012;2012:481806. https://doi.org/10.1155/2012/481806. Epub 2012 Mar 22. PMID: 22536238; PMCID: PMC3321462.
64. Bierman SM, Reuter KL, Hunter RE. Meigs syndrome and ovarian fibroma: CT findings. J Comput Assist Tomogr. 1990;14(5):833–4. https://doi.org/10.1097/00004728-199009000-00035.
65. Sawyer RW, Vick CW, Walsh JW, McClure PH. Computed tomography of benign ovarian masses. J Comput Assist Tomogr. 1985;9(4):784–9.
66. Micco M, Sala E, Lakhman Y, Hricak H, Vargas HA. Role of imaging in the pretreatment evaluation of common gynecological cancers. Womens Health. 2014;10:299–321.
67. Heilbrun ME, Olpin J, Shaaban A. Imaging of benign adnexal masses: characteristic presentations on ultrasound, computed tomography, and magnetic resonance imaging. Clin Obstet Gynecol. 2009;52(1):21–39. https://doi.org/10.1097/GRF.0b013e318195834b.
68. Koutras A, Perros P, Prokopakis I, Ntounis T, Fasoulakis Z, Pittokopitou S, Samara AA, Valsamaki A, Douligeris A, Mortaki A, Sapantzoglou I, Katrachouras A, Pagkalos A, Symeonidis P, Palios VC, Psarris A, Theodora M, Antsaklis P, Makrydimas G, Chionis A, Daskalakis G, Kontomanolis EN. Advantages and limitations of ultrasound as a screening test for ovarian cancer. Diagnostics (Basel). 2023;13(12):2078. https://doi.org/10.3390/diagnostics13122078. PMID: 37370973; PMCID: PMC10297553.
69. Hu X, Li W, Li X, Li D, Cai J, Wang P. 18F-FDG PET/CT features of Meigs syndrome induced by ovarian sex cord stromal tumors: a retrospective clinical study. Sci Rep. 2024;14(1).
70. Lee ES, Kim TS, Yoo CW, Seo SS, Kim S. A case of Meigs' syndrome: the 18F-FDG PET/CT findings. Nucl Med Mol Imaging. 2011;45(3):229–32.
71. Roberts ME, Rahman NM, Maskell NA, Bibby AC, Blyth KG, Corcoran JP, et al. British Thoracic Society guideline for pleural disease. Thorax. 2023;78(Suppl 3):s1–42.
72. Ferreiro L, José ES, Antelo JS, Valdés L. Bilateral pleural effusion: a proposed diagnostic decision algorithm. PubMed. 2016;13(10):1865–7.
73. Martinez-Zayas G, Molina S, Ost DE. Sensitivity and complications of thoracentesis and thoracoscopy: a meta-analysis. Eur Respir Rev. 2022;31(166).
74. Neustadt JE. Hemorrhagic pleural effusion in Meigs' syndrome. JAMA. 1968 Apr 1;204(1):81.

75. Broaddus VC, Light RW. Chapter 79: Pleural effusion. In: Murray and Nadel's textbook of respiratory medicine. 6th ed. Philadelphia: Elsevier; 2016.
76. Mitsuboshi S, Matsumoto T, Isaka T, Kumakiri J, Yamamoto T, Kanzaki M. A case of unexplained pleural effusion diagnosed as Meigs' syndrome. DOAJ (DOAJ: Directory of Open Access Journals). 2019.
77. Simson JNL. Amylase levels in pleural and peritoneal fluid in Meigs' syndrome. J R Soc Med. 1987;80(10):661.
78. Harvey JJ, Prentice R, George J. Diagnostic and therapeutic abdominal paracentesis. Med J Aust. 2023;218(1):18–21. https://doi.org/10.5694/mja2.51795. Epub 2022 Nov 30. PMID: 36450339; PMCID: PMC10099762.
79. Runyon BA. Care of patients with ascites. N Engl J Med. 1994;330(5):337–42.
80. O'Connell GJ, Ryan E, Murphy KJ, Prefontaine M. Predictive value of CA 125 for ovarian carcinoma in patients presenting with pelvic masses. Obstet Gynecol. 1987;70(6):930–2.
81. Mezger J, Wilmanns W, Lamerz R. Elevated serum CA 125 levels in patients with benign ascitic or pleural effusions. Tumour Biol. 1988;9(1):47–52.
82. Timmerman D, Moerman P, Vergote I. Meigs' syndrome with elevated serum CA 125 levels: two case reports and review of the literature. Gynecol Oncol. 1995;59(3):405–8.
83. Patsner B. Meigs syndrome and "false positive" preoperative serum CA-125 levels: analysis of ten cases. Eur J Gynaecol Oncol. 2000;21(4):362–3.
84. Hou YY, Li P, Zhou M. Meigs syndrome with pleural effusion as initial manifestation: a case report. World J Clin Cases. 2021;9(21):5972–9.
85. Liou JH, Tzu Cheng S, Hsu JC. Meigs' syndrome with elevated serum cancer antigen 125 levels in a case of ovarian sclerosing stromal tumor. Taiwan J Obstet Gynecol. 2011;50(2):196–200.
86. Parwate NS, Patel SM, Arora R, Gupta M. Ovarian fibroma: a clinico-pathological study of 23 cases with review of literature. J Obstet Gynecol India. 2015;66(6):460–5.
87. Im SS, Gordon AN, Buttin BM, Leath CA 3rd, Gostout BS, Shah C, Hatch KD, Wang J, Berman ML. Validation of referral guidelines for women with pelvic masses. Obstet Gynecol. 2005;105(1):35–41. https://doi.org/10.1097/01.AOG.0000149159.69560.ef.
88. Long AE. Hemothorax in relation to benign pelvic tumors. Calif Med. 1948;68(5):383–7. PMID: 18731450; PMCID: PMC1643259.
89. Stabile G, Zinicola G, Romano F, Laganà AS, Dal Pozzolo C, Ricci G. Pelvic mass, ascites, hydrothorax: a malignant or benign condition? Meigs syndrome with high levels of CA 125. Menopause Rev. 2021;20(2):103–7. https://doi.org/10.5114/pm.2021.106100.
90. Abad A, Cazorla E, Ruiz F, Aznar I, Asins E, Llixiona J. Meigs' syndrome with elevated CA 125: case report and review of the literature. Eur J Obstet Gynecol Reprod Biol. 1999;82(1):97–9. https://doi.org/10.1016/S0301-2115(98)00220-7.

11 Post-cardiac Injury Syndrome

Douglas Frenia and Anum Qadri

Introduction

Post-cardiac injury syndrome (PCIS) is an inflammatory condition affecting the pericardium, pleura, or lung tissues that occurs after a myocardial infarction, cardiac surgery, or thoracic trauma. The first mention of post-cardiac injury syndrome appeared in the literature in 1952, as described by Janton and Glover [1]. A report involving 100 cases of mitral commissurotomy found that 30% of patients experienced post-surgical pleuropericardial chest pain, which was called post-commissurotomy syndrome. The nature of the pain was unusual compared to typical chest pain after thoracotomy. It was reported to occur about 2 weeks after surgery, sometimes recur, and last up to 6 months. Some patients also developed pericardial and pleural effusions. In 1956, Dr. William Dressler famously described ten cases of pericarditis, pleuritis, and/or pneumonitis that appeared after a myocardial infarction. Seven of these cases developed pleural effusions. Leukocytosis and relapsing fever were also observed in several cases. These findings are now commonly known as Dressler syndrome [2]. In 1966, Aronstam and Cox reported similar observations in ten cases, eight following open or closed cardiac surgery, and two after penetrating trauma. They suggested that in all cases, a likely trigger was the presence of residual blood in the pericardial sac or pleura, leading to an inflammatory response [3]. These causes, including post-myocardial infarction, post-pericardiotomy, and thoracic trauma, are collectively called post-cardiac injury syndrome [4].

D. Frenia (✉)
Department of Pulmonary and Critical Care, Saint Peter's University Hospital, New Brunswick, NJ, USA
e-mail: dfrenia@saintpetersuh.com

A. Qadri
Department of Pulmonary and Critical Care, Washington University School of Medicine, Saint Louis, MI, USA
e-mail: aqadri@saintpetersuh.com

Epidemiology

PCIS occurs due to injury of the pericardium or myocardium following myocardial infarction, post-pericardiotomy, or iatrogenic and non-iatrogenic thoracic trauma. Awareness of post-cardiac injury syndrome has significantly increased due to more frequent and complex cardiac procedures performed on an aging population [4]. One large study identified PCIS as the cause of pericarditis in 21% of patients [5]. The incidence of PCIS varies significantly by etiology. Differences in reported incidences may result from variable diagnostic criteria and underlying causes. Cardiac surgery is the most common cause of PCIS, with rates around 10–40%. Trauma from iatrogenic injury has been observed following procedures such as central venous catheter insertion, pacemaker and cardioverter-defibrillator

F. Ido (ed.), *Rare Pleural Diseases*, https://doi.org/10.1007/978-3-032-14873-5_11

placement, percutaneous coronary intervention, and arrhythmia ablation [4, 5]. PCIS has been shown to occur after 1–5% of pacemaker device insertions and about 0.2% of percutaneous interventions [6, 7]. Recent studies indicate that Dressler syndrome has become increasingly rare, with incidence rates below 1% [8]. The decline may be due to the advent of percutaneous coronary intervention. Procedures involving greater cardiac injury, such as open valve replacement, are more likely to lead to PCIS than coronary artery bypass grafting [9]. Evidence suggests that pleural incision increases the risk of developing PCIS, with one study reporting it as the most common risk factor, showing a hazard ratio of 4.31 [10]. In post-pericardiotomy syndrome, nearly 80% of cases occur within the first month after surgery, with the remaining cases occurring in the second (13%) and third (7.4%) months [10]. Pleural effusions of all types have been seen within 28 days after coronary artery bypass grafting and valvular surgery, with reported incidences of 63% and 45%, respectively [11]. However, pleural effusions in post-pericardiotomy syndrome specifically are reported to occur in nearly 93% of cases [10].

Pathophysiology

The mechanism for the development of PCIS remains unclear but likely involves both innate and adaptive immune responses. The initiating event is presumed to be damage to the mesothelial lining of the pericardium or pleura, accompanied by blood accumulation within the serosal membranes [12]. Additionally, damage to cardiac cells exposes intracellular antigens, which are believed to form complexes with circulating antibodies. These antibodies deposit in the pericardium, pleura, and lungs, triggering a hypersensitivity immune response [13]. The autoimmune mechanism is supported by the detection of anti-myosin and anti-actin antibodies, both systemically and within pleural fluid [9]. Furthermore, the autoantibody titer has been shown to correlate positively with the severity of PCIS [8]. However, the exact role of these antibodies is not fully understood, as a small study demonstrated negative testing for anti-heart antibodies (AHA) at the time of PCIS diagnosis, but subsequent positive AHA testing within 14 days [14]. This finding raises the question of whether AHA antibodies are a consequence of PCIS rather than its primary cause.

Recently, the involvement of the innate immune system has emerged as a potential requirement for developing pericarditis. A cytosolic macrostructure known as NLRP3 (NACHT, LRR, and pyrin domain-containing protein-3) is an inflammasome located within immune cells, specifically macrophages and neutrophils [15]. The expression of NLRP3 triggers the release of inflammatory cytokines IL-1β and IL-18 [16]. This process results in the recruitment of additional immune cells to the injury site, leading to tissue damage and serosal inflammation. Human subjects and mouse models have shown increased activation of the NLRP3 inflammasome following pericardial injury, resulting in pericarditis [17].

Clinical Features

The diagnosis of PCIS requires a latency period, with approximately 80% of cases exhibiting symptoms within the first month [15]. Pleuritic chest pain is the most common symptom, occurring in 55% to 80% of cases [4, 16]. It is typically a sharp, stabbing pain that worsens with deep breathing, swallowing, and while in the supine position, but improves when sitting upright [18]. Low-grade fever and dyspnea are present in about 50–60% of cases [4]. During physical examination, a pericardial rub may be auscultated in 30–60% of cases [4, 16]. Rales were found in nearly 51% of cases [19]. The absence of breath sounds due to a pleural effusion, or crackles due to pleural inflammation, may be observed in 83% of patients [18]. Pleural effusion and pericardial effusion can be visible in 92.6% and 88.9%, respectively.

Diagnosis

A diagnostic criterion for PCIS has been proposed, requiring multiple features following cardiac injury and the exclusion of alternative causes. Since the latency period varies, no precise time frame has been established. Diagnosis is based on meeting at least two of the following five criteria: (i) fever without an alternative cause, (ii) pleuritic or pericarditic pain, (iii) presence of a pericardial or pleural friction rub on physical exam, (iv) evidence of pericardial effusion, and/or (v) pleural effusion with an elevated C-reactive protein (CRP) [19]. PCIS should be differentiated from mechanical complications causing pleural effusion in the early postoperative period after cardiac surgery, such as bleeding and atelectasis [12].

Laboratory abnormalities are common, including leukocytosis on a complete blood count, elevated erythrocyte sedimentation rate (ESR), and CRP, which occur in 70–80% of cases [13]. Cardiac troponins T or I are also usually elevated but may reflect the initial cardiac injury rather than the development of PCIS. Normal or stable levels, followed by a rise after a latency period, can support the diagnosis of PCIS [20]. Anti-myosin, anti-actin, and anti-heart antibodies are not primary diagnostic tools for PCIS, though they can serve as supporting indicators when combined with other clinical evidence. Although their elevation supports the autoimmune hypothesis, the significance of these antibodies in PCIS remains unclear and is currently under investigation [21]. Therefore, measuring antibody levels is not routinely performed in clinical practice. Although not routinely performed, a pleural biopsy can demonstrate chronic inflammation along with non-necrotizing granulomas (Fig. 11.1b) [40].

Data on pleural fluid analysis remains limited. A study involving 70 cases of PCIS-related pleural effusions showed that 76% involved less than or equal to one-third of the hemithorax, 18% affected half of the hemithorax, and 6% extended to at least two-thirds of the hemithorax. All cases where pleural effusion occupied more than two-thirds of the hemithorax occurred after coronary

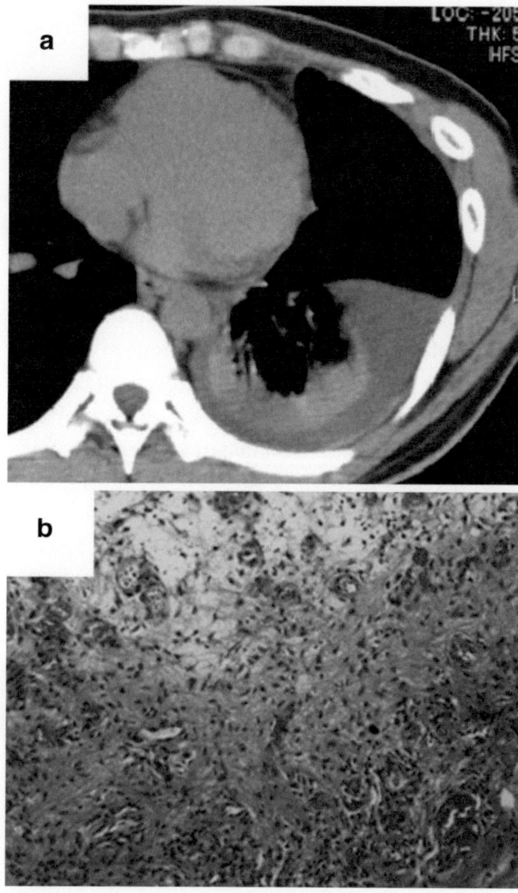

Fig. 11.1 Radiologic and histopathologic findings in post-cardiac injury syndrome following radiofrequency ablation for paroxysmal atrial fibrillation (**a**) Chest computed tomography demonstrates a recurrent left-sided pleural effusion associated with diffuse parietal pleural thickening (**b**) Hematoxylin and eosin-stained section of the left parietal pleura showing chronic pleuritis with a non-necrotizing granulomatous inflammatory reaction Attribution: Reprinted from *Respiratory Medicine Case Reports*, Vol 15, Yukumi S., Ichiki H., Funada J., Suzuki H., Morimoto M., Fujita T., Izumi N., Abe M., "Postcardiac injury syndrome following vascular interventional radiofrequency ablation for paroxysmal atrial fibrillation," pp. 89–91, Copyright © 2015 Elsevier Inc. Reproduced by permission of Elsevier through RightsLink License No. 6133221077689 for *Rare Pleural Disease* (Springer Nature, 2026). All rights reserved. No further reproduction or distribution is permitted without permission from Elsevier

artery bypass graft (CABG) procedures. In Dressler syndrome cases, 95% of pleural effusions involved no more than one-third of the hemithorax. The pleural effusions linked to PCIS were mainly left-sided (55%), though right-sided (12%) and bilateral effusions (33%) were also observed. Subgroup analysis showed that pleural effusions were left-sided in 63% of post-cardiac surgery cases, 48% in Dressler syndrome, and 33% following pacemaker implantation. Bilateral pleural effusions were more prevalent in Dressler syndrome (52%) and post-pacemaker placement (50%) compared to post-cardiac surgery cases (20%). Pleural fluid was classified as exudative in 97% of cases according to Light's criteria, with an average total protein level of 3.8 g/dL and a lactate dehydrogenase level of 385 U/L. The red blood cell count in PCIS pleural fluid exceeded 10,000/μL in 57% of cases, especially in post-cardiac surgery (73%), Dressler syndrome (26%), and post-pacemaker placement (67%). The pleural fluid was predominantly lymphocytic in 74% of PCIS cases, with all three categories ranging from 62% to 83%. Pleural fluid analysis performed within 10 days of symptom onset usually shows a predominance of polymorphonuclear cells, shifting to mononuclear cells after 20 days from symptom development [19]. Notably, none of the pleural effusions in PCIS had a pH of ≤ 7.2 [18]. Pleural fluid glucose was always reported as greater than 60 mg/100 mL [19].

There is a limited amount of information available about electrocardiogram changes in PCIS overall. ECG findings in PCIS due to late post-myocardial infarction (Dressler's syndrome) appear in about 60% of patients and include T wave inversions, diffuse concave ST elevations, PR depression in limb and precordial leads (V2–V6), and PR elevation along with ST depression in aVR (± V1) [22, 23]. Recognizing and interpreting these findings can be complicated by the underlying condition that triggered Dressler's syndrome [12]. Electrical alternans or low-voltage QRS complexes may also be seen if a pericardial effusion occurs.

In a single study, a chest X-ray was reportedly abnormal in 94% of cases. Pleural effusion was the most common abnormality, present in 83% of cases. Pulmonary infiltrate was observed in 74% of cases, with 62% involving the left lower lobe. Additionally, 49% of cases also demonstrated an enlarged cardiac silhouette [19]. The overall sensitivity and specificity for detecting pericardial effusion by chest radiography are 71% and 41%, respectively [24].

Ultrasound can detect even small amounts of pericardial and pleural fluid. Additionally, echocardiography and thoracic ultrasound can provide insight into the quality of serosal fluid and provide details regarding septations, loculations, and the precise location of the accumulations [24]. Pleural effusions can be effectively visualized on chest computed tomography (CT), which also permits evaluation for a concurrent pericardial effusion, a finding that is observed in approximately two-thirds of patients with post-cardiac injury syndrome (Fig. 11.1a). Pericardial effusions larger than 1 cm in thickness have been observed after cardiac surgery (27%), in cases of Dressler syndrome (41%), and following pacemaker implantation (17%) [20]. Cardiac CT and cardiac magnetic resonance imaging (MRI) have also been used to evaluate pericardial inflammation, such as that seen in PCIS [25, 26]. Moreover, cardiac CT and MRI can help differentiate between acute and chronic pericarditis [21].

Prevention and Treatment

The management mirrors that of acute pericarditis, focusing on anti-inflammatory therapy as the primary intervention. Combination therapy with colchicine and aspirin or a nonsteroidal anti-inflammatory drug (NSAID) is considered the first-line treatment. Systemic corticosteroids, including dexamethasone and methylprednisolone, may be used in refractory cases, though evidence supporting their efficacy remains limited. Medical management with NSAIDs, colchicine, and corticosteroids is recommended prior to pleural fluid drainage, as invasive procedures carry risks of hemorrhage, pneumothorax, and infection [27]. Therapeutic thoracentesis should be reserved for large, symptomatic, or refractory pleural effusions. If the effusion reaccumulates, repeat drainage via tube thoracostomy may be indicated [18].

The use of aspirin has been shown to be effective in resolving acute pericarditis, though data specific to PCIS are lacking. Prophylactic aspirin did not reduce the incidence of PCIS when administered at 20–50 mg daily for 6 weeks following atrial septal defect surgery [28]. NSAIDs, such as ibuprofen and indomethacin, have demonstrated efficacy in achieving symptomatic resolution within 48 h in patients with post-pericardiotomy syndrome, and were also associated with a nearly 50% reduction in recurrence rates [29]. Additionally, the prophylactic use of indomethacin in patients undergoing aortic surgery was associated with a reduced incidence of pericardial effusion at 6 weeks [30].

Both methylprednisolone and dexamethasone have been evaluated for the prevention of PCIS, with at least two studies showing no significant difference in outcomes compared to controls [31, 32]. However, one trial demonstrated that a single intraoperative dose of methylprednisolone significantly reduced the incidence of post-pericardiotomy syndrome [33]. Colchicine is highly effective in preventing the development of PCIS when administered pre- and post-operatively [27, 34–36]. It has also been shown to reduce the volume of pleural effusion associated with post-pericardiotomy syndrome [35]. Recently, interleukin-1 inhibitors, such as anakinra and rilonacept, have shown benefit in preventing recurrences of pericarditis in patients refractory to colchicine and corticosteroids, suggesting potential applicability in resistant cases of PCIS [37, 38].

Prognosis

The overall prognosis is generally favorable, with most cases resolving spontaneously within weeks to months. The reported recurrence rate ranges between 10% and 15% [35]. Only a limited number of studies have evaluated the impact of PCIS on long-term mortality, but one investigation demonstrated a 72% increase in first-year mortality following cardiac surgery among patients diagnosed with PCIS [9]. Factors associated with poorer outcomes include recurrent episodes, female sex, treatment with corticosteroids, and a history of cardiotomy [39].

References

1. Janton OH, Glover RP, O'Neill TJE, Gregory JE, Froio GF. Results of the surgical treatment for mitral stenosis: analysis of one hundred consecutive cases. Circulation. 1952;6(3):321–33. https://doi.org/10.1161/01.CIR.6.3.321.
2. Dressler W. A post-myocardial-infarction syndrome: preliminary report of a complication resembling idiopathic, recurrent, benign pericarditis. JAMA. 1956;160(16):1379–83. https://doi.org/10.1001/jama.1956.02960510005002.
3. Aronstam EM, Cox WA. A new concept of the pleuropericardial syndrome. Postpericardiotomy or post-cardiotomy syndrome. J Thorac Cardiovasc Surg. 1966;51(3):341–5.
4. Imazio M, Hoit BD. Review: post-cardiac injury syndromes. An emerging cause of pericardial diseases. Int J Cardiol. 2013;168:648–52.
5. Gouriet F, Levy PY, Casalta JP, Zandotti C, Collart F, Lepidi H, et al. Etiology of pericarditis in a prospective cohort of 1162 cases. Am J Med. 2015;128(7):784.e1–8.
6. Troughton RW, Asher CR, Klein AL. Pericarditis. Lancet. 2004;363(9410):717–27.
7. Imazio M, Hoit BD. Post-cardiac injury syndromes. An emerging cause of pericardial diseases. Int J Cardiol. 2013;168(2):648–52.
8. Imazio M, Negro A, Belli R, Beqaraj F, Forno D, Giammaria M, et al. Frequency and prognostic significance of pericarditis following acute myocardial infarction treated by primary percutaneous coronary intervention. Am J Cardiol. 2009;103(11):1525–9.
9. Lehto J, Kiviniemi T, Gunn J, Airaksinen J, Rautava P, Kytö V. Occurrence of postpericardiotomy syndrome: association with operation type and postoperative mortality after open-heart operations. J Am Heart Assoc. 2018;7(22):e010269.
10. Imazio M, Brucato A, Rovere ME, Gandino A, Cemin R, Ferrua S, et al. Contemporary features, risk factors, and prognosis of the post-pericardiotomy syndrome. Am J Cardiol. 2011;108(8):1183–7.
11. Light RW, Rogers JT, Moyers JP, Lee YCG, Rodriguez RM, Alford WC, et al. Prevalence and clinical course of pleural effusions at 30 days after coronary artery and cardiac surgery. Am J Respir Crit Care Med. 2002;166(12 I):1567–71.
12. Sasse T, Eriksson U. Post-cardiac injury syndrome: aetiology, diagnosis, and treatment. E-J Cardiol Pract. 2017;15(21).

13. Lai R, Xu T. Update for diagnosis and treatment of syndrome after cardiac injury: a mini-review. Front Cardiovasc Med. 2025;12:1526671.
14. Hoffman M, Fried M, Jabareen F, Vardinon N, Turner D, Burke M, et al. Anti-heart antibodies in postpericardiotomy syndrome: cause or epiphenomenon? A prospective, longitudinal pilot study. Autoimmunity. 2002;35(4):241–5.
15. Vecchié A, Del Buono MG, Chiabrando GJ, Dentali F, Abbate A, Bonaventura A. Interleukin-1 and the NLRP3 inflammasome in pericardial disease. Curr Cardiol Rep. 2021;23(11):157.
16. Yang Y, Wang H, Kouadir M, Song H, Shi F. Recent advances in the mechanisms of NLRP3 inflammasome activation and its inhibitors. Cell Death Dis. 2019;10:128.
17. Mauro AG, Bonaventura A, Vecchié A, Mezzaroma E, Carbone S, Narayan P, et al. The role of NLRP3 inflammasome in pericarditis: potential for therapeutic approaches. JACC Basic Transl Sci. 2021;6(2):137–50.
18. Jaworska-Wilczyńska M, Kuśmierczyk M, Abramczuk E, Hryniewiecki T. Post-cardiac injury syndrome. Pol J Cardio-Thoracic Surg. 2013;1:20–6.
19. Adler Y, Charron P, Imazio M, Badano L, Barón-Esquivias G, Bogaert J, et al. 2015 ESC guidelines for the diagnosis and management of pericardial diseases. Eur Heart J. 2015;36:2921–64.
20. Köhler I, Saraiva PJ, Wender OB, Zago Porto Alegre AJ. Behavior of inflammatory markers of myocardial injury in cardiac surgery. Laboratory correlation with the clinical picture of postpericardiotomy syndrome. Arq Bras Cardiol. 2003;81:285–90.
21. Malik J, Zaidi SMJ, Rana AS, Haider A, Tahir S. Post-cardiac injury syndrome: an evidence-based approach to diagnosis and treatment. Am Heart J Plus. 2021;12
22. Michael GS, Bryan VCF, Pragnesh PP, Peter PM, Charles BJ. Peri-myocardial infarction pericarditis: current concepts. Clin Cardiol Cardiovasc Med. 2019:23–6.
23. Ibanez B, James S, Agewall S, Antunes MJ, Bucciarelli-Ducci C, Bueno H, et al. 2017 ESC guidelines for the management of acute myocardial infarction in patients presenting with ST-segment elevation. Eur Heart J. 2018;39(2):119–77.
24. Eisenberg MJ, Dunn MM, Kanth N, Gamsu G, Schiller NB. Diagnostic value of chest radiography for pericardial effusion. J Am Coll Cardiol. 1993;22(2):588–93.
25. Verma BR, Chetrit M, Gentry Iii JL, Noll A, Bafadel A, Khayata M, et al. Multimodality imaging in patients with post-cardiac injury syndrome. Heart. 2020;106(9):639–46.
26. Bogaert J, Francone M. Pericardial disease: value of CT and MR imaging. Radiology. 2013;267(2):340–56.
27. Giacinto O, Minati A, Lusini M, Cardetta F, Saltarocchi S, D'Abramo M, et al. Treatment and prophylaxis of post-pericardiotomy syndrome in cardiac surgery patients: a systematic review. Cardiovasc Drugs Ther. 2023;37:771–9.
28. Gill PJ, Forbes K, Coe JY. The effect of short-term prophylactic acetylsalicylic acid on the incidence of postpericardiotomy syndrome after surgical closure of atrial septal defects. Pediatr Cardiol. 2009;30(8):1061–7.
29. Horneffer PJ, Miller RH, Pearson TA, Rykiel MF, Reitz BA, Gardner TJ. The effective treatment of postpericardiotomy syndrome after cardiac operations. A randomized placebo-controlled trial. J Thorac Cardiovasc Surg. 1990;100(2):292–6.
30. Inan MB, Yazcoglu L, Erylmaz S, Srlak M, Cetntas D, Kaya B, et al. Effects of prophylactic indomethacin treatment on postoperative pericardial effusion after aortic surgery. J Thorac Cardiovasc Surg. 2011;141(2):578–82.
31. Mott AR, Fraser CD, Kusnoor AV, Giesecke NM, Reul GJ, Drescher KL, et al. The effect of short-term prophylactic methylprednisolone on the incidence and severity of postpericardiotomy syndrome in children undergoing cardiac surgery with cardiopulmonary bypass. 2001.
32. Bunge JJH, van Osch D, Dieleman JM, Jacob KA, Kluin J, van Dijk D, et al. Dexamethasone for the prevention of postpericardiotomy syndrome: a dexamethasone for cardiac surgery substudy. Am Heart J. 2014;168(1):126–31.e1.
33. Sevuk U, Baysal E, Altindag R, Yaylak B, Adiyaman MS, Ay N, et al. Role of methylprednisolone in the prevention of postpericardiotomy syndrome after cardiac surgery. Eur Rev Med Pharmacol Sci. 2016;20(3):514–9.
34. Martinon F, Pétrilli V, Mayor A, Tardivel A, Tschopp J. Gout-associated uric acid crystals activate the NALP3 inflammasome. Nature. 2006;440(7081):237–41.
35. Imazio M, Trinchero R, Brucato A, Rovere ME, Gandino A, Cemin R, et al. COlchicine for the prevention of the post-pericardiotomy syndrome (COPPS): a multicentre, randomized, double-blind, placebo-controlled trial. Eur Heart J. 2010;31(22):2749–54.
36. Imazio M, Belli R, Brucato A, Cemin R, Ferrua S, Beqaraj F, et al. Efficacy and safety of colchicine for treatment of multiple recurrences of pericarditis (CORP-2): a multicentre, double-blind, placebo-controlled, randomised trial. Lancet. 2014;383(9936):2232–7.
37. Imazio M, Andreis A, De Ferrari GM, Cremer PC, Mardigyan V, Maestroni S, et al. Anakinra for corticosteroid-dependent and colchicine-resistant pericarditis: the IRAP (international registry of

Anakinra for pericarditis) study. Eur J Prev Cardiol. 2020;27(9):956–64.
38. Klein AL, Imazio M, Cremer P, Brucato A, Abbate A, Fang F, et al. Phase 3 trial of interleukin-1 trap rilonacept in recurrent pericarditis. N Engl J Med. 2021;384(1):31–41.
39. Agrawal A, Berglund F, Kumar AK, Yesilyaprak A, Verma BR, Mahalwar G, et al. Adverse prognosis in patients with postcardiac injury syndrome–related recurrent pericarditis. JACC Adv. 2023;2(4):100330.
40. Yukumi S, Ichiki H, Funada J, Suzuki H, Morimoto M, Fujita T, Izumi N, Abe M. Postcardiac injury syndrome following vascular interventional radiofrequency ablation for paroxysmal atrial fibrillation. Respir Med Case Rep. 2015;15:89–91. https://doi.org/10.1016/j.rmcr.2015.03.008.

12 Benign Asbestos Pleural Effusion

Luke Simmons, Firas Ido, and Mohamed Turki

Introduction

Benign asbestos pleural effusion (BAPE) refers to a pleural effusion associated with significant active or past asbestos exposure, with no other identifiable cause [1–6]. Asbestos, a naturally occurring heat-insulating fiber, has been used since ancient times, but its clinical importance has only been recognized over the last 125 years [7, 8]. In the early 1900s, exposure levels were much higher due to the lack of regulations on asbestos concentrations in workplaces. A 1930 report by Merewether and Price established the relationship between asbestos exposure duration and concentration with pulmonary fibrosis, regardless of age and sex, which prompted increased regulation [9]. During this period, the link between asbestos exposure and pleural disease was also established; however, the first documented case of BAPE was not reported until 1964 [1–3, 10–12].

The implementation of regulatory guidelines on asbestos manufacturing and handling in the 1940s and 1950s reduced overall exposure. As a result, patients may develop symptoms after longer latency periods [1–5, 10, 13]. Diagnostic criteria have been established since 1982; however, advancements in diagnostic technologies, such as CT imaging and fluid analysis, have enhanced the accuracy of diagnoses [14, 15]. In 2020, Kishimoto and Fujimoto established a checklist comprising six criteria for diagnosing BAPE. These include a documented occupational history of asbestos exposure; confirmation of an exudative pleural effusion according to Light's criteria; exclusion of pleural fluid malignancy; exclusion of rheumatic and infectious causes; absence of malignancy on radiologic imaging; and either negative thoracoscopic biopsies or clear follow-up imaging at 3 months to rule out the development of malignancy [14].

The risk of BAPE is positively associated with the extent of asbestos exposure [14–20]. Although asbestos exposure is required, standardized threshold levels for predicting the onset of BAPE have not yet been established [2, 5, 14, 19, 21–26]. In 1982, a study on BAPE epidemiology was published, classifying patients based on severe, indirect, and peripheral exposure [6]. The prevalence of severe exposure was estimated to be 7%, indirect exposure was 3.7%, and peripheral exposure was 0.2%. The corresponding incidence rates were 9.2 effusions per 1000 person-years in the severe exposure group, 3.9 in the indirect group, and 0.7 in the peripheral group. Notably, the latency period for BAPE is shorter than that of

L. Simmons · F. Ido · M. Turki (✉)
Department of Pulmonary and Critical Care Medicine, St. Luke's University Health Network, Bethlehem, PA, USA
e-mail: luke.simmons@sluhn.org; firas.ido@sluhn.org; Mohamed.turki@sluhn.org

F. Ido (ed.), *Rare Pleural Diseases*, https://doi.org/10.1007/978-3-032-14873-5_12

other asbestos-related pulmonary diseases, with effusions typically developing within 10–20 years following exposure. However, cases have been recorded up to 50 years post-exposure [2, 15, 18, 22]. BAPE accounts for 21% of all asbestos-related lung diseases [7]. The incidence and prevalence of BAPE might vary in the twenty-first century due to evolving workplace exposure and asbestos regulations [8–11].

Asbestos exposure is the sole risk factor for developing BAPE [12]. Current evidence indicates that the risk of BAPE does not inherently vary across different ethnic groups or sexes [4, 8, 13, 27]. Historically, the incidence of asbestos-related lung diseases has been highest among Caucasian males, attributed primarily to occupational exposure rather than genetic predisposition. The underdiagnosis of these conditions in non-Caucasian patients is associated with barriers to healthcare access [28].

In the era of unregulated asbestos exposure, cases were often diagnosed during the third or fourth decade of life [3, 13, 29]. However, due to exposure limitations and enhanced safety protocols, prolonged exposure to lower levels has led to a delayed onset of symptoms [14, 18, 19, 30, 31]. A review reported a mean age at presentation of 53.5 years, with a range from 18 to 73 years. The median duration of exposure was 38 years (range: 2–55 years), while the mean exposure time was also reported to be as low as 5.5 years [2]. Historically, BAPE was primarily observed among Caucasian males, corresponding to the demographic composition within specific occupational sectors. The median age at diagnosis was 79 years, with a range of 60 to 93 years. Occupations most frequently associated with the condition included shipbuilding, construction, insulation work, and employment in the asbestos mining industry. Exposure may also result from natural disasters or active conflict zones, where the destruction of asbestos-containing buildings leads to significant aerosolization of asbestos [23, 32–35]. Individuals residing in these environments for extended periods have demonstrated an increased incidence of asbestos-related pulmonary diseases in later life [34–36].

Pathophysiology

The pathophysiology of BAPE remains incompletely characterized. The capacity of asbestos fibers to reach the alveoli is a primary determinant in the development of BAPE. This capability is influenced mainly by the physical attributes, specifically, the shape and size of the fibers [4, 21, 37–39]. Chrysotile fibers, recognized for their elongated and serpentine morphology, are frequently retained within the conducting airways and eliminated through mucociliary clearance [8]. Conversely, crocidolite and other amphibole fibers (including tremolite, anthophyllite, amosite, and actinolite) tend to be smaller and more linear, which facilitates their entry into the distal bronchioles and alveoli [13, 40, 41].

Upon arrival at the alveoli, the surface molecules of asbestos fibers initiate redox reactions that generate reactive oxygen species, resulting in injury to type I pneumocytes [37, 42–48]. This process leads to alveolitis and subsequently attracts macrophages, which are tasked with phagocytosing and removing the asbestos fibers. The act of phagocytosis by macrophages induces the release of TGF-β, TNF-α, and IL-1β, thereby promoting fibrogenesis [37, 49–52]. As a result, mucopolysaccharides are synthesized and deposited onto the asbestos fibers, which can be visualized microscopically as dumbbell-shaped structures known as asbestos bodies [39, 45, 49, 51–57]. This pathognomonic feature, indicative of asbestos exposure, is confined to the alveoli and is not present within the pleural space.

Clinical Features

Approximately 60% of patients present without symptoms, with effusions being identified incidentally, leading to referral to pulmonology [14, 18, 19]. No specific signs or symptoms are pathognomonic for the diagnosis of BAPE; presentations are generally nonspecific and overlap with those of other respiratory conditions, such as emphysema, pulmonary fibrosis, and pulmonary edema. When symptoms occur, progressive dyspnea is reported in 35% of cases and a nonproductive cough in 10–15% [18]. Less common but documented manifestations include chest pain, fever, weight loss, wheezing, palpitations, and back pain [18]. Physical examination typically reveals diminished, and at times coarse, breath sounds at the bases of affected lungs, with dullness to percussion over areas of effusion.

Diagnosis

There is currently no single definitive test for the diagnosis of BAPE. A thorough occupational history is essential to document potential asbestos exposure [2, 3, 14, 15, 19, 24, 58, 59]. While imaging studies play a critical role in the diagnostic process, they are not sufficient by themselves to confirm the disease. Evaluation of pleural fluid to rule out infection and malignancy, combined with stable findings on follow-up imaging, contributes to establishing the diagnosis [14, 19, 58, 60].

Pulmonary function testing to assess dyspnea does not contribute to the diagnosis of BAPE; however, results commonly indicate a reduction in vital capacity to less than 60% of predicted values or a decrease in the forced expiratory volume in 1 s (FEV1) to below 50% of predicted [61]. Ultrasonography serves primarily to quantify the volume of fluid present in cases of BAPE. Certain ultrasonographic features may also be observed with pleural plaques, which frequently co-occur with BAPE. Calcified pleural plaques may display a comet-tail sign, with or without linear artifacts, though these are considered nonspecific findings [62, 63].

Chest radiographs typically reveal pleural effusions in patients with the condition. The volume of effusion generally measures less than 1000 mL, although reported values range from 200 to 2000 mL [4, 15, 22, 24, 59]. BAPE most frequently presents with unilateral effusions; however, one review noted that 27% of cases involved bilateral effusions [64]. Pleural plaques, predominantly affecting the parietal pleura, are observed in approximately 90% of BAPE cases, and about 75% of these plaques exhibit calcifications [18]. Diffuse pleural thickening, characterized by substantial thickening of both the parietal and visceral pleura with partial obliteration of the pleural space, is present in roughly 25% of cases [11, 18]. Rounded atelectasis is identified in 37% of BAPE cases [18].

Computed tomography (CT) provides enhanced visualization of features identified on chest radiographs and offers greater diagnostic detail for distinguishing between conditions such as mesothelioma and benign asbestos pleural effusion (BAPE) (Fig. 12.1a, b). Mediastinal pleural plaques, which typically do not occur in BAPE, have a positive predictive value of 89% for mesothelioma when present [65, 66]. Intraparenchymal pleural plaques are observed in 55% of mesothelioma cases [65]. Pleural nodularity on CT imaging is also indicative of malignancy rather than BAPE [67]. Additionally, contrast-enhanced CT is useful for detecting prominent lymphadenopathy, further supporting the diagnosis of mesothelioma over BAPE.

Positron emission tomography (PET) is valuable for assessing pleural effusions and identifying pleural irregularities to help exclude malignancy [14, 68]. Effusions associated with benign asbestos pleural effusion generally present with low standard uptake values (SUV), typically less than 0.8, whereas mesothelioma-associated effusions exhibit SUV values greater than 2 [68, 69]. When using an SUV threshold of greater than 2.2, PET imaging achieves a sensitivity of 94% and a specificity approaching 100% in differentiating mesothelioma from BAPE [68].

Evaluation of pleural fluid is essential for accurate diagnosis, with exudative fluid being characteristic of BAPE. The presence of a transudate effectively excludes BAPE from consideration. In most cases (approximately 79%), the pleural fluid is grossly bloody, though it may also appear serosanguinous or serous [1, 3, 22, 59, 70]. Analysis typically reveals a lymphocyte-predominant white blood cell differential; however, neutrophils or eosinophils may predominate in certain instances [14, 18, 22, 24]. Notably, the absence of eosinophilia does not exclude a diagnosis of BAPE.

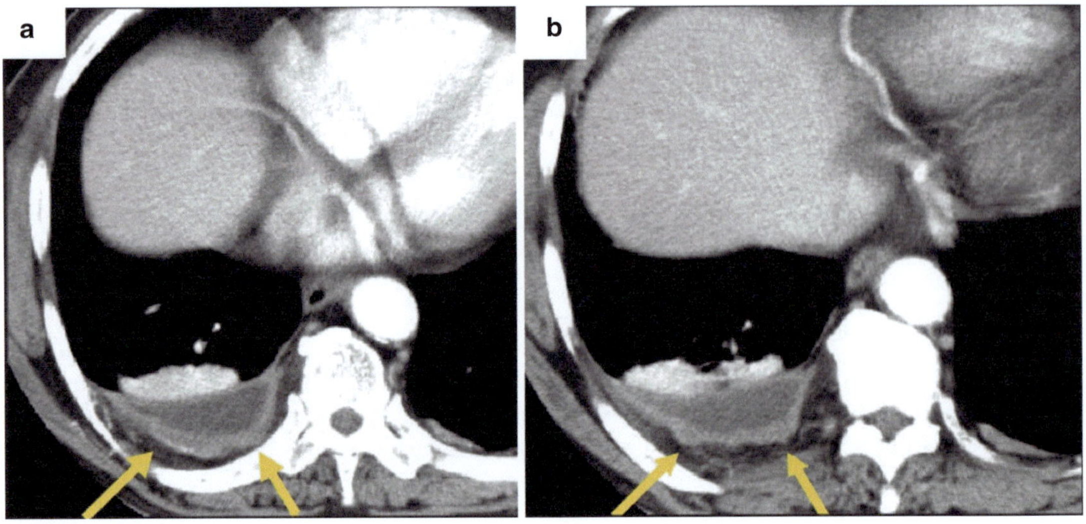

Fig. 12.1 Radiologic evolution of benign asbestos pleural effusion (BAPE)
(**a**) Axial computed tomography (CT) at diagnosis showing irregular pleural thickening (yellow arrows) with an associated small pleural effusion and adjacent compressive atelectasis
(**b**) Follow-up axial CT obtained 5 years later at the same level, demonstrating persistent irregular pleural thickening (yellow arrows) with no interval progression
Attribution: Reprinted from *European Journal of Radiology*, Vol 85(9), Kato K., Gemba K., Fujimoto N., Aoe K., Takeshima Y., Inai K., Kishimoto T., "Pleural irregularities and mediastinal pleural involvement in early stages of malignant pleural mesothelioma and benign asbestos pleural effusion," pp. 1594–1600, Copyright © 2016 Elsevier Ireland Ltd. Reproduced by permission of Elsevier through RightsLink License No. 6132630356063 for *Rare Pleural Disease* (Springer Nature, 2026). All rights reserved. No further reproduction or distribution is permitted without permission from Elsevier

Cultures should be obtained from all samples to exclude infectious etiologies. Adenosine deaminase (ADA) levels may show slight elevation, but values exceeding 35 IU/L are more indicative of tuberculosis infection [71]. Pleural fluid cytology also helps differentiate between BAPE and malignancy. However, negative cytology alone is insufficient, as the diagnostic yield for initial thoracentesis in malignant effusions is approximately 60%, and even lower for mesothelioma at 30% [70, 72–75].

Biomarkers indicative of malignancy can also be identified in pleural fluid. An elevated carcinoembryonic antigen (CEA) level may indicate the presence of malignancy [71]. Furthermore, intrapleural hyaluronic acid (HA) concentrations can be markedly increased in mesothelioma, often exceeding 70,000 ng/mL, but can also be elevated in BAPE [71, 76]. Soluble mesothelin-related peptide (SMRP) levels may be elevated in mesothelioma and in BAPE [77, 78].

Secretory leukocyte peptidase inhibitor (SLPI) has emerged as a valuable biomarker for differentiating benign asbestos pleural effusion from mesothelioma and other malignant effusions. SLPI is typically present in mucosal epithelial cells, where it plays a role in protecting tissues from excessive inflammatory damage while preserving antimicrobial defense. Elevated SLPI levels have been observed in cancer physiology, potentially shielding malignant cells from immune-mediated destruction. In BAPE effusions, SLPI concentrations are modestly increased (57.8 ± 25.7 ng/mL). In contrast, higher levels are noted in mesothelioma (173 ± 134.5 ng/mL), lung cancer effusions (103.5 ± 85.7 ng/mL), and non-lung cancer effusions (124.8 ± 12.9 ng/mL) [79]. While SLPI shows promise as a tool to distinguish BAPE from malignant conditions, its application remains primarily research-based, and clinical testing is not yet widely accessible.

To ensure an accurate diagnosis of BAPE, it is necessary to exclude underlying malignancy. Patients with BAPE often have pleural irregularities, and it is recommended to obtain a pleural biopsy [14, 19]. Histological evaluation of BAPE typically reveals pleural fibrosis accompanied by inflammatory cell infiltration and fibroblast proliferation [2, 19]. Image-guided biopsy techniques, such as thoracoscopy, either direct or video-assisted thoracoscopic surgery, are preferred over blind pleural biopsy to exclude malignancy [80, 81]. Image-guided needle biopsies achieve diagnostic yields nearing 85% for mesothelioma [80]. Thoracoscopy, both video-assisted and direct, is considered the gold standard for pleural tissue sampling, with a yield approaching 97% [73, 75, 82, 83]. Thoracotomy is not advised for pleural biopsy as it does not improve diagnostic yield and carries increased risk of complications [84]. Once malignancy has been initially excluded, repeat imaging should be performed after 3 months [14]. Features suggestive of malignancy include progressive pleural thickening, new involvement of the mediastinal pleura, or plaques that appear to encase the ipsilateral thorax. Patients exhibiting these findings should be considered for tissue sampling [14, 19, 85].

Treatment

Management of BAPE effusions following diagnosis has demonstrated variability. Initial thoracentesis provides both diagnostic clarification and therapeutic relief. Approximately 30% of patients experience resolution of BAPE after this initial procedure [2]. In instances of fluid re-accumulation, recurrence typically occurs within 4–6 months post-drainage, and effusions may return at similar or increased volumes [2]. Notably, evacuating the pleural space in BAPE does not improve overall patient outcomes; fluid drainage is indicated solely for symptom alleviation. Drainage is not recommended in asymptomatic individuals.

The use of intrapleural catheters for symptomatic pleural effusions has expanded to benign etiologies beyond malignancy [82, 86]; however, there is currently insufficient evidence regarding their efficacy or safety in BAPE specifically. Persistent symptoms associated with recurrent effusion warrant a thorough evaluation for additional pathologies such as trapped lung, heart failure, or renal failure, given that BAPE typically does not accumulate rapidly. Pleurodesis has been employed to reduce recurrence in other benign effusions [75, 87, 88]. Nevertheless, patients exposed to asbestos at levels sufficient to develop BAPE remain at elevated risk for mesothelioma.

Prognosis

The prognosis for patients diagnosed with Benign Asbestos Pleural Effusion is generally favorable. In many cases, effusions resolve spontaneously within 4–12 months [2]. Initial drainage typically suffices for permanent resolution; however, recurrence rates of 28–36% have been reported [2, 15]. Radiologic surveillance over a 2-year period is recommended for optimal management [89]. Individuals with BAPE frequently present with other pulmonary conditions attributable to asbestos exposure and are at elevated risk for developing diffuse pleural thickening, which may lead to respiratory compromise and mortality [11, 18, 90]. A case series indicated a median post-diagnosis survival of 103 months, though causes of death were unrelated directly to the effusion [2].

Historical research on asbestos-related effusions preceding the establishment of BAPE as a distinct diagnosis followed patients over varying periods, averaging 6 years [2, 3, 5, 15, 17, 18, 22, 61]. In a series of 56 observed individuals, only one patient developed mesothelioma, which was not directly linked to the effusion [2, 15]. Once benign pleura has been confirmed surrounding the fluid, repeated sampling for malignancy offers no clinical benefit in the absence of imaging changes [14, 18]. The diagnosis of BAPE does not independently increase the risk of subsequent mesothelioma or lung cancer; any increased risk of malignancy is attributable solely to asbestos exposure rather than the effusion itself. Comparisons between cancer risk among

BAPE patients and those exposed to asbestos without BAPE are limited by insufficient sample sizes.

References

1. Eisenstadt HB. Asbestos pleurisy. Dis Chest. 1964;46(1):78–81.
2. Robinson BW, Musk AW. Benign asbestos pleural effusion: diagnosis and course. Thorax. 1981;36(12):896–900.
3. Gaensler E, Kaplan A. Asbestos pleural effusions. Ann Intern Med. 1971;74:2.
4. Myers R. Asbestos-related pleural disease. Curr Opin Pulm Med. 2012;18(4):377–81.
5. Ferrer J, Balcells E, Orriols R, Villarino MA, Drobnic Z, Morell F. Benign asbestos pleural effusion. Report of a first series in Spain. Med Clin (Barc). 1996;107(14):535–8.
6. Fishwick D, Barber CM. Non-malignant asbestos-related diseases: a clinical view. Clin Med. 2014;14(1):68–71.
7. Cooke WE. Fibrosis of the lungs due to the inhalation of asbestos dust. BMJ. 1924;2(3317):147–0.
8. Wagner GR. Asbestosis and silicosis. Lancet. 1997;349(9061):1311–5.
9. Merewether ERA, Price CW. Report on effects of asbestos on the lungs and dust suppression in dust the asbestos industry. London; 1930.
10. Elmes PC. The epidemiology and clinical features of asbestosis and related diseases. Postgrad Med J. 1966;42(492):623–35.
11. McLoud T, Woods B, Carrington C, Epler G, Gaensler E. Diffuse pleural thickening in an asbestos-exposed population: prevalence and causes. Am J Roentgenol. 1985;144(1):9–18.
12. Brodkin CA, Barnhart S, Anderson G, Checkoway H, Omenn GS, Rosenstock L. Correlation between respiratory symptoms and pulmonary function in asbestos-exposed workers. Am Rev Respir Dis. 1993;148(1):32–7.
13. Jamrozik E, de Klerk N, Musk AW. Asbestos-related disease. Intern Med J. 2011;41(5):372–80.
14. Kishimoto T, Fujimoto N, Mizuhashi K, Kozawa S, Miura M. Retrospective investigation on diagnostic process for benign asbestos pleural effusion (BAPE) using checklist. J Occup Health. 2020;62(1).
15. Epler GR, McLoud TC, Gaensler EA. Prevalence and incidence of benign asbestos pleural effusion in a working population. JAMA. 1982;247(5):617–22.
16. Hughes JM, Weill H. Asbestos exposure – quantitative assessment of risk 1– 3. Am Rev Respir Dis. 1986;133(1):5–13.
17. Cvitanović S, Znaor L, Konsa T, Ivancević Z, Perić I, Erceg M, et al. Malignant and non-malignant asbestos-related pleural and lung disease: 10-year follow-up study. Croat Med J. 2003;44(5):618–25.
18. Fujimoto N, Gemba K, Aoe K, Kato K, Yokoyama T, Usami I, et al. Clinical investigation of benign asbestos pleural effusion. Pulm Med. 2015;2015:1–6.
19. Luo W, Zeng Y, Shen P, Wu X, Wang J, Zhang X. A multidisciplinary approach for the diagnosis of benign asbestos pleural effusion: a single-center experience. J Thorac Dis. 2020;12(8):4338–46.
20. Kishimoto T, Okahara M, Chikamori K, Ozaki S, Aoe K, Ohke M, et al. Clinical evaluation of benign asbestos pleurisy. Nihon Kokyuki Gakkai Zasshi. 1998;36(1):18–22.
21. Musk AW, de Klerk N, Reid A, Hui J, Franklin P, Brims F. Asbestos-related diseases. Int J Tuberc Lung Dis. 2020;24(6):562–7.
22. Hillerdal G, Ozesmi M. Benign asbestos pleural effusion: 73 exudates in 60 patients. Eur J Respir Dis. 1987;71(2):113–21.
23. Goldberg M, Luce D. The health impact of nonoccupational exposure to asbestos: what do we know? Eur J Cancer Prev. 2009;18(6):489–503.
24. Martensson G, Hagberg S, Pettersson K, Thiringer G. Asbestos pleural effusion: a clinical entity. Thorax. 1987;42(9):646–51.
25. Cookson WO, De Klerk NH, Musk AW, Glancy JJ, Armstrong BK, Hobbs MS. Benign and malignant pleural effusions in former Wittenoom crocidolite millers and miners. Aust NZ J Med. 1985;15(6):731–7.
26. Dement J. Estimation of dose and evalueation of dose-response in a retrospective cohort mortality study of chrysotile asbestos textile workers. University of North Carolina at Chapel Hill; 1980.
27. Prazakova S, Thomas PS, Sandrini A, Yates DH. Asbestos and the lung in the 21st century: an update. Clin Respir J. 2014;8(1):1–10.
28. Juon HS, Hong A, Pimpinelli M, Rojulpote M, McIntire R, Barta JA. Racial disparities in occupational risks and lung cancer incidence: analysis of the National Lung Screening Trial. Prev Med (Baltim). 2021;143:106355.
29. Ernst P, Zejda J. Mineral fibers and health. Boca Raton: CRC; 1991. 121–34 p.
30. Occupational Safety and Health Standards. 1910 Subpart Z May 14, 2019.
31. Belackova L, Verbeek JH, Hoving JL, van der Molen HF, Gagliardi D, Curti S, et al. Personal protective equipment for preventing asbestos exposure in workers. Cochrane Database Syst Rev. 2024;2024(5)
32. Marsh GM, Riordan AS, Keeton KA, Benson SM. Non-occupational exposure to asbestos and risk of pleural mesothelioma: review and meta-analysis. Occup Environ Med. 2017;74(11):838–46.
33. Hansen J, de Klerk NH, Musk AW, Hobbs MST. Environmental exposure to crocidolite and mesothelioma. Am J Respir Crit Care Med. 1998;157(1):69–75.
34. Lee EK, Kim JS, Kim Y, Park JS. CT findings in people who were environmentally exposed to asbestos in Korea. J Korean Med Sci. 2015;30(12):1896.

35. Balbay EG, Kayalar Ö, Balbay Ö, Dikensoy Ö, Arbak P, Bayram H. Impact of earthquakes on lung health. Thoracic Res Pract. 2024;25(2):89–98.
36. Visonà SD, Capella S, Borrelli P, Villani S, Favaron C, Kurzhunbaeva Z, et al. Asbestos burden in lungs of non-occupationally exposed women from Broni (Pavia, Italy): a postmortem SEM-EDS study. J Thorac Dis. 2023;15(12):6555–69.
37. Liu G, Cheresh P, Kamp DW. Molecular basis of asbestos-induced lung disease. Annu Rev Pathol Mech Dis. 2013;8(1):161–87.
38. Mishra A, Hogan SP, Brandt EB, Rothenberg ME. An etiological role for aeroallergens and eosinophils in experimental esophagitis. J Clin Invest. 2001;107(1):83–90.
39. Kalomenidis I, Light RW. Pathogenesis of the eosinophilic pleural effusions. Curr Opin Pulm Med. 2004;10(4):289–93.
40. Frank AL. Global problems from exposure to asbestos. Environ Health Perspect. 1993;101(suppl 3):165–7.
41. U.S. Environmental Protection Agency. Risk evaluation for asbestos: part 2 – supplemental evaluation including legacy uses and associated disposals of asbestos. Washington (DC): U.S. EPA; 2024.
42. Mossman BT, Churg A. Mechanisms in the pathogenesis of asbestosis and silicosis. Am J Respir Crit Care Med. 1998;157(5 Pt 1):1666–80.
43. Kumagai-Takei N, Yamamoto S, Lee S, Maeda M, Masuzzaki H, Sada N, et al. Inflammatory alteration of human t cells exposed continuously to asbestos. Int J Mol Sci. 2018;19(2):504.
44. Peacock C, Copley SJ, Hansell DM. Asbestos-related benign pleural disease. Clin Radiol. 2000;55(6):422–32.
45. Rosmus J, Vančíková O, Marc J, Deyl Z. Studies on the structure of collagen V. The site of binding of trivalent iron on collagen. Experientia. 1967;23(11):898.
46. Poser I, Rahman Q, Lohani M, Yadav S, Becker HH, Weiss DG, et al. Modulation of genotoxic effects in asbestos-exposed primary human mesothelial cells by radical scavengers, metal chelators and a glutathione precursor. Mutat Res Genet Toxicol Environ Mutagen. 2004;559(1–2):19–27.
47. Ghio AJ, Soukup JM, Dailey LA, Richards JH, Tong H. The biological effect of asbestos exposure is dependent on changes in iron homeostasis. Inhal Toxicol. 2016;28(14):698–705.
48. Ghio AJ, Stewart M, Sangani RG, Pavlisko EN, Roggli VL. Asbestos and iron. Int J Mol Sci. 2023;24(15):12390.
49. Shukla A, Ramos-Nino M, Mossman B. Cell signaling and transcription factor activation by asbestos in lung injury and disease. Int J Biochem Cell Biol. 2003;35(8):1198–209.
50. Kumagai-Takei N, Lee S, Srinivas B, Shimizu Y, Sada N, Yoshitome K, et al. The effects of asbestos fibers on human T cells. Int J Mol Sci. 2020;21(19):6987.
51. Chen F, Sun S, Kuhn DC, Gaydos LJ, Shi X, Lu Y, et al. Involvement of NF-kappaB in silica-induced cyclooxygenase II gene expression in rat alveolar macrophages. Am J Phys Lung Cell Mol Phys. 1997;272(4):L779–86.
52. Bunda S, Kaviani N, Hinek A. Fluctuations of intracellular iron modulate elastin production. J Biol Chem. 2005;280(3):2341–51.
53. Gardi C, Arezzini B, Fortino V, Comporti M. Effect of free iron on collagen synthesis, cell proliferation and MMP-2 expression in rat hepatic stellate cells. Biochem Pharmacol. 2002;64(7):1139–45.
54. Ikeda H, Wu GY, Wu CH. Evidence that an iron chelator regulates collagen synthesis by decreasing the stability of procollagen mRNA. Hepatology. 1992;15(2):282–7.
55. Kinberger GA, Taulane JP, Goodman M. Fe (III) -binding collagen mimetics. Inorg Chem. 2006;45(3):961–3.
56. Sannes PL. Cytochemical visualization of anions in collagenous and elastic fiber-associated connective tissue matrix in neonatal and adult rat lungs using iron-containing stains. Histochemistry. 1986;84(1):49–56.
57. Churg AM, Warnock ML. Asbestos and other ferruginous bodies: their formation and clinical significance. Am J Pathol. 1981;102(3):447–56.
58. Guidotti TL, Miller A, Christiani D, Wagner G, Balmes J, Harber P, et al. Diagnosis and initial management of nonmalignant diseases related to asbestos. Am J Respir Crit Care Med. 2004;170:691–715.
59. Rosenstock L, Hudson LD. The pleural manifestations of asbestos exposure. Occup Med. 1987;2(2):383–407.
60. Luo W, Zeng Y, Shen P, He J, Wang J. Diagnostic procedure for idiopathic eosinophilic pleural effusion: a single-center experience. BMC Pulm Med. 2020;20(1):82.
61. Kishimoto T, Kato K, Ashizawa K, Kurihara Y, Tokuyama T, Sakai F. A retrospective study on radiological findings of diffuse pleural thickening with benign asbestos pleural effusion in Japanese cases. Ind Health. 2022;60(5):429–35.
62. Morgan RA, Pickworth FE, Dubbins PA, McGavin CR. The ultrasound appearance of asbestos-related pleural plaques. Clin Radiol. 1991;44(6):413–6.
63. Smargiassi A, Pasciuto G, Pedicelli I, Lo Greco E, Calvello M, Inchingolo R, et al. Chest ultrasonography in health surveillance of asbestos-related lung diseases. Toxicol Ind Health. 2017;33(6):537–46.
64. Jeebun V, Stenton SC. The presentation and natural history of asbestos-induced diffuse pleural thickening. Occup Med (Chic Ill). 2012;62(4):266–8.
65. Araki T, Yanagawa M, Sun FJ, Dupuis J, Nishino M, Yamada Y, et al. Pleural abnormalities in the Framingham heart study: prevalence and CT image features. Occup Environ Med. 2017;74(10):756–61.
66. Yamada A, Taiji R, Nishimoto Y, Itoh T, Marugami A, Yamauchi S, et al. Pictorial review of pleural disease: multimodality imaging and differential diagnosis. Radiographics. 2024;44(4).

67. Traill ZC, Davies RJO, Gleeson FV. Thoracic computed tomography in patients with suspected malignant pleural effusions. Clin Radiol. 2001;56(3):193–6.
68. Yildirim H, Metintas M, Entok E, Ak G, Ak I, Dundar E, et al. Clinical value of Fluorodeoxyglucose-positron emission tomography/computed tomography in differentiation of malignant mesothelioma from asbestos-related benign pleural disease: an observational pilot study. J Thorac Oncol. 2009;4(12):1480–4.
69. Kruse M, Sherry SJ, Paidpally V, Mercier G, Subramaniam RM. FDG PET/CT in the management of primary pleural tumors and pleural metastases. Am J Roentgenol. 2013;201(2):W215–26.
70. American Thoracic Society. Diagnosis and initial management of nonmalignant diseases related to asbestos. Am J Respir Crit Care Med. 2004;170(6):691–715.
71. Kishimoto T, Kojima Y, Fujimoto N. Significance of secretory leukocyte peptidase inhibitor in pleural fluid for the diagnosis of benign asbestos pleural effusion. Sci Rep. 2021;11(1):12965.
72. Brun C, Gay P, Cottier M, Karpathiou G, Patoir A, Tiffet O, et al. Comparison of cytology, chest computed and positron emission tomography findings in malignant pleural effusion from lung cancer. J Thorac Dis. 2018;10(12):6903–11.
73. Asciak R, Rahman NM. Malignant Pleural Effusion. Clin Chest Med. 2018;39(1):181–93.
74. Porcel JM, Hernández P, Martínez-Alonso M, Bielsa S, Salud A. Accuracy of fluorodeoxyglucose-PET imaging for differentiating benign from malignant pleural effusions. Chest. 2015;147(2):502–12.
75. Dixit R, Agarwal K, Gokhroo A, Patil C, Meena M, Shah N, et al. Diagnosis and management options in malignant pleural effusions. Lung India. 2017;34(2):160.
76. Fujimoto N, Gemba K, Asano M, Fuchimoto Y, Wada S, Ono K, et al. Hyaluronic acid in the pleural fluid of patients with malignant pleural mesothelioma. Respir Investig. 2013;51(2):92–7.
77. Gao R, Wang F, Wang Z, Wu Y, Xu L, Qin Y, et al. Diagnostic value of soluble mesothelin-related peptides in pleural effusion for malignant pleural mesothelioma. Medicine. 2019;98(14):e14979.
78. Fujimoto N, Gemba K, Asano M, Wada S, Ono K, Ozaki S, et al. Soluble mesothelin-related protein in pleural effusion from patients with malignant pleural mesothelioma. Exp Ther Med. 2010;1(2):313–7.
79. Nugteren S, Samsom JN. Secretory leukocyte protease inhibitor (SLPI) in mucosal tissues: protects against inflammation, but promotes cancer. Cytokine Growth Factor Rev. 2021;59:22–35.
80. Maskell N, Gleeson F, Davies R. Standard pleural biopsy versus CT-guided cutting-needle biopsy for diagnosis of malignant disease in pleural effusions: a randomised controlled trial. Lancet. 2003;361(9366):1326–30.
81. Maturu VN, Dhooria S, Bal A, Singh N, Aggarwal AN, Gupta D, et al. Role of medical thoracoscopy and closed-blind pleural biopsy in undiagnosed exudative pleural effusions. J Bronchol Interv Pulmonol. 2015;22(2):121–9.
82. Agrawal A, Murgu S. Multimodal approach to the management of malignant pleural effusions: role of thoracoscopy with pleurodesis and tunneled indwelling pleural catheters. J Thorac Dis. 2020;12(5):2803–11.
83. Wrightson JM, Davies HE. Outcome of patients with nonspecific pleuritis at thoracoscopy. Curr Opin Pulm Med. 2011;17(4):242–6.
84. Shojaee S, Lee HJ. Thoracoscopy: medical versus surgical-in the management of pleural diseases. J Thorac Dis. 2015;7(Suppl 4):S339–51.
85. Scherpereel A, Opitz I, Berghmans T, Psallidas I, Glatzer M, Rigau D, et al. ERS/ESTS/EACTS/ESTRO guidelines for the management of malignant pleural mesothelioma. Eur Respir J. 2020;55(6):1900953.
86. Patil M, Dhillon SS, Attwood K, Saoud M, Alraiyes AH, Harris K. Management of benign pleural effusions using indwelling pleural catheters. Chest. 2017;151(3):626–35.
87. Medford A, Maskell N. Pleural effusion. Postgrad Med J. 2005;81(961):702–10.
88. Gibson PG, Abramson M, Wood-Baker R, Volmink J, Hensley M, Costabel U, editors. Evidence-based respiratory medicine. Wiley; 2005.
89. Bintcliffe OJ, Lee GYC, Rahman NM, Maskell NA. The management of benign non-infective pleural effusions. Eur Respir Rev. 2016;25(141):303–16.
90. Hara R, Yano Y, Okabe F, Kuge T, Mori M, Urasaki K. Radiographic change over 11 years in a patient with asbestos-related pleural disease. Respirol Case Rep. 2020;8(7).

Lymphomatous Pleural Effusion

13

Benjamin Fleming and Toribiong Uchel

Introduction

Lymphomas are among the most common hematologic malignancies associated with pleural disease, frequently presenting with pleural effusion [1]. Lymphoma-related pleural effusion (LPE) can occur at any stage of the lymphoproliferative process and is more prevalent in non-Hodgkin lymphoma (NHL), affecting up to 20% of cases, compared with an incidence of approximately 7% in Hodgkin lymphoma (HL) [2, 3]. In NHL, the pleural effusion may even represent the initial manifestation of disease [4]. Both HL and NHL can produce malignant or benign effusions, particularly in cases involving mediastinal lymph node enlargement [2]. Of all malignant pleural effusions, nearly 10% are attributable to either HL or NHL [2, 5]. The mechanisms underlying LPE include direct malignant infiltration, lymphatic obstruction, or secondary pulmonary infection [5].

Most lymphomatous effusions are exudative, although transudative effusions have occasionally been reported. In a retrospective study spanning 1993–2002, Ahmed et al. demonstrated that 88% of patients with lymphoproliferative disease and pleural effusion had exudative effusions [5]. In addition, lymphoma, particularly NHL, is a well-recognized cause of chylothorax, which requires targeted management to reduce chyle formation and pleural accumulation, alongside disease-directed therapy [6]. Indeed, malignancy remains the leading cause of nontraumatic chylothorax, with lymphoma accounting for approximately 70% of cases [7].

Two distinct lymphoma subtypes are particularly associated with pleural involvement, primary effusion lymphoma (PEL), and pyothorax-associated lymphoma (PAL). Both are rare, aggressive B-cell NHL variants that typically present as serous cavity effusions without a solid mass [8]. PEL, formerly known as *body cavity lymphoma*, is characterized by malignant effusions within the pleural, pericardial, or peritoneal spaces and occurs predominantly in immunocompromised individuals, especially those with advanced acquired immunodeficiency syndrome (AIDS) and human herpesvirus-8 (HHV-8) infection. PAL, first described in 1987, develops in patients with long-standing pyothorax, most often secondary to therapeutic pneumothorax for tuberculous pleuritis [9]. It has been identified during thoracoscopic evaluation as a pleural mass with plasmablastic lymphoma morphology. Unlike PEL, PAL is typically mass-forming and demonstrates a greater tendency for local invasion and dissemination [10].

B. Fleming
Department of Pulmonary and Critical Care, Rochester General Hospital, Rochester, NY, USA

T. Uchel (✉)
Division of Pulmonary and Critical Care, Department of Internal Medicine, Virginia Commonwealth University, Richmond, VA, USA
e-mail: uchelt@vcu.edu

F. Ido (ed.), *Rare Pleural Diseases*, https://doi.org/10.1007/978-3-032-14873-5_13

Pathophysiology

Lymphoma-related pleural effusions are predominantly exudative, though they may occasionally present as transudates in cases of venous or lymphatic obstruction [2]. Lower-grade lymphomas can cause transudative effusions secondary to extrathoracic manifestations such as hypoalbuminemia, renal dysfunction, or congestive heart failure [2].

Exudative effusions in lymphomatous malignancies are most often attributed to impaired lymphatic drainage caused by mediastinal lymphadenopathy or thoracic duct obstruction [11]. Direct pleural involvement, particularly in non-Hodgkin lymphoma, represents the primary pathogenic mechanism of effusion formation. NHL-related pleural effusions are typically exudative and may result from malignant pleural infiltration, chylothorax, impaired lymphatic return, or secondary infection [12]. Pleural fluid analysis commonly demonstrates a lymphocyte-predominant profile, closely resembling that of tuberculous effusions [13]. Chylothorax occurs more frequently in NHL than in Hodgkin lymphoma and usually results from thoracic duct obstruction [14]. Mediastinal lymphadenopathy from lymphoproliferative disease can also compress central lymphatic channels, impeding chyle flow and leading to chylous accumulation within the pleural space [7].

The precise mechanism of effusion formation in primary effusion lymphoma remains uncertain. Aoki and Tosato proposed that markedly elevated vascular endothelial growth factor (VEGF) levels, up to 50,000 times more potent than histamine, induce increased vascular permeability, thereby promoting effusion formation. Elevated VEGF production is stimulated by human herpesvirus-8 infection of Kaposi sarcoma-like spindle cells, which drives VEGF secretion [15].

Pyothorax-associated lymphoma was initially described in Japanese patients who had undergone therapeutic pneumothoraces for pulmonary tuberculosis, later developing chronic pyothorax persisting for over two decades [9]. PAL is strongly associated with Epstein–Barr virus (EBV) infection and is hypothesized to result from p53 mutation in EBV-infected lymphocytes within the chronically inflamed pleural cavity. The loss of tumor suppressor p53 function permits uncontrolled B-lymphocyte proliferation and survival, driving lymphomagenesis in this setting [16].

Epidemiology

Lung and breast carcinomas account for approximately 50–65% of malignant pleural effusions (MPEs); however, lymphoma represents the third most common etiology, occurring in about 20% of patients with lymphoma [2, 5]. In both non-Hodgkin lymphoma and Hodgkin lymphoma, pleural effusion is often present at the time of diagnosis and typically reflects widespread lymphatic involvement. Notably, up to 90% of HL patients with pleural effusion also demonstrate mediastinal lymphadenopathy, while in NHL, the presence of effusion frequently indicates advanced, disseminated nodal disease [2].

Pleural effusion occurs in approximately 20% of patients with NHL [2]. Among lymphoma-associated effusions, primary effusion lymphoma is exceedingly rare, representing about 4% of HIV-associated NHL cases and <1% of non-HIV-associated lymphomas [17, 18]. Patients with PEL are predominantly male and often have HIV infection or other immunosuppressive conditions, including cirrhosis or solid-organ transplantation [18]. Epstein–Barr virus coinfection is also common in these patients.

Pyothorax-associated lymphoma was first described in Japanese patients with chronic pyothorax persisting for 20–64 years [9]. Subsequent cases have been reported globally, including in France and Italy. While most PAL cases followed artificial pneumothorax therapy for pulmonary tuberculosis, nontuberculous cases and even one associated with pulmonary asbestosis have been documented. PAL exhibits a marked male predominance, and over 50% of patients present with a large pleural mass exceeding 10 cm in diameter [9].

Clinical Presentation

Symptoms of lymphoma-related pleural disease vary depending on the lymphoma subtype, disease burden, and tumor aggressiveness. The classic B symptoms, fever, night sweats, and unintentional weight loss, may be present, reflecting systemic inflammatory activity. Many patients exhibit non-tender, firm lymphadenopathy, which is often generalized or localized to the mediastinum. Intrathoracic involvement should be suspected when respiratory symptoms, such as dyspnea or cough, develop, whereas pleuritic chest pain typically suggests direct pleural infiltration.

Bulky mediastinal disease can lead to airway compression, manifesting as localized wheezing near the site of obstruction, tachypnea, or stridor. Superior vena cava (SVC) syndrome may occur secondary to mediastinal venous obstruction, resulting in facial plethora, distended neck veins, and upper extremity edema.

In cases of chylothorax, rapid loss of chyle into the pleural cavity can precipitate hypovolemia and dyspnea. With chronic losses, patients may develop malnutrition due to depletion of macronutrients, vitamins, and electrolytes [7]. Furthermore, immunoglobulin loss through the chyle predisposes patients to opportunistic infections as a result of secondary immunosuppression [19].

Diagnosis

The diagnostic process for lymphomatous pleural effusion typically begins with the identification of pleural fluid on chest radiography. In Hodgkin lymphoma, effusions are almost invariably accompanied by mediastinal lymphadenopathy [20]. In contrast, non-Hodgkin lymphoma effusions are generally unilateral and left-sided, though bilateral presentations can occur [21]. Chylothorax, however, is usually right-sided because the thoracic duct predominantly traverses the right hemithorax. The duct crosses to the left at the T4–T6 vertebral level, and thus obstruction at or above this crossover can lead to left-sided or bilateral chylothorax [19]. On chest radiograph, mediastinal widening suggests lymphadenopathy, while pleural thickening and parenchymal opacities may also be evident [22]. Although radiographic differentiation between HL and NHL is not feasible, their patterns of involvement differ: HL often presents with bulky superior mediastinal masses, whereas NHL may involve pulmonary parenchyma without central lymphadenopathy. Cases of NHL presenting solely with pleural effusion are uncommon [22].

Chest radiograph typically demonstrates a unilateral, small to moderate pleural effusion, situated within the dependent portions of the lung (Fig. 13.1a). Computed tomography (CT) provides greater anatomic resolution than radiography and may reveal peribronchovascular thickening, pleural or parenchymal nodules or thickening, or masses (Fig. 13.1b). Contrast-enhanced CT is preferred for precise delineation of lymph nodes, enabling accurate measurement and differentiation from adjacent vascular structures [23]. Multiple abnormalities are often identified, though CT attenuation values cannot distinguish between transudative and exudative effusions. Nonetheless, features such as fluid loculation, pleural thickening, and pleural nodularity are more suggestive of exudates. In chylothorax, CT attenuation of chyle does not reliably differentiate it from other effusions; however, visualization of thoracic duct compression strongly supports the diagnosis. CT lymphangiography, involving direct contrast injection into the cisterna chyli, may precisely identify the site of chyle leakage [19].

Positron emission tomography-computed tomography (PET/CT) with F-18 fluorodeoxyglucose (FDG) is integral to the diagnostic workup and staging of lymphoma. PET/CT facilitates visualization of metabolically active sites, including lymph nodes, pulmonary parenchyma, and the pleural lining, which are frequently involved in LPE [23, 24].

Thoracic ultrasound offers additional evaluation of pleural fluid characteristics. Transudates typically appear anechoic (noncomplex), while exudates may appear echogenic or complex, occasionally demonstrating septations, pleural

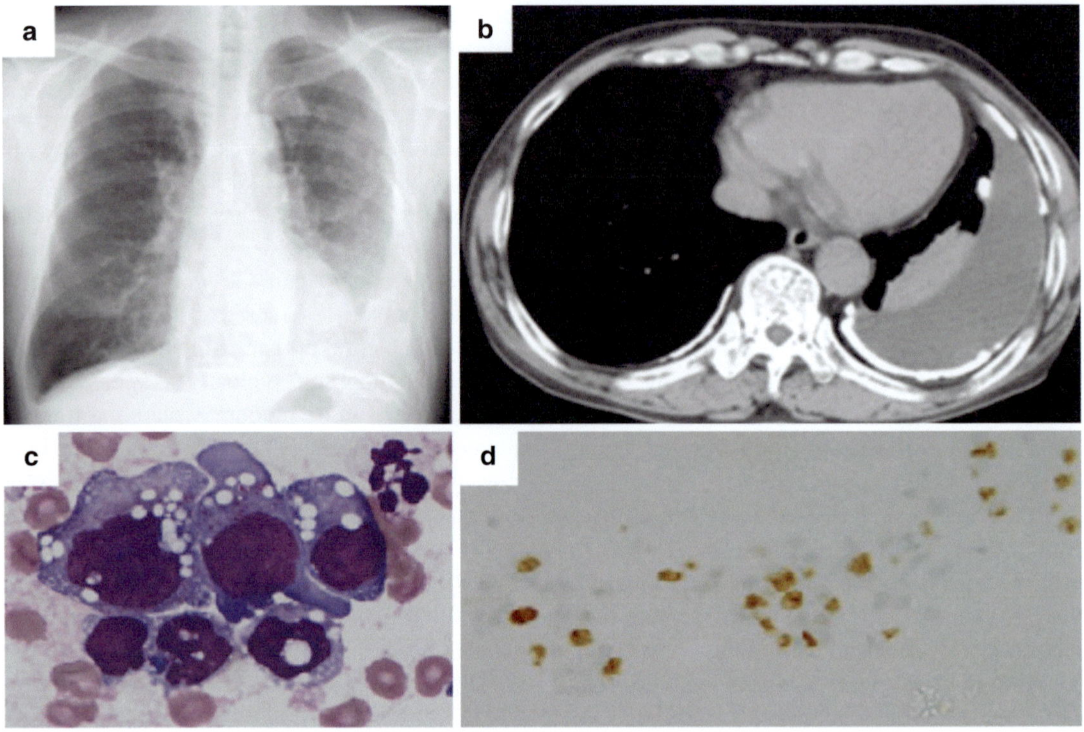

Fig. 13.1 Radiologic and cytopathologic findings of lymphomatous pleural effusion in a patient with prior asbestos exposure and diffuse large B-cell lymphoma. (**a**) Chest radiograph showing an irregular left basal opacity and blunting of the costodiaphragmatic angle consistent with a pleural effusion. (**b**) Axial contrast-enhanced computed tomography (CT) image demonstrating a homogeneous left pleural effusion with adjacent pleural thickening and scattered calcifications. (**c**) Cytologic analysis of the pleural fluid showing large atypical lymphoid cells with distinct nucleoli and a high nucleus-to-cytoplasm ratio (hematoxylin and eosin stain, ×40). (**d**) Immunohistochemical staining revealing CD20-positive lymphoid cells (×10), confirming a B-cell phenotype. (Attribution: Reprinted from *Respiratory Medicine Case Reports*, Vol 16, Hara N., Fujimoto N., Miyamoto Y., Yamagishi T., Asano M., Fuchimoto Y., Wada S., Ozaki S., Kishimoto T., "Lymphoproliferative disorder in pleural effusion in a subject with past asbestos exposure," pp. 169–171, Copyright © 2015 Elsevier Inc. Reproduced by permission of Elsevier through RightsLink License No. 6133221416444 for *Rare Pleural Disease* (Springer Nature, 2026). All rights reserved. No further reproduction or distribution is permitted without permission from Elsevier)

thickening, or nodularity, all suggestive of malignant or inflammatory etiologies [25]. Although ultrasound cannot distinguish chylothorax from other effusion types, it remains invaluable for guiding thoracentesis and pleural biopsy [19].

Pleural fluid analysis commonly demonstrates a lymphocyte-predominant differential. However, cytologic diagnosis of lymphoma can be difficult due to sparse malignant cells or reactive lymphocyte mimicry (Fig. 13.1c). Therefore, ancillary studies such as flow cytometry and immunocytochemistry are essential for diagnostic confirmation and lymphoma subtyping (Fig. 13.1d) [26].

Additional pleural fluid markers, including pH < 7.3 and glucose <60 mg/dL, have been shown to improve the diagnostic yield of cytology [27]. Light's criteria remain the standard for differentiating exudates, defined by a pleural fluid-to-serum protein ratio >0.5, LDH ratio >0.6, or pleural fluid LDH > two-thirds the upper limit of normal [13]. Combined diagnostic approaches yield cytologic detection rates of approximately 61–75% [1]. If cytology is nondiagnostic and clinical suspicion persists, medical thoracoscopy with pleural biopsy is indicated [27, 28].

Chylous effusions are classically milky or opalescent in appearance, though fasting may render them serous, and empyemas can also appear milky, making gross inspection unreliable. The biochemical hallmark of chylothorax is a pleural fluid triglyceride concentration >110 mg/dL. Levels <50 mg/dL effectively exclude the diagnosis, while intermediate levels (50–110 mg/dL) warrant lipoprotein electrophoresis to confirm the presence of chylomicrons [19].

Treatment

Management of lymphomatous pleural effusion primarily focuses on treating the underlying malignancy, as most effusions resolve or significantly improve with effective chemotherapy due to the disease's chemosensitivity. In some instances, intrapleural therapy may be warranted for persistent or symptomatic effusions [29]. When effusions fail to resolve despite systemic therapy, palliative interventions are considered to alleviate dyspnea and enhance quality of life. These measures parallel the management of other malignant pleural effusions and include repeated therapeutic thoracenteses, chemical pleurodesis, or placement of an indwelling pleural catheter (IPC). In a study by Faiz et al., pleurodesis was achieved at a median of 180 days following IPC placement, attributed to combined systemic therapy and aggressive pleural drainage, which likely promoted inflammatory adhesion of pleural surfaces [30].

Chylothorax associated with lymphoma generally improves following chemotherapy, although adjunctive management is often necessary even after disease control. Treatment approaches may be medical, surgical, or hybrid, necessitating a multidisciplinary strategy to individualize care. Lymphoma-related chylothorax is typically low output (<1 L/day) and may respond to conservative therapy, which includes dietary restriction of long-chain triglycerides to reduce chyle formation, coupled with medium-chain triglyceride (MCT) supplementation, as MCTs are directly absorbed into the portal venous system rather than lymphatics.

If dietary modification fails, total parenteral nutrition (TPN) may be implemented to further minimize chyle flow. Pharmacologic agents such as somatostatin and its synthetic analog octreotide can be administered alongside dietary measures to reduce lymphatic output and facilitate closure of the leak [19]. Symptomatic relief can be provided by therapeutic thoracentesis, intercostal chest tube drainage, or indwelling pleural catheter insertion for recurrent effusions.

Surgical intervention is reserved for refractory chylothorax. Thoracic duct ligation remains the most definitive approach, whereas thoracic duct embolization (TDE), performed by interventional radiology, is a less invasive alternative. TDE involves lymphangiography to localize the site of chyle leakage, followed by coil or glue embolization of the thoracic duct to occlude the flow. In cases resistant to all other therapies, pleuroperitoneal shunting may be employed. This procedure utilizes a fenestrated catheter system that connects the pleural and peritoneal cavities and is equipped with a subcutaneous pump to recirculate chyle and maintain fluid balance [31].

Prognosis

The prognostic significance of lymphomatous pleural effusions remains incompletely defined, although their presence is frequently correlated with advanced-stage disease and higher tumor burden [11]. Prognosis varies considerably based on the lymphoma subtype, extent of pleural involvement, and treatment responsiveness. Notably, an elevated pleural fluid-to-serum lactate dehydrogenase ratio has been associated with adverse outcomes [5]. This parameter is included in the LENT prognostic score, a validated tool used to estimate survival in patients with malignant pleural effusions, emphasizing the clinical relevance of pleural LDH levels in prognostication. The outlook for primary effusion lymphoma is particularly poor, with a median survival of approximately 6 months, and it accounts for less than 1% of non-HIV-associated lymphomas [17, 32, 33]. However, in HIV-positive patients receiving antiretroviral therapy, survival outcomes may improve substantially, and case reports have described complete or partial remissions achieved through antiviral therapy alone [17]. By comparison, pyothorax-associated lymphoma demonstrates a relatively better, though still guarded, prognosis, with five-year survival rates of approximately 20% [34]. The poorer outcomes associated with both PEL and PAL underscore the importance of early recognition, targeted oncologic therapy, and comprehensive supportive management in improving overall survival and quality of life in affected patients.

References

1. Bashoura L, Eapen GA, Faiz SA. Pulmonary manifestations of lymphoma and leukemia. Clin Chest Med. 2017;38:187–200.
2. Alexandrakis MG, Passam FH, Kyriakou DS, Bouros D. Pleural effusions in hematologic malignancies. Chest. 2004;125(4):1546–55. https://doi.org/10.1378/chest.125.4.1546.
3. Gastesi A, Kapadia D. Primary pleural lymphoma. Respir Med Case Rep. 2024;50:102046.
4. Berkman N, Breuer R. Pulmonary involvement in lymphoma. Respir Med. 1993;87:85.
5. Ahmed S, Shahid RK, Rimawi R, Siddiqui AK, Rossoff L, Sison CP, et al. Malignant pleural effusions in lymphoproliferative disorders. Leuk Lymphoma. 2005;46(7):1039–44.
6. Hillerdal G. Effusions from lymphatic disruptions. In: Light R, Lee YG, editors. Textbook of pleural diseases. 2nd ed. London: Hodder Arnold; 2008. p. 389–95.
7. McGrath EE, Blades Z, Anderson PB. Chylothorax: aetiology, diagnosis and therapeutic options. Respir Med. 2010;104:1–8.
8. Gathers DA, Galloway E, Kelemen K, Rosenthal A, Gibson SE, Munoz J. Primary effusion lymphoma: a clinicopathologic perspective. Cancers (Basel). 2022;14:722.
9. Aozasa K, Takakuwa T, Nakatsuka SI. Pyothorax-associated lymphoma a lymphoma developing in chronic inflammation. Adv Anat Pathol. 2005;12:324.
10. Welcker K, Nakashima M, Diemel K, Welker L, Galle J, Merz H, Branscheid D. Pyothorax-associated lymphoma (PAL): report and review of a rare entity. Thorac Surg Sci. 2004;1:Doc03.
11. Weick JK, Kiely JM, Harrison EG, Carr DT, Scanlon PW. Pleural effusion in lymphoma. Cancer. 1973;31(4):848–53.
12. Elis A, Blickstein D, Mulchanov I, Manor Y, Radnay J, Shapiro H, et al. Pleural effusion in patients with non-Hodgkin's lymphoma: a case-controlled study. Cancer. 1998;83(8):1607–11.
13. Rodriguez-Panadero F. Effusions from malignancy. In: Light R, Lee YG, editors. Textbook of pleural diseases. 2nd ed. London: Hodder Arnold; 2008. p. 330–1.
14. Berkman N, Breuer R, Kramer MR, Polliack A. Pulmonary involvement in lymphoma. Leuk Lymphoma. 1996;20(3–4):229–37.
15. Aoki Y, Tosato G. Role of vascular endothelial growth factor/vascular permeability factor in the pathogenesis of Kaposi's sarcoma-associated herpesvirus-infected primary effusion lymphomas. Blood. 1999;94(12):4247–54.
16. Wang X, Medeiros L, Bueso-Ramos C, Tang G, Wang S, Oki Y, Desai P, Khoury J, Miranda R, Tang Z, Reddy N, Li S. P53 expression correlates with poorer survival and augments the negative prognostic effect of MYC rearrangement, expression or concurrent MYC/BCL2 expression in diffuse large B-cell lymphoma. Mod Pathol. 2017;30:194–203.
17. Conconi A, Carbone A. Primary effusion lymphoma. In: Extranodal lymphomas: pathology and management. Boca Raton: CRC Press; 2008. p. 299–305.
18. Narkhede M, Arora S, Ujjani C. Primary effusion lymphoma: current perspectives. OncoTargets Ther. 2018;11:3747–54.
19. Bhatnagar M, Fisher A, Ramsaroop S, Carter A, Pippard B. Chylothorax: pathophysiology, diagnosis, and management, a comprehensive review. J Thorac Dis. 2024;16:1645–61.
20. Au V, Leung AN. Pictorial essay radiologic manifestations of lymphoma in the thorax. AJA. 1997; Available from: www.ajronline.org
21. Basuthakur S, Sarkar A, Burman S, Dandale R. A rare case of pleural lymphoma. Lung India. 2008;25(4):160–2.
22. Celikoglu E, Teirstein AS, Krellenstein DJ, Strauchen JA. Pleural effusion in non-Hodgkin's lymphoma. CHEST. 1992;101:1357–60.
23. Mhlanga J, Alazraki A, Cho S, Lai H, Nadel H, Pandit-Taskar N, Qi J, Rajderkar D, Voss S, Watal P, McCarten K. Imaging recommendations in pediatric lymphoma: a COG diagnostic imaging committee/SPR oncology committee white paper. Pediatr Blood Cancer. 2022;70(Suppl 4):e29968.
24. Jahanshahi A, Hiradfar A, Zarrintan A, Mirza-Aghazadeh-Attari M. Primary pleural lymphoma of T cell origin in a paediatric patient with a focus on radiological findings—a case report and review of literature. Pol J Radiol. 2019;84:e353–9.
25. Wang T, Du G, Fang L, Bai Y, Liu Z, Wang L. Value of ultrasonography in determining the nature of pleural effusion: analysis of 582 cases. Medicine (Baltimore). 2022;101(33):e30119.
26. Das DK. Serous effusions in malignant lymphomas: a review. Diagn Cytopathol. 2006;34(5):335–47.
27. Official Statement of ATS. Management of malignant pleural effusions. Am J Respir Crit Care Med. 2000;162:1987–2001.
28. He X, Yu F, Guo T, Xiang F, Tao X, Zhang J, Zhou Q. T-cell lymphoblastic lymphoma presenting with

pleural effusion: a case report. Respir Med Case Rep. 2014;12:55–8.
29. Islam A, Takita H. Malignant pleural effusion and advanced-stage low-grade non-Hodgkin's lymphoma successfully treated with intrapleural instillation of rituximab. Blood. 2012;120(21):4891.
30. Faiz S, Pathania P, Song J, et al. Indwelling pleural catheters for patients with hematologic malignancies. A 14-year, single-center experience. Ann Am Thorac Soc. 2017;14(6):976–85.
31. Thomas JM, Musani AI. Malignant pleural effusions. A review. Clin Chest Med. 2013;34:459–71.
32. Karpathiou G, Peoc'h M. Pleura revisited: from histology and pathophysiology to pathology and molecular biology. Clin Respir J. 2019;13:3–13.
33. Kaplan LD. Human herpesvirus-8: Kaposi sarcoma, multicentric Castleman disease, and primary effusion lymphoma. Hematology Am Soc Hematol Educ Program. 2013;2013:103–8. https://doi.org/10.1182/asheducation-2013.1.103.
34. Narimatsu H, Ota Y, Kami M, Takeuchi K, Suzuki R, Matsuo K, Matsumura T, Yuji K, Kishi Y, Hamaki T, Sawada U, Miyata S, Sasaki T, Tobinai K, Kawabata M, Atsuta Y, Tanaka Y, Ueda R, Nakamura S. Clinicopathological features of pyothorax-associated lymphoma; a retrospective survey involving 98 patients. Ann Oncol. 2007;18(1):122–8.

Part IV

Rare Pleural Neoplasms

14 Malignant Pleural Mesothelioma

Kaitlin Nguyen, Santo Longo, Firas Ido, and William Burfeind

Introduction

Malignant mesothelioma (MM) represents a rare, progressive, and often times, fatal malignancy that originates from the mesothelial cells of serosal membranes [1–3]. Pleural mesothelioma (PM) accounts for approximately 85-90% of all MM cases. Diffuse pleural mesothelioma (DPM) is most frequently observed, encompassing likely over 90–95% of cases, while the remainder is characterized by localized disease [4]. Other primary sites of MM include the peritoneum (15%), pericardium (<1%), and tunica vaginalis (<1%) [1–3]. The most significant risk factor associated with the development of MM is asbestos exposure, unaffected by an individual's smoking status [1, 5].

K. Nguyen
Department of General Surgery, St. Luke's University Health Network, Bethlehem, PA, USA
e-mail: kaitlin.nguyen@sluhn.org

S. Longo
Department of Pathology, St. Luke's University Health Network, Bethlehem, PA, USA
e-mail: santo.longo@sluhn.org

F. Ido
Department of Pulmonary and Critical Care Medicine, St. Luke's University Health Network, Bethlehem, PA, USA
e-mail: firas.ido@sluhn.org

W. Burfeind (✉)
Department of Thoracic Surgery, St. Luke's University Health Network, Bethlehem, PA, USA
e-mail: William.Burfeind@sluhn.org

The three histologic subtypes of pleural mesothelioma are epithelioid (50%), biphasic (30%), and sarcomatoid (15–20%), each exhibiting significant prognostic differences [1, 3]. The epithelioid type, characterized by squamous and/or cuboidal-appearing malignant cells, is associated with the most favorable prognosis. The sarcomatoid subtype is the most aggressive and is composed of elongated, malignant, spindle-shaped cells. The biphasic subtype encompasses varying percentages of both epithelioid and sarcomatoid patterns, requiring a minimum of 10% of the sarcomatoid pattern to be present. The greater the proportion of sarcomatoid features, the poorer the prognosis [6].

Epidemiology

General Epidemiology

In 2020, mesothelioma accounted for 0.016% of all cancers worldwide, with 30,870 new reported cases [7]. In the United States between 2004 and 2020, the incidence of diffuse pleural mesothelioma was approximately 0.25%, with an average of 2417 cases per year [8]. The incidence rate is significantly higher in states with asbestos-related industries than in those without, with rates of 1 per 100,000 compared to 2–3 per 100,000, respectively [9–11]. The reported median age at diagnosis is 72–78 years, with

F. Ido (ed.), *Rare Pleural Diseases*, https://doi.org/10.1007/978-3-032-14873-5_14

patients recorded between 18 and 90 years of age [8, 12, 13]. The highest incidence of malignant pleural mesothelioma is among Caucasian males (74%) [12]. In males, the cumulative risk between 0 and 74 years of age has been calculated as 0.05%, compared to 0.02% in females [7]. Between 2004 and 2020 in the United States, the majority of patients diagnosed with malignant pleural mesothelioma were Caucasian (93.3%), compared to African American (5.0%), Asian (0.9%), or of other racial identity (0.8%). Male patients comprised 73.2% of this population, compared to 26.8% females. The gender distribution remained consistent through this period [8]. This disparity is thought to reflect historical gender differences in occupations with asbestos exposure. However, there is a higher incidence in females in countries such as Italy and the United Kingdom (0.6 per 100,000), compared to the United States (0.3 per 100,000) or Europe as a whole (0.4 per 100,000). This suggests the potential presence of nonoccupational asbestos exposures in these populations [14].

Risk Factors: Asbestos

Exposure to asbestos, a naturally occurring mineral fiber, is the most well-established risk factor for the development of malignant pleural mesothelioma, associated with up to 80% of cases [15]. This causal relationship was first established in 1960, with a series of 33 histologically proven cases of pleural mesothelioma in South Africa. Out of 33, 28 patients had known exposure to the asbestos mining operations, four had industry-related asbestos exposure, and one patient had no confirmed exposure to asbestos [5].

Asbestos contains six different mineral fibers used in industries such as shipbuilding, insulation manufacturing, and various cement products [1, 6]. The morphology and dimensions of asbestos fibers are categorized into two subtypes, serpentine and amphibole. Chrysotile, which represents the exclusive serpentine fiber utilized in commercial applications, exhibits a more efficient clearance from the lungs. Of the remaining five types of fibers in the amphibole category, crocidolite and amosite are the most extensively used commercially [6, 16]. Crocidolite has the strongest association with the development of malignant pleural mesothelioma [17].

By the 1980s, the United States and several other countries had enacted regulations to minimize asbestos exposure in mining and product manufacturing. Several decades later, the incidence of mesothelioma remains essentially unchanged, suggesting that the population-wide effects of asbestos exposure persist despite decreased frequency of new exposures [1, 18, 19]. The continued high incidence may in part reflect the prolonged latency period between asbestos exposure and the development of malignant pleural mesothelioma. The estimated mean latency period is 32 years, with a documented range of 13–17 years, and 96% of cases are diagnosed 20 or more years after exposure [17]. No minimum threshold of asbestos exposure has been established that correlates with the development of pleural mesothelioma. However, epidemiologic models demonstrate a clear correlation between the intensity, duration, and frequency of asbestos exposure and the likelihood of pleural mesothelioma development [20]. Although asbestos is a clear risk factor, an estimated 20-50% of malignant pleural mesothelioma cases develop in patients without a documented history of asbestos exposure, suggesting additional risk factors [1].

Risk Factors: Genetic

Mutations in BRCA-associated protein 1 (BAP1) have been linked to an increased susceptibility to mesothelioma, irrespective of asbestos exposure [21, 22]. Genetic analyses of patients with malignant mesothelioma identified a germline BAP1 mutation in 60% of cases. It is noteworthy that BAP1 mutations have been observed in the predisposition to uveal melanoma, basal cell carcinoma, renal cell carcinoma, and lung adenocarcinoma [23–30]. Additional genes implicated in the development of MM include SETD2, PBRM1, and SMARCCI [1, 31].

Pathophysiology

The inhalation of asbestos fibers that reach the alveoli triggers a macrophage phagocytic inflammatory response. These fibers translocate into the pleural space and are deposited near the lymphatic stomata of the parietal pleura [1, 28, 29]. Consequently, mesothelial cells and macrophages release reactive oxygen species (ROS) that induce DNA damage [32, 33]. Additionally, TNFα activates the NF-κB pathway. In combination, these processes are believed to promote the conversion of the chronic adaptive hyperplastic mesothelial cells to malignant mesothelioma [34–37].

Clinical Features

The most common presenting symptom of pleural mesothelioma is dyspnea. Additional symptoms include dull or pleuritic chest pain, dry cough, fatigue, early satiety, and unintentional weight loss [16, 38, 39]. Commonly, on physical examination, diminished breath sounds occur on the affected side. The use of accessory respiratory muscles and dullness to percussion are often encountered in the presence of a pleural effusion [38].

Diagnosis

Imaging

Imaging studies, categorically, when used alone in the initial evaluation, are insufficient for diagnosing pleural mesothelioma or determining the histological subtype. However, various imaging modalities can effectively indicate the extent of intrathoracic disease, including involvement of the lung parenchyma, the presence of pleural effusions, and invasion of adjacent extrapleural structures. Imaging provides helpful information regarding distant metastasis, which guides management. Additionally, imaging is essential in monitoring disease progression and the response to treatment [40]. The imaging findings may include any or all of the following: pleural thickening (nodular or diffuse), ipsilateral pleural effusion, mediastinal lymphadenopathy, mediastinal shift, loss of lung volume, pleural calcifications, tumor extension into extrapleural structures (chest wall, mediastinum, pericardium, diaphragm), as well as distal metastases (Fig. 14.1a–c) [41–44]. Chest X-ray is the initial assessment tool for patients presenting with respiratory symptoms. Although pleural effusion, masses, and pleural plaques can be routinely visualized with standard radiography, it is limited in detecting mediastinal lymphadenopathy, the extent of invasion of adjacent structures, and extrapleural metastasis. Contrast-enhanced computed tomography (CT) is superior in visualizing features of advanced pleural mesothelioma, including nodal involvement, differentiating pleural thickening from adjacent effusions and/or compressive atelectasis, and delineating vasculature [40, 42–45]. CT of the thorax routinely extends to the upper abdomen, providing the assessment of the transdiaphragmatic extent of the disease [41]. Perfusion CT, a functional imaging technique, serves as an adjunct that can effectively delineate the microvasculature of the tumor, provide physiological data regarding blood flow, and evaluate the response to treatment [45].

When deemed necessary, thoracic magnetic resonance imaging (MRI) can provide a more precise definition and extent of local tumor invasion. The enhanced metabolic activity of tumor cells within metastases can be detected using positron-emission tomography (PET/CT) (Fig. 14.1d–f) [41, 43, 44]. On PET/CT, DPM shows fluorodeoxyglucose (FDG) avidity with standardized uptake value (SUV) above 2.0–2.2 [46–48]. These modalities provide objective information regarding anatomic staging, prognosis, surgical planning, and monitoring treatment response [44, 49–51].

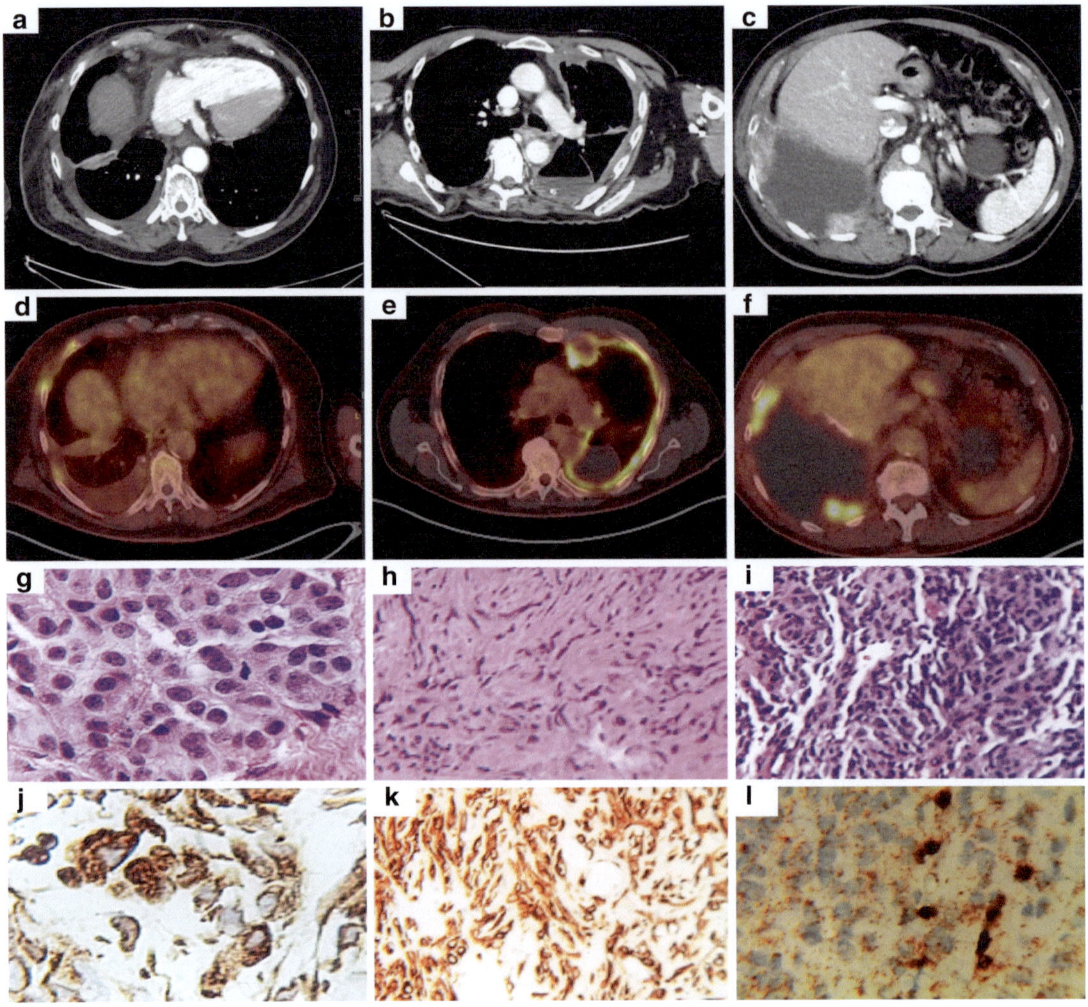

Fig. 14.1 Spectrum of imaging and histopathologic findings in malignant pleural mesothelioma

(**a**) Epithelioid mesothelioma: Irregular nodular thickening of the right pleura with extension into the interlobar fissure

(**b**) Sarcomatoid mesothelioma: Circumferential thickening of the left pleura, including the mediastinal pleura, with a loculated effusion in the dependent zone

(**c**) Biphasic mesothelioma: Patchy nodular thickening involving the right lower-lobe pleura

(**d**) Epithelioid mesothelioma: Positron-emission tomography (PET) with increased FDG uptake in nodular pleural thickening

(**e**) Sarcomatoid mesothelioma: Diffuse circumferential FDG avidity involving the pleura and interlobar fissures, extending to the mediastinum

(**f**) Biphasic mesothelioma: Focal increased FDG avidity of nodular pleural thickening along the right lower lobe with an associated non-avid pleural effusion

(**g**) Epithelioid subtype (H&E × 400): Tumor cells with bland round nuclei and pink, glassy cytoplasm consistent with well-to moderately differentiated epithelial carcinoma

(**h**) Sarcomatoid subtype (H&E × 400): Clusters of pleomorphic spindle-shaped tumor cells embedded within dense fibrous stroma, consistent with sarcomatoid malignancy

(**i**) Biphasic subtype (H&E × 400): Tumor composed of intermixed clusters of malignant epithelioid cells abutting fascicles of pleomorphic spindle cells

(**j**) Epithelioid mesothelioma: Patchy WT-1 nuclear immunostaining

(**k**) Sarcomatoid mesothelioma: Diffuse cytoplasmic pankeratin immunoreactivity

(**l**) Malignant mesothelioma: Characteristic loss of BAP1 nuclear expression on immunohistochemistry

Attribution: Panels A–F courtesy of Dr. Firas Ido. Panels G–L courtesy of Dr. Santo Longo. All images are original and unpublished, reproduced here with permission of the respective authors

Pathology

To the general pathologist, the diagnosis of malignant pleural mesothelioma can be most challenging. This difficulty reflects the rarity of the tumor, suboptimal tissue sampling, and histologic similarities resembling other malignancies [1]. In addition to routine histologic assessment, immunohistochemistry (IHC) must be performed. In some instances, further molecular testing may be required to distinguish pleural mesothelioma from metastatic carcinoma or reactive mesothelial cells [3]. In comparison to lung cancers, the genetic mutational burden of malignant mesothelioma is relatively low. The detection of known genomic mutations in tumor suppressor proteins in malignant mesothelioma serves a diagnostic purpose, but there are no established therapeutic targets. These mutations help differentiate malignant mesothelioma from other reactive mesothelial proliferations [52].

Biopsy

For the diagnosis of pleural mesothelioma, histologic specimens are preferred over cytologic samples, as tissue architecture is essential for accurate subtyping and differentiation from other pleural malignancies. Although pleural fluid cytology often serves as the initial diagnostic test in patients presenting with an undifferentiated pleural effusion, cytology alone is frequently insufficient to confirm diffuse pleural mesothelioma due to sampling limitations and a high false-negative rate [3].

The diagnostic yield for biopsy samples is directly related to both the number and size of biopsy specimens, two factors that determine the total tissue volume obtained. In a study assessing concordance between pre-surgical thoracoscopic or core biopsies to the final diagnosis following definitive surgical resections, the diagnostic agreement approached 100% when more than nine biopsy samples were collected [53]. Among the three histologic subtypes of malignant pleural mesothelioma, sarcomatoid mesothelioma demonstrates the highest diagnostic accuracy, while epithelioid mesothelioma shows the lowest. In contrast, biphasic mesothelioma exhibits low sensitivity (50.4%) but high specificity (96.3%) for concordant histologic diagnosis between biopsy and surgical specimens [53]. When using closed percutaneous biopsy techniques, either blind or CT-guided, the biopsy size significantly influences diagnostic success. Specimens measuring greater than 10 mm in diameter yield a definitive diagnosis in 75% of cases, compared to only 8% when the sample is smaller than 10 mm [54]. To reduce the likelihood of sampling error, biopsies should be obtained from multiple accessible regions of the pleural abnormality. Thoracoscopic biopsy remains the preferred diagnostic approach, offering a sensitivity of 88–95% and a specificity of 100% [54–57]. However, all pleural interventions, particularly biopsy procedures, carry a risk of tumor tract seeding, with the highest incidence observed following thoracotomy incisions [58, 59]. Consequently, when selecting a biopsy approach, the trajectory should be aligned with potential future surgical incisions, allowing for en bloc excision of the biopsy tract during definitive resection if necessary.

Histologic Criteria

Establishing the diagnosis of pleural mesothelioma requires confirming that the lesion is of mesothelial origin and malignant. Although pleural mesothelioma is most commonly diffuse, localized or solitary pleural mesotheliomas have been reported and are generally associated with a more favorable prognosis. Correlation with clinical presentation and imaging findings is essential to determine if the neoplasm fulfills the criteria for diffuse disease [60, 61]. While mesothelioma may share histopathologic features with other pleural malignancies, immunohistochemical and molecular analyses reliably distinguish its mesothelial lineage. The final diagnostic requirement is demonstration of malignancy, differentiating mesothelioma from reactive mesothelial proliferations. Hallmarks of malignancy include involvement of the full-thickness pleura, formation of expansile nodules, and, particularly, invasion into adjacent tissues, which remains the most definitive indicator of malignant mesothelioma [60, 62].

Macroscopic Features

Macroscopically, diffuse pleural mesothelioma is characterized by circumferential pleural thickening often accompanied by firm, tan to white nodules and plaques distributed along the pleural surface. The tumor commonly extends into the interlobar fissures, encasing the lung and restricting its expansion. During surgical exploration, tumoral invasion of adjacent structures, including the chest wall, diaphragm, and pericardium, may be apparent. In advanced cases, direct extension into the underlying lung parenchyma has also been reported [54, 60].

Microscopic Features

The three principal histologic subtypes of malignant pleural mesothelioma, epithelioid, sarcomatoid, and biphasic, are defined by their distinct cytomorphologic characteristics. In general, malignant pleural mesothelioma is composed of cellular clusters exhibiting irregular, scalloped borders, reflecting its infiltrative growth pattern. The cytoplasm of neoplastic mesothelial cells often appears two-toned, characterized by a dense, eosinophilic inner zone and a paler peripheral rim. Cytologically, mesothelioma cells display hallmarks of malignancy, including nuclear irregularity, pleomorphism, and prominent nucleoli. Acinar formation or smooth cellular contours, in contrast, are features more typical of adenocarcinoma and help distinguish it from mesothelioma. In comparison, benign pleural effusions are generally hypocellular, consisting of small, flat aggregates of mesothelial cells without significant atypia or architectural complexity [3].

Epithelioid mesothelioma, the most common subtype of malignant pleural mesothelioma, is composed of epithelioid to polygonal cells arranged in a variety of architectural patterns, including tubulopapillary, trabecular, solid, and acinar formations. Multiple growth patterns are often observed within the same specimen, reflecting the tumor's morphological heterogeneity (Fig. 14.1g) [60, 63, 64]. Sarcomatoid mesothelioma is characterized by spindle-shaped tumor cells that are typically organized in interlacing fascicles or broad sheets [60, 64]. Histologic variants include the lymphohistiocytoid and desmoplastic patterns (Fig. 14.1h) [64]. The desmoplastic subtype may mimic reactive fibrous tissue; however, it can be distinguished by the presence of bland collagen necrosis and infiltration into submesothelial adipose tissue [54]. Biphasic mesothelioma, accounting for approximately 30% of all malignant pleural mesothelioma cases, demonstrates both epithelioid and sarcomatoid components, each comprising at least 10% of the total tumor volume (Fig. 14.1I) [60, 64]. Other neoplasms that may display a biphasic appearance in the pleura and should be considered in the differential diagnosis include synovial sarcoma, carcinosarcoma, and pulmonary blastoma [64]. In addition to these three principal histologic types, rare variants of pleural mesothelioma have been described. Identified primarily through immunohistochemical analysis, these include the clear cell, deciduoid, rhabdoid, signet-ring cell, and small cell subtypes [3].

Immunohistochemistry plays a critical role in differentiating mesothelioma from morphologically similar entities such as reactive mesothelial proliferations and metastatic adenocarcinoma [3]. Diagnostic IHC panels typically include both mesothelial and epithelial markers. Mesothelial markers such as WT1, calretinin, and pankeratin (CK5/6) usually demonstrate nuclear and cytoplasmic positivity, confirming mesothelial differentiation (Fig. 14.1j, k). Conversely, carcinoma-associated markers, including TTF-1, CEA, and p63, are generally negative in mesothelioma but positive in adenocarcinoma, aiding in the exclusion of metastatic disease. The concurrent positivity for at least one mesothelial marker and negativity for carcinoma markers is considered ideal for establishing the diagnosis of mesothelioma [1, 3].

Loss of expression of BAP1 and MTAP on IHC further supports a diagnosis of malignant mesothelioma (Fig. 14.11). BAP1, a tumor suppressor gene frequently mutated in mesothelioma, shows loss of nuclear staining in approximately 60–70% of epithelioid mesotheliomas but retains nuclear positivity in reactive mesothelial cells [3]. Similarly, MTAP, which encodes methylthioadenosine phosphorylase, is often co-deleted with CDKN2A, and its loss of cytoplasmic staining is highly specific for mesothelioma. In addition to IHC, fluorescence in situ hybridization (FISH) or polymerase chain reaction (PCR) may be employed to detect deletions or mutations involving these genes, thereby providing further diagnostic confirmation [3, 65].

Staging

Historically, several staging systems have been proposed for diffuse pleural mesothelioma [66–69]. However, owing to the rarity of the disease, these systems demonstrated considerable variability, often lacked external validation, and provided limited prognostic value [68, 70, 71]. In 1994, the International Association for the Study of Lung Cancer (IASLC) International Mesothelioma Interest Group (IMIG) established a TNM-based staging system, which was subsequently adopted by both the Union for International Cancer Control (UICC) and the American Joint Committee on Cancer (AJCC) [72]. Over time, the system underwent multiple refinements through international, multi-institutional collaboration. The ninth edition of the TNM classification was released in 2024, incorporating updated descriptors and definitions [71, 73–78].

Unlike most solid tumors, for which the T descriptor is based primarily on lesion size, the T categories for DPM reflect the degree of local extension from the pleura to adjacent structures [70]. The AJCC/UICC ninth edition defines both clinical (cT) and pathological (pT) T categories. Clinical staging utilizes quantitative imaging assessments of pleural thickness, including maximal measurements along the fissures (Fmax), diaphragm (Dmax), and pleural surfaces (Pmax). Statistically significant differences in overall survival have been observed among the various clinical T categories. Pathologic T classification, relevant only to surgically treated patients, is determined by qualitative evaluation of tumor invasion into adjacent structures [76].

The presence and anatomical distribution of lymph node metastases define the N descriptor. Both clinically and pathologically, node-positive disease (N1 or N2) is associated with significantly reduced overall survival compared with node-negative status (N0). No significant difference in survival has been demonstrated between single-station and multi-station nodal involvement. Furthermore, the incidence of lymph node metastasis increases with advancing T category. Future refinements are expected to focus on improving the radiologic identification of nodal involvement, thereby enhancing concordance between clinical (cN) and pathological (pN) staging [77, 79].

The M descriptor denotes the presence (M1) or absence (M0) of distant metastasis, with overall survival markedly worse in patients with metastatic disease [73, 78]. Clinical stage groupings derived from these descriptors continue to demonstrate prognostic variability, emphasizing the need for ongoing validation and refinement [75].

Treatment

Establishing a standardized treatment protocol for diffuse pleural mesothelioma has been hindered by the disease's rarity, its aggressive clinical course, and the resulting scarcity of randomized controlled trials. Nevertheless, the most widely accepted therapeutic strategy remains a trimodality approach, incorporating surgery, systemic therapy, and radiation. This requires an experienced, multidisciplinary team that includes surgeons, medical oncologists, radiation oncologists, pathologists, and pulmonologists. Treatment is tailored to the individual patient but may include a combination of surgery, systemic therapy, and radiation [80].

Surgery

Surgical treatment for DPM aims to achieve macroscopic complete resection via extrapleural pneumonectomy (EPP) or pleurectomy/decortication (P/D). This is often difficult to achieve despite resecting portions of adjacent anatomic structures. Therefore, adjuvant chemotherapy and radiation are typically employed to manage microscopic residual disease and improve local control [80–82].

Because DPM frequently presents at an advanced stage, surgical resection is not feasible for all patients. Contraindications to operative intervention include rib or mediastinal invasion, multilevel chest wall involvement, contralateral pleural disease, distant metastases, sarcomatoid or biphasic histologic subtype, contralateral or supraclavicular lymph node involvement (N2), and poor functional status that precludes major thoracic surgery [83]. To address inconsistencies in surgical terminology, the International Mesothelioma Interest Group (IMIG) and the International Association for the Study of Lung Cancer (IASLC) Mesothelioma Domain have established standardized definitions for surgical procedures. Extrapleural pneumonectomy (EPP) refers to the en bloc resection of the parietal and visceral pleura, ipsilateral lung, and, when indicated, the pericardium and/or diaphragm if directly invaded by tumor. Pleurectomy/decortication involves the removal of both the visceral and parietal pleura with resection of all visible tumors while preserving the underlying lung. Extended pleurectomy/decortication (EPD) includes additional resection of the diaphragm and/or pericardium when these structures are involved by tumor [84]. EPP is a technically challenging and highly invasive procedure, performed traditionally for patients with locally advanced mesothelioma. Complications have been reported with a rate of 60.4% in patients undergoing EPP, including atrial fibrillation (44.2%), prolonged intubation (7.9%), myocardial infarction (1.5%), technical complications (6.1%), deep vein thrombosis (6.4%), pulmonary embolus (1.5%), and empyema (2.4%) [85]. Reported perioperative mortality rates range from 2.2% to 7% across multiple institutional series [81, 85–93]. Despite these risks, EPP has been associated with symptomatic improvement, including reductions in dyspnea, chest pain, cough, and fever, leading to measurable enhancements in quality of life among appropriately selected patients [94]. Distant recurrence following EPP is more common than local recurrence (66% vs. 31%), which can be attributed to extensive cytoreduction combined with high-dose postoperative radiation of the hemithorax [81].

Pleurectomy/decortication aims to achieve macroscopic complete resection of both the visceral and parietal pleura while preserving the ipsilateral lung. Traditionally, this approach has been indicated for patients with early-stage disease or for those deemed at excessive surgical risk for extrapleural pneumonectomy. The most frequently encountered complications include hemorrhage and prolonged air leak, occurring in approximately 4–10% of cases, with reported perioperative mortality ranging between 1% and 5% [81, 82, 86, 95, 96]. Pleurectomy/decortication also provides substantial palliative benefit in most patients, with documented improvement in dyspnea, cough, pain, and control of pleural effusion [96].

The selection between extrapleural pneumonectomy and pleurectomy/decortication has traditionally been guided by factors such as baseline pulmonary function, tumor morphology, and the extent of intrathoracic disease involvement [81]. In recent years, there has been a discernible shift toward favoring P/D over EPP, primarily due to its reduced physiological impact and lower perioperative mortality rates [80, 86]. However, a definitive survival advantage of P/D compared with EPP has not yet been clearly established [80, 81, 86]. When performed in conjunction with extrapleural pneumonectomy or pleurectomy/decortication, heated intraoperative chemotherapy (HIOC) may enhance local disease control. During HIOC, cisplatin is circulated within the ipsilateral hemithorax at a temperature of approximately 42 °C for 1 h [97, 98]. Among patients with epithelioid diffuse pleural mesothelioma and a low predicted risk of early recurrence or mortality—defined by a tumor volume < 500 cm^3, normal hemoglobin levels in men, and female sex—HIOC has been associated with prolonged time to recurrence and improved overall survival. This benefit appears to be more pronounced in patients with N1 or N2 nodal disease who do not subsequently receive postoperative radiotherapy [99]. Intraoperative pleural lavage using hyperthermic povidone-iodine has also been described as part of multimodal treatment strategies; however, its independent therapeutic efficacy remains unproven [100, 101].

In patients with malignant pleural effusion secondary to diffuse pleural mesothelioma (DPM), symptomatic relief of dyspnea can be achieved through talc pleurodesis or the placement of an indwelling pleural catheter. When fluorodeoxyglucose positron-emission tomography/computed tomography (FDG PET/CT) is indicated, it should ideally be performed prior to pleurodesis, as the subsequent pleural inflammation may confound imaging interpretation [83]. In cases where future surgical intervention remains a possibility, the use of an indwelling pleural catheter is preferred over pleurodesis [102].

Chemotherapy

Systemic therapy for DPM encompasses both chemotherapy and immunotherapy, with specific regimens tailored according to histologic subtype, disease resectability, molecular tumor profile, and individual patient factors [103]. The current first-line chemotherapy regimen combines the platinum-based alkylating agent cisplatin with the folate analog metabolic inhibitor pemetrexed [104]. In a pivotal randomized trial, the addition of pemetrexed to cisplatin significantly improved outcomes compared with cisplatin alone, resulting in increased median overall survival (12.1 months vs. 9.3 months), median time to disease progression, and objective response rates. To minimize treatment-related toxicity, supplementation with folic acid and vitamin B12 is recommended throughout therapy [104]. For patients unable to tolerate cisplatin, most commonly due to nephrotoxicity or other dose-limiting adverse effects, carboplatin may be substituted with comparable efficacy [87, 105]. Additional chemotherapeutic regimens that have demonstrated activity include cisplatin with gemcitabine, pemetrexed monotherapy, and vinorelbine-based therapy [106–109]. Depending on disease stage and treatment objectives, patients may receive induction chemotherapy prior to surgical resection, proceed directly to definitive surgery, or undergo adjuvant chemotherapy followed by postoperative radiotherapy as part of a multimodality treatment approach.

Immunotherapy

Recent investigations regarding monoclonal antibodies in the treatment of DPM have shown promising results [110–113]. The CheckMate 743 trial, a multicenter, randomized, phase III study published in 2021, established dual immune checkpoint inhibition with ipilimumab and nivolumab as an approved first-line therapy for previously unresectable DPM in adult patients with good performance status. Compared with standard platinum–pemetrexed chemotherapy, the combination of nivolumab and ipilimumab significantly prolonged median overall survival (OS) (18.1 vs. 14.1 months) and improved two-year survival rates (41% vs. 27%) [114]. Extended follow-up demonstrated a durable survival benefit, with three-year progression-free survival (PFS) rates of 14% for immunotherapy compared with 1% for chemotherapy [115].

Additional immunotherapy has been explored with varying degrees of success. The antiangiogenic monoclonal antibody bevacizumab, when added to cisplatin and pemetrexed, was associated with a modest improvement in overall survival (18.8 vs. 16.1 months) but at the cost of increased adverse events, including hypertension and thrombotic complications [116].

Radiation Therapy

Radiation therapy (RT) plays a role in the management of DPM both as an adjuvant modality to target residual postoperative disease and as a palliative treatment for unresectable tumors. The primary technical challenge of RT lies in delivering high-dose radiation to the extensive hemithoracic volume while minimizing toxicity to adjacent vital structures such as the spinal cord, kidneys, and contralateral lung [117, 118].

As surgical management of DPM has shifted toward lung-sparing procedures, such as P/D, increasing emphasis has been placed on defining optimal adjuvant radiation regimens to improve local control and survival outcomes. However, the efficacy of adjuvant radiotherapy following P/D has been inconsistently demonstrated in the literature. Early studies evaluating P/D combined with adjuvant hemithoracic radiation reported less favorable median overall survival (OS) compared with patients undergoing EPP followed by adjuvant RT, 13.5 months versus 17–19 months, respectively [89, 117, 119, 120].

Subsequent clinical trials integrating pemetrexed-based chemotherapy with radical hemithoracic radiation (RHR) have demonstrated more favorable outcomes. In patients with DPM who underwent lung-sparing surgery combined with systemic chemotherapy (carboplatin or cisplatin plus pemetrexed), RHR was associated with a significant improvement in overall survival compared to palliative radiation therapy. It achieved two-year survival rates of 58% versus 28%, respectively, and a corresponding reduction in local recurrence. Notably, the survival benefit was independent of patient age, surgical technique, or TNM stage [121]. In a separate study evaluating image-guided RHR following P/D, the median overall survival was reported as 33 months, underscoring the potential value of advanced radiotherapy techniques in optimizing outcomes for patients treated with lung-sparing approaches [118, 122].

Radiotherapy has also been utilized following invasive diagnostic or therapeutic pleural procedures with the intent of preventing procedure-tract metastases (PTM). However, clinical studies have demonstrated no significant benefit of this practice in reducing PTM incidence, improving overall survival, enhancing quality of life, or providing symptomatic relief. In light of these findings and the availability of routine imaging follow-up, prophylactic procedure-tract radiation is no longer routinely recommended [123].

Prognosis

Despite the best available treatment, the overall prognosis for patients with DPM remains poor, with a 17–25 month median survival. For unresectable pleural mesothelioma, median survival is less than a year [124]. When stratified by disease stage, histologic subtype, and tumor grade, improved survival outcomes have been reported in patients receiving combined tumor-directed surgery and radiation therapy compared with those treated with either modality alone or with nonsurgical, non-radiation approaches [12]. The incorporation of pemetrexed into platinum-based chemotherapy regimens, as well as the introduction of immune checkpoint inhibitors, has modestly prolonged survival in selected patient populations [104, 114]. Despite these advances, median overall survival remains limited, ranging from 17 to 25 months in patients with resectable disease and 9 to 12 months in those with unresectable disease [124].

Histologic subtype is among the strongest prognostic determinants. Patients with epithelioid tumors experience the most favorable outcomes, whereas those with sarcomatoid tumors have the poorest prognosis; biphasic tumors demonstrate intermediate survival [6, 63]. For patients with stage I–III DPM, reported median survival durations are 14 months for the epithelioid subtype, 10 months for the biphasic subtype, and 4 months for the sarcomatoid subtype. Surgical intervention confers a survival benefit, particularly in patients with epithelioid histology [125]. Additional negative prognostic factors include advanced age at diagnosis, male sex, high tumor grade, advanced clinical stage, and the absence of surgical or radiotherapeutic treatment [12].

Acknowledgements The authors thank Jeffrey S. Mayro, MD, Radiologist, St. Luke's University Health Network, for his expert review of the imaging section of this chapter.

References

1. Carbone M, Yang H. Mesothelioma: recent highlights. Ann Transl Med. 2017;5(11):238.
2. WHO Classification of Tumours Editorial Board. WHO classification of tumours: thoracic tumours. 5th ed. Lyon: International Agency for Research on Cancer; 2021.
3. Rao N, Wei S. Mesothelioma. Cytojournal. 2022;19:10.
4. Nakano T, Hamanaka R, Oiwa K, Nakazato K, Masuda R, Iwazaki M. Localized malignant pleural mesothelioma. Gen Thorac Cardiovasc Surg. 2012;60(7):468–74.
5. Wagner JC, Sleggs CA, Marchand P. Diffuse pleural mesothelioma and asbestos exposure in the North Western Cape Province. Occup Environ Med. 1960;17(4):260–71.
6. Attanoos RL, Gibbs AR. Pathology of malignant mesothelioma. Histopathology. 1997;30(5):403–18.
7. Sung H, Ferlay J, Siegel RL, Laversanne M, Soerjomataram I, Jemal A, et al. Global cancer statistics 2020: GLOBOCAN estimates of incidence and mortality worldwide for 36 cancers in 185 countries. CA Cancer J Clin. 2021;71(3):209–49.
8. Bou-Samra P, Chang A, Azari F, Kennedy G, Segil A, Guo E, et al. Epidemiological, therapeutic, and survival trends in malignant pleural mesothelioma: a review of the National Cancer Database. Cancer Med. 2023;12(11):12208–20.
9. Baumann F, Ambrosi JP, Carbone M. Asbestos is not just asbestos: an unrecognised health hazard. Lancet Oncol. 2013;14(7):576–8.
10. Carbone M, Kanodia S, Chao A, Miller A, Wali A, Weissman D, et al. Consensus report of the 2015 Weinman international conference on mesothelioma. J Thorac Oncol. 2016;11(8):1246–62.
11. Baumann F, Carbone M. Environmental risk of mesothelioma in the United States: an emerging concern epidemiological issues. J Toxicol Environ Health Part B. 2016;19(5–6):231–49.
12. Milano MT, Zhang H. Malignant pleural mesothelioma: a population-based study of survival. J Thorac Oncol. 2010;5(11):1841–8.
13. Beebe-Dimmer J, Fryzek J, Yee C, Dalvi T, Garabrant D, Schwartz A, et al. Mesothelioma in the United States: a surveillance, epidemiology, and end results (SEER) Medicare investigation of treatment patterns and overall survival. Clin Epidemiol. 2016;8:743–50.
14. Alpert N, Gerwen MV, Taioli E. Epidemiology of mesothelioma in the 21st century in Europe and the United States, 40 years after restricted/banned asbestos use. Transl Lung Cancer Res. 2020;9(S1):S28–38.
15. Robinson B. Malignant pleural mesothelioma: an epidemiological perspective. Ann Cardiothorac Surg. 2012;1(4):491–6.
16. Carbone M, Adusumilli PS, Alexander HR, Baas P, Bardelli F, Bononi A, et al. Mesothelioma: scientific clues for prevention, diagnosis, and therapy. CA Cancer J Clin. 2019;69(5):402–29.
17. Lanphear B, Buncher CR. Latent period for malignant mesothelioma of occupational origin. J Occup Med. 1992;34(7):718–21.
18. Henley S, Larson TC, Wu M, Antao VCS, Lewis M, Pinheiro GA, et al. Mesothelioma incidence in 50 states and the District of Columbia, United States, 2003–2008. Int J Occup Environ Health. 2013;19(1):1–10.
19. Neumann V, Löseke S, Nowak D, Herth FJF, Tannapfel A. Malignant pleural mesothelioma: incidence, etiology, diagnosis, treatment, and occupational health. Dtsch Arztebl Int. 2013;110(18):319–26. https://doi.org/10.3238/arztebl.2013.0319.
20. Klebe S, Hocking AJ, Soeberg M, Leigh J. The significance of short latency in mesothelioma for attribution of causation: report of a case with predisposing germline mutations and review of the literature. Int J Environ Res Public Health. 2021;18(24):13310.
21. Testa JR, Cheung M, Pei J, Below JE, Tan Y, Sementino E, et al. Germline BAP1 mutations predispose to malignant mesothelioma. Nat Genet. 2011;43(10):1022–5.
22. Napolitano A, Pellegrini L, Dey A, Larson D, Tanji M, Flores EG, et al. Minimal asbestos exposure in germline BAP1 heterozygous mice is associated with deregulated inflammatory response and increased risk of mesothelioma. Oncogene. 2016;35(15):1996–2002.
23. Cebulla CM, Binkley EM, Pilarski R, Massengill JB, Rai K, Liebner DA, et al. Analysis of BAP1 germline gene mutation in young uveal melanoma patients. Ophthalmic Genet. 2015;36(2):126–31.
24. De La Fouchardière A, Cabaret O, Savin L, Combemale P, Schvartz H, Penet C, et al. Germline BAP1 mutations predispose also to multiple basal cell carcinomas. Clin Genet. 2015;88(3):273–7.
25. Popova T, Hebert L, Jacquemin V, Gad S, Caux-Moncoutier V, Dubois-d'Enghien C, et al. Germline BAP1 mutations predispose to renal cell carcinomas. Am J Hum Genet. 2013;92(6):974–80.
26. Wadt KAW, Aoude LG, Johansson P, Solinas A, Pritchard A, Crainic O, et al. A recurrent germline BAP1 mutation and extension of the BAP1 tumor predisposition spectrum to include basal cell carcinoma. Clin Genet. 2015;88(3):267–72.
27. Abdel-Rahman MH, Pilarski R, Cebulla CM, Massengill JB, Christopher BN, Boru G, et al. Germline BAP1 mutation predisposes to uveal melanoma, lung adenocarcinoma, meningioma, and other cancers. J Med Genet. 2011;48(12):856–9.
28. Peña-Llopis S, Vega-Rubín-de-Celis S, Liao A, Leng N, Pavía-Jiménez A, Wang S, et al. BAP1 loss defines a new class of renal cell carcinoma. Nat Genet. 2012;44(7):751–9.

29. Farley MN, Schmidt LS, Mester JL, Peña-Llopis S, Pavia-Jimenez A, Christie A, et al. A novel germline mutation in BAP1 predisposes to familial clear-cell renal cell carcinoma. Mol Cancer Res. 2013;11(9):1061–71.
30. Wiesner T, Obenauf AC, Murali R, Fried I, Griewank KG, Ulz P, et al. Germline mutations in BAP1 predispose to melanocytic tumors. Nat Genet. 2011;43(10):1018–21.
31. Yoshikawa Y, Emi M, Hashimoto-Tamaoki T, Ohmuraya M, Sato A, Tsujimura T, et al. High-density array-CGH with targeted NGS unmask multiple noncontiguous minute deletions on chromosome 3p21 in mesothelioma. Proc Natl Acad Sci. 2016;113(47):13432–7.
32. An X, Li-Jun W, Santella RM, Hei TK. Role of oxyradicals in mutagenicity and DNA damage induced by crocidolite asbestos in mammalian cells. Cancer Res. 1999;59(23):5922–6.
33. Xu A, Zhou H, Yu DZ, Hei TK. Mechanisms of the genotoxicity of crocidolite asbestos in mammalian cells: implication from mutation patterns induced by reactive oxygen species. Environ Health Perspect. 2002;110(10):1003–8.
34. Suarez JS, Novelli F, Goto K, Ehara M, Steele M, Kim JH, et al. HMGB1 released by mesothelial cells drives the development of asbestos-induced mesothelioma. Proc Natl Acad Sci. 2023;120(39):e2307999120.
35. Xue J, Patergnani S, Giorgi C, Suarez J, Goto K, Bononi A, et al. Asbestos induces mesothelial cell transformation via HMGB1-driven autophagy. Proc Natl Acad Sci. 2020;117(41):25543–52.
36. Yang H, Bocchetta M, Kroczynska B, Elmishad AG, Chen Y, Liu Z, et al. TNF-α inhibits asbestos-induced cytotoxicity via a NF-κB-dependent pathway, a possible mechanism for asbestos-induced oncogenesis. Proc Natl Acad Sci. 2006;103(27):10397–402.
37. Yang H, Rivera Z, Jube S, Nasu M, Bertino P, Goparaju C, et al. Programmed necrosis induced by asbestos in human mesothelial cells causes high-mobility group box 1 protein release and resultant inflammation. Proc Natl Acad Sci. 2010;107(28):12611–6.
38. Mott FE. Mesothelioma: a review. Ochsner J. 2012;12(1):70–9.
39. Moore AJ, Parker RJ, Wiggins J. Malignant mesothelioma. Orphanet J Rare Dis. 2008;3(1):34.
40. Hassan M, Touman AA, Grabczak EM, Skaarup SH, Faber K, Blyth KG, et al. Imaging of pleural disease. Breathe. 2024;20(1):230172.
41. Gill RR. Imaging of mesothelioma. In: Tannapfel A, editor. Malignant mesothelioma, Recent results in cancer research, vol. 189. Berlin/Heidelberg: Springer; 2011. p. 27–43. https://doi.org/10.1007/978-3-642-10862-4_2.
42. Gill RR, Gerbaudo VH, Sugarbaker DJ, Hatabu H. Current trends in radiologic management of malignant pleural mesothelioma. Semin Thorac Cardiovasc Surg. 2009;21(2):111–20.
43. Metintas M, Ucgun I, Elbek O, Erginel S, Metintas S, Kolsuz M, et al. Computed tomography features in malignant pleural mesothelioma and other commonly seen pleural diseases. Eur J Radiol. 2002;41(1):1–9.
44. Gill RR, Tsao AS, Kindler HL, Richards WG, Armato SG, Francis RJ, et al. Radiologic considerations and standardization of malignant pleural mesothelioma imaging within clinical trials: consensus statement from the NCI thoracic malignancy steering committee – International Association for the Study of Lung Cancer – mesothelioma applied research foundation clinical trials planning meeting. J Thorac Oncol. 2019;14(10):1718–31.
45. Drevs J, Schneider V. The use of vascular biomarkers and imaging studies in the early clinical development of anti-tumour agents targeting angiogenesis. J Intern Med. 2006;260(6):517–29.
46. Yildirim H, Metintas M, Entok E, Ak G, Ak I, Dundar E, et al. Clinical value of fluorodeoxyglucose-positron emission tomography/computed tomography in differentiation of malignant mesothelioma from asbestos-related benign pleural disease: an observational pilot study. J Thorac Oncol. 2009;4(12):1480–4.
47. Bénard F, Sterman D, Smith RJ, Kaiser LR, Albelda SM, Alavi A. Metabolic imaging of malignant pleural mesothelioma with fluorodeoxyglucose positron emission tomography. Chest. 1998;114(3):713–22.
48. Kruse M, Sherry SJ, Paidpally V, Mercier G, Subramaniam RM. FDG PET/CT in the management of primary pleural tumors and pleural metastases. Am J Roentgenol. 2013;201(2):W215–26.
49. Nowak AK, Francis RJ, Phillips MJ, Millward MJ, Van Der Schaaf AA, Boucek J, et al. A novel prognostic model for malignant mesothelioma incorporating quantitative FDG-PET imaging with clinical parameters. Clin Cancer Res. 2010;16(8):2409–17.
50. Klabatsa A, Chicklore S, Barrington SF, Goh V, Lang-Lazdunski L, Cook GJR. The association of 18F-FDG PET/CT parameters with survival in malignant pleural mesothelioma. Eur J Nucl Med Mol Imaging. 2014;41(2):276–82.
51. Incerti E, Broggi S, Fodor A, Cuzzocrea M, Samanes Gajate AM, Mapelli P, et al. FDG PET-derived parameters as prognostic tool in progressive malignant pleural mesothelioma treated patients. Eur J Nucl Med Mol Imaging. 2018;45(12):2071–8.
52. Churg A. New developments in mesothelial pathology. Histopathology. 2024;84(1):136–52.
53. Chirieac LR, Hung YP, Foo WC, Hofer MD, VanderLaan PA, Richards WG, et al. Diagnostic value of biopsy sampling in predicting histology in patients with diffuse malignant pleural mesothelioma. Cancer. 2019;125(23):4164–71.

54. Attanoos RL, Gibbs AR. The comparative accuracy of different pleural biopsy techniques in the diagnosis of malignant mesothelioma. Histopathology. 2008;53(3):340–4.
55. Fletcher SV, Clark RJ. The Portsmouth thoracoscopy experience, an evaluation of service by retrospective case note analysis. Respir Med. 2007;101(5):1021–5.
56. Blanc FX, Atassi K, Bignon J, Housset B. Diagnostic value of medical thoracoscopy in pleural disease. Chest. 2002;121(5):1677–83.
57. Medford ARL, Agrawal S, Free CM, Bennett JA. A local anaesthetic video-assisted thoracoscopy service: prospective performance analysis in a UK tertiary respiratory Centre. Lung Cancer. 2009;66(3):355–8.
58. Metintas M, Ak G, Parspour S, Yildirim H, Erginel S, Alatas F, et al. Local recurrence of tumor at sites of intervention in malignant pleural mesothelioma. Lung Cancer. 2008;61(2):255–61.
59. Lee C, Bayman N, Swindell R, Faivre-Finn C. Prophylactic radiotherapy to intervention sites in mesothelioma: a systematic review and survey of UK practice. Lung Cancer. 2009;66(2):150–6.
60. Hung YP, Chirieac LR. Pathology of malignant pleural mesothelioma. Thorac Surg Clin. 2020;30(4):367–82.
61. Marchevsky AM, Khoor A, Walts AE, Nicholson AG, Zhang YZ, Roggli V, et al. Localized malignant mesothelioma, an unusual and poorly characterized neoplasm of serosal origin: best current evidence from the literature and the international mesothelioma panel. Mod Pathol. 2020;33(2):281–96.
62. Churg A, Galateau-Salle F. The separation of benign and malignant mesothelial proliferations. Arch Pathol Lab Med. 2012;136(10):1217–26.
63. Tischoff I, Neid M, Neumann V, Tannapfel A. Pathohistological diagnosis and differential diagnosis. In: Tannapfel A, editor. Malignant mesothelioma, Recent results in cancer research, vol. 189. Berlin/Heidelberg: Springer; 2011. p. 57–78. https://doi.org/10.1007/978-3-642-10862-4_4.
64. Allen TC. Recognition of histopathologic patterns of diffuse malignant mesothelioma in differential diagnosis of pleural biopsies. Arch Pathol Lab Med. 2005;129(11):1415–20.
65. Cheng YY, Yuen ML, Rath EM, Johnson B, Zhuang L, Yu TK, et al. CDKN2A and MTAP are useful biomarkers detectable by droplet digital PCR in malignant pleural mesothelioma: a potential alternative method in diagnosis compared to fluorescence in situ hybridisation. Front Oncol. 2020;10:579327.
66. Tammilehto L, Kivisaari L, Salminen US, Maasilta P, Mattson K. Evaluation of the clinical TNM staging system for malignant pleural mesothelioma: an assessment in 88 patients. Lung Cancer. 1995;12(1–2):25–34.
67. Butchart EG, Ashcroft T, Barnsley WC, Holden MP. Pleuropneumonectomy in the management of diffuse malignant mesothelioma of the pleura. Experience with 29 patients. Thorax. 1976;31(1):15–24.
68. Rusch VW, Venkatraman E. The importance of surgical staging in the treatment of malignant pleural mesothelioma. J Thorac Cardiovasc Surg. 1996;111(4):815–26.
69. Sugarbaker DJ, Strauss GM, Lynch TJ, Richards W, Mentzer SJ, Lee TH, et al. Node status has prognostic significance in the multimodality therapy of diffuse, malignant mesothelioma. J Clin Oncol. 1993;11(6):1172–8.
70. Euhus CJ, Ripley RT. The staging of malignant pleural mesothelioma. Thorac Surg Clin. 2020;30(4):425–33.
71. Pass H, Giroux D, Kennedy C, Ruffini E, Cangir AK, Rice D, et al. The IASLC mesothelioma staging project: improving staging of a rare disease through international participation. J Thorac Oncol. 2016;11(12):2082–8.
72. Rusch V. A proposed new international TNM staging system for malignant pleural mesothelioma. Chest. 1995;108(4):1122–8.
73. Rusch VW, Chansky K, Kindler HL, Nowak AK, Pass HI, Rice DC, et al. The IASLC mesothelioma staging project: proposals for the M descriptors and for revision of the TNM stage groupings in the forthcoming (eighth) edition of the TNM classification for mesothelioma. J Thorac Oncol. 2016;11(12):2112–9.
74. Wolf AS, Eisele M, Giroux DJ, Gill R, Nowak AK, Bille A, et al. The international association for the study of lung cancer pleural mesothelioma staging project: expanded database to inform revisions in the ninth edition of the TNM classification of pleural mesothelioma. J Thorac Oncol. 2024;19(8):1242–52.
75. Nowak AK, Giroux DJ, Eisele M, Rosenthal A, Bille A, Gill RR, et al. The International Association for the Study of Lung Cancer pleural mesothelioma staging project: proposal for revision of the TNM stage groupings in the forthcoming (ninth) edition of the TNM classification for pleural mesothelioma. J Thorac Oncol. 2024;19(9):1339–51.
76. Gill RR, Nowak AK, Giroux DJ, Eisele M, Rosenthal A, Kindler H, et al. The International Association for the Study of Lung Cancer mesothelioma staging project: proposals for revisions of the "T" descriptors in the forthcoming ninth edition of the TNM classification for pleural mesothelioma. J Thorac Oncol. 2024;19(9):1310–25.
77. Bille A, Ripley RT, Giroux DJ, Gill RR, Kindler HL, Nowak AK, et al. The International Association for the Study of Lung Cancer mesothelioma staging project: proposals for the "N" descriptors in the forthcoming ninth edition of the TNM classification for pleural mesothelioma. J Thorac Oncol. 2024;19(9):1326–38.
78. Kindler HL, Rosenthal A, Giroux DJ, Nowak AK, Billè A, Gill RR, et al. The International Association for the Study of Lung Cancer mesothelioma stag-

ing project: proposals for the m descriptors in the forthcoming ninth edition of the TNM classification for pleural mesothelioma. J Thorac Oncol. 2024;19(11):1564–77.
79. Rice D, Chansky K, Nowak A, Pass H, Kindler H, Shemanski L, et al. The IASLC mesothelioma staging project: proposals for revisions of the N descriptors in the forthcoming eighth edition of the TNM classification for pleural mesothelioma. J Thorac Oncol. 2016;11(12):2100–11.
80. Song KJ, Flores RM, Wolf AS. Effective multimodal approaches for malignant pleural mesothelioma. Thorac Surg Clin. 2020;30(4):481–7.
81. Flores RM, Pass HI, Seshan VE, Dycoco J, Zakowski M, Carbone M, et al. Extrapleural pneumonectomy versus pleurectomy/decortication in the surgical management of malignant pleural mesothelioma: results in 663 patients. J Thorac Cardiovasc Surg. 2008;135(3):620–626.e3.
82. Sugarbaker DJ, Wolf AS. Surgery for malignant pleural mesothelioma. Expert Rev Respir Med. 2010;4(3):363–72.
83. Kindler HL, Ismaila N, Armato SG, Bueno R, Hesdorffer M, Jahan T, et al. Treatment of malignant pleural mesothelioma: American Society of Clinical Oncology clinical practice guideline. J Clin Oncol. 2018;36(13):1343–73.
84. Rice D, Rusch V, Pass H, Asamura H, Nakano T, Edwards J, et al. Recommendations for uniform definitions of surgical techniques for malignant pleural mesothelioma: a consensus report of the International Association for the Study of Lung Cancer international staging committee and the international mesothelioma interest group. J Thorac Oncol. 2011;6(8):1304–12.
85. Sugarbaker DJ, Jaklitsch MT, Bueno R, Richards W, Lukanich J, Mentzer SJ, et al. Prevention, early detection, and management of complications after 328 consecutive extrapleural pneumonectomies. J Thorac Cardiovasc Surg. 2004;128(1):138–46.
86. Taioli E, Wolf AS, Flores RM. Meta-analysis of survival after pleurectomy decortication versus extrapleural pneumonectomy in mesothelioma. Ann Thorac Surg. 2015;99(2):472–80.
87. Santoro A, O'Brien ME, Stahel RA, Nackaerts K, Baas P, Karthaus M, et al. Pemetrexed plus cisplatin or pemetrexed plus carboplatin for chemonaïve patients with malignant pleural mesothelioma: results of the international expanded access program. J Thorac Oncol. 2008;3(7):756–63.
88. Yan TD, Boyer M, Tin MM, Wong D, Kennedy C, McLean J, et al. Extrapleural pneumonectomy for malignant pleural mesothelioma: outcomes of treatment and prognostic factors. J Thorac Cardiovasc Surg. 2009;138(3):619–24.
89. Rusch VW, Rosenzweig K, Venkatraman E, Leon L, Raben A, Harrison L, et al. A phase II trial of surgical resection and adjuvant high-dose hemithoracic radiation for malignant pleural mesothelioma. J Thorac Cardiovasc Surg. 2001;122(4):788–95.
90. Weder W, Stahel RA, Bernhard J, Bodis S, Vogt P, Ballabeni P, et al. Multicenter trial of neo-adjuvant chemotherapy followed by extrapleural pneumonectomy in malignant pleural mesothelioma. Ann Oncol. 2007;18(7):1196–202.
91. De Perrot M, Feld R, Cho BCJ, Bezjak A, Anraku M, Burkes R, et al. Trimodality therapy with induction chemotherapy followed by extrapleural pneumonectomy and adjuvant high-dose hemithoracic radiation for malignant pleural mesothelioma. J Clin Oncol. 2009;27(9):1413–8.
92. Krug LM, Pass HI, Rusch VW, Kindler HL, Sugarbaker DJ, Rosenzweig KE, et al. Multicenter phase II trial of neoadjuvant pemetrexed plus cisplatin followed by extrapleural pneumonectomy and radiation for malignant pleural mesothelioma. J Clin Oncol. 2009;27(18):3007–13.
93. Flores RM, Zakowski M, Venkatraman E, Krug L, Rosenzweig K, Dycoco J, et al. Prognostic factors in the treatment of malignant pleural mesothelioma at a large tertiary referral center. J Thorac Oncol. 2007;2(10):957–65.
94. Ambrogi V, Mineo D, Gatti A, Pompeo E, Mineo TC. Symptomatic and quality of life changes after extrapleural pneumonectomy for malignant pleural mesothelioma. J Surg Oncol. 2009;100(3):199–204.
95. Rusch VW. Pleurectomy/decortication and adjuvant therapy for malignant mesothelioma. Chest. 1993;103(4):382S–4S.
96. Soysal O. Pleurectomy/decortication for palliation in malignant pleural mesothelioma: results of surgery. Eur J Cardiothorac Surg. 1997;11(2):210–3.
97. Baldini EH, Richards WG, Gill RR, Goodman BM, Winfrey OK, Eisen HM, et al. Updated patterns of failure after multimodality therapy for malignant pleural mesothelioma. J Thorac Cardiovasc Surg. 2015;149(5):1374–81.
98. Tilleman TR, Richards WG, Zellos L, Johnson BE, Jaklitsch MT, Mueller J, et al. Extrapleural pneumonectomy followed by intracavitary intraoperative hyperthermic cisplatin with pharmacologic cytoprotection for treatment of malignant pleural mesothelioma: a phase II prospective study. J Thorac Cardiovasc Surg. 2009;138(2):405–11.
99. Sugarbaker DJ, Gill RR, Yeap BY, Wolf AS, DaSilva MC, Baldini EH, et al. Hyperthermic intraoperative pleural cisplatin chemotherapy extends interval to recurrence and survival among low-risk patients with malignant pleural mesothelioma undergoing surgical macroscopic complete resection. J Thorac Cardiovasc Surg. 2013;145(4):955–63.
100. Bille A, Jhala H, Ashrafian L, Allison L, Russell M, Fleck R, et al. Does hyperthermic povidone-iodine lavage increase the apoptotic rate of residual cancer cell in patients with malignant pleural mesothelioma? – A prospective pilot study. Transl Lung Cancer Res. 2023;12(7):1384–90.
101. Lang-Lazdunski L, Bille A, Papa S, Marshall S, Lal R, Galeone C, et al. Pleurectomy/decortication, hyperthermic pleural lavage with povidone-iodine,

prophylactic radiotherapy, and systemic chemotherapy in patients with malignant pleural mesothelioma: a 10-year experience. J Thorac Cardiovasc Surg. 2015;149(2):558–66.
102. Feller-Kopman DJ, Reddy CB, DeCamp MM, Diekemper RL, Gould MK, Henry T, et al. Management of malignant pleural effusions. An official ATS/STS/STR clinical practice guideline. Am J Respir Crit Care Med. 2018;198(7):839–49.
103. Leal JL, Peters G, Szaumkessel M, Leong T, Asadi K, Rivalland G, et al. NTRK and ALK rearrangements in malignant pleural mesothelioma, pulmonary neuroendocrine tumours and non-small cell lung cancer. Lung Cancer. 2020;146:154–9.
104. Vogelzang NJ, Rusthoven JJ, Symanowski J, Denham C, Kaukel E, Ruffie P, et al. Phase III study of pemetrexed in combination with cisplatin versus cisplatin alone in patients with malignant pleural mesothelioma. J Clin Oncol. 2003;21(14):2636–44.
105. Castagneto B, Botta M, Aitini E, Spigno F, Degiovanni D, Alabiso O, et al. Phase II study of pemetrexed in combination with carboplatin in patients with malignant pleural mesothelioma (MPM). Ann Oncol. 2008;19(2):370–3.
106. Nowak AK, Byrne MJ, Williamson R, Ryan G, Segal A, Fielding D, et al. A multicentre phase II study of cisplatin and gemcitabine for malignant mesothelioma. Br J Cancer. 2002;87(5):491–6.
107. Van Haarst JMW, Baas P, Manegold CH, Schouwink JH, Burgers JA, De Bruin HG, et al. Multicentre phase II study of gemcitabine and cisplatin in malignant pleural mesothelioma. Br J Cancer. 2002;86(3):342–5.
108. Taylor P, Castagneto B, Dark G, Marangolo M, Scagliotti GV, Van Klaveren RJ, et al. Single-agent pemetrexed for chemonaïve and pretreated patients with malignant pleural mesothelioma: results of an international expanded access program. J Thorac Oncol. 2008;3(7):764–71.
109. Muers MF, Stephens RJ, Fisher P, Darlison L, Higgs CM, Lowry E, et al. Active symptom control with or without chemotherapy in the treatment of patients with malignant pleural mesothelioma (MS01): a multicentre randomised trial. Lancet. 2008;371(9625):1685–94.
110. Scherpereel A, Mazieres J, Greillier L, Lantuejoul S, Dô P, Bylicki O, et al. Nivolumab or nivolumab plus ipilimumab in patients with relapsed malignant pleural mesothelioma (IFCT-1501 MAPS2): a multicentre, open-label, randomised, non-comparative, phase 2 trial. Lancet Oncol. 2019;20(2):239–53.
111. Disselhorst MJ, Quispel-Janssen J, Lalezari F, Monkhorst K, De Vries JF, Van Der Noort V, et al. Ipilimumab and nivolumab in the treatment of recurrent malignant pleural mesothelioma (INITIATE): results of a prospective, single-arm, phase 2 trial. Lancet Respir Med. 2019;7(3):260–70.
112. Fennell DA, Ewings S, Ottensmeier C, Califano R, Hanna GG, Hill K, et al. Nivolumab versus placebo in patients with relapsed malignant mesothelioma (CONFIRM): a multicentre, double-blind, randomised, phase 3 trial. Lancet Oncol. 2021;22(11):1530–40.
113. De Gooijer CJ, Borm FJ, Scherpereel A, Baas P. Immunotherapy in malignant pleural mesothelioma. Front Oncol. 2020;10:187.
114. Baas P, Scherpereel A, Nowak AK, Fujimoto N, Peters S, Tsao AS, et al. First-line nivolumab plus ipilimumab in unresectable malignant pleural mesothelioma (CheckMate 743): a multicentre, randomised, open-label, phase 3 trial. Lancet. 2021;397(10272):375–86.
115. Peters S, Scherpereel A, Cornelissen R, Oulkhouir Y, Greillier L, Kaplan MA, et al. First-line nivolumab plus ipilimumab versus chemotherapy in patients with unresectable malignant pleural mesothelioma: 3-year outcomes from CheckMate 743. Ann Oncol. 2022;33(5):488–99.
116. Zalcman G, Mazieres J, Margery J, Greillier L, Audigier-Valette C, Moro-Sibilot D, et al. Bevacizumab for newly diagnosed pleural mesothelioma in the mesothelioma Avastin cisplatin Pemetrexed study (MAPS): a randomised, controlled, open-label, phase 3 trial. Lancet. 2016;387(10026):1405–14.
117. Gupta V, Mychalczak B, Krug L, Flores R, Bains M, Rusch VW, et al. Hemithoracic radiation therapy after pleurectomy/decortication for malignant pleural mesothelioma. Int J Radiat Oncol. 2005;63(4):1045–52.
118. Minatel E, Trovo M, Polesel J, Baresic T, Bearz A, Franchin G, et al. Radical pleurectomy/decortication followed by high dose of radiation therapy for malignant pleural mesothelioma. Final results with long-term follow-up. Lung Cancer. 2014;83(1):78–82.
119. Forster KM, Smythe WR, Starkschall G, Liao Z, Takanaka T, Kelly JF, et al. Intensity-modulated radiotherapy following extrapleural pneumonectomy for the treatment of malignant mesothelioma: clinical implementation. Int J Radiat Oncol. 2003;55(3):606–16.
120. Sugarbaker DJ, Flores RM, Jaklitsch MT, Richards WG, Strauss GM, Corson JM, et al. Resection margins, extrapleural nodal status, and cell type determine postoperative long-term survival in trimodality therapy of malignant pleural mesothelioma: results in 183 patients. J Thorac Cardiovasc Surg. 1999;117(1):54–65.
121. Trovo M, Relevant A, Polesel J, Muraro E, Barresi L, Drigo A, et al. Radical hemithoracic radiotherapy versus palliative radiotherapy in non-metastatic malignant pleural mesothelioma: results from a phase 3 randomized clinical trial. Int J Radiat Oncol. 2021;109(5):1368–76.
122. Minatel E, Trovo M, Polesel J, Rumeileh IA, Baresic T, Bearz A, et al. Tomotherapy after pleurectomy/decortication or biopsy for malignant pleural mesothelioma allows the delivery of high dose of radiation in patients with intact lung. J Thorac Oncol. 2012;7(12):1862–6.

123. Clive AO, Taylor H, Dobson L, Wilson P, De Winton E, Panakis N, et al. Prophylactic radiotherapy for the prevention of procedure-tract metastases after surgical and large-bore pleural procedures in malignant pleural mesothelioma (SMART): a multicentre, open-label, phase 3, randomised controlled trial. Lancet Oncol. 2016;17(8):1094–104.
124. Tsao AS, Lindwasser OW, Adjei AA, Adusumilli PS, Beyers ML, Blumenthal GM, et al. Current and future management of malignant mesothelioma: a consensus report from the National Cancer Institute thoracic malignancy steering committee, International Association for the Study of Lung Cancer, and Mesothelioma Applied Research Foundation. J Thorac Oncol. 2018;13(11):1655–67.
125. Meyerhoff RR, Yang CFJ, Speicher PJ, Gulack BC, Hartwig MG, D'Amico TA, et al. Impact of mesothelioma histologic subtype on outcomes in the surveillance, epidemiology, and end results database. J Surg Res. 2015;196(1):23–32.

Primary Pleural Synovial Sarcoma

15

Daniel Kapadia and Peter Boshara

Introduction

Primary pleural synovial sarcoma (PPSS) is an aggressive neoplasm originating from submesothelial, undifferentiated mesenchymal cells. First documented in the early 1900s, the neoplasm was observed to originate from or near joint spaces. Microscopically, the cells displayed similarities to syncytiocytes. Since the pleural membrane does not naturally contain synovial tissue, it is now believed that the cells derive from undifferentiated mesenchymal cells capable of differentiating into synovial tissue. Nonetheless, the term has persisted as a misnomer [1, 2].

Synovial sarcoma of the lungs and pleura most frequently presents as metastatic disease originating from the extremities and soft tissues [3, 4]. Primary pulmonary synovial sarcoma is far more uncommon and was first documented in a case series of 25 patients in 1995. Subsequently, Gaertner et al. reported primary pleural synovial sarcoma the following year, also as a case series of five patients [5, 6]. This neoplasm is exceedingly uncommon, accounting for approximately 16% of pulmonary sarcomas, which themselves represent about 0.5% of all primary lung neoplasms [7]. Fewer than 100 cases have been documented in the literature, thereby limiting the capacity for comprehensive study and comparison of various treatment modalities and patient outcomes [8]. Pulmonary synovial sarcoma most often affects young to middle-aged adults, typically between 30 and 50 years of age, with a median presentation age of 47 years [9, 10]. There is no evident gender predilection, as the incidence is similar in both sexes [3]. Due to the extreme rarity of this condition, no known risk factors, ethnic, or geographic patterns have been established in the literature to date. PPSS can originate from either the visceral or parietal pleura, or both, and may locally invade adjacent structures, including the chest wall, lung parenchyma, and even the central airways [11, 12]. Although it generally presents as a solid, localized, pleural-based soft-tissue tumor, PPSS can, less frequently, manifest as extensive pleural thickening [13].

Clinical Features

The symptoms of PPSS can be nonspecific, and patients may present with chest pain, dyspnea, nonproductive cough, and constitutional symptoms, including fatigue, low-grade fever, or weight loss [14, 15]. Hemoptysis is a less common complaint [11]. Most patients are symptomatic at the time of diagnosis. However, many are asymptomatic, with no respiratory or constitu-

D. Kapadia (✉)
Interventional Pulmonology, Henry Ford Health, Detroit, MI, USA
e-mail: Dkapadi1@hfhs.org

P. Boshara
Department of Interventional Pulmonology, University of Illinois Chicago, Chicago, IL, USA

F. Ido (ed.), *Rare Pleural Diseases*, https://doi.org/10.1007/978-3-032-14873-5_15

tional complaints, and PPSS is discovered incidentally on routine chest imaging [15, 16]. In a case series of 19 patients with PPSS, chest pain was the most common presenting symptom, followed by dyspnea and cough [17]. Pleural effusion is a common coexisting finding, and the presence of an accompanying pleural effusion may result in severe dyspnea and hypoxemia [14, 18]. In the setting of PPSS with a malignant pleural effusion, physical exam findings can include decreased unilateral breath sounds and dullness to percussion [14]. PPSS can also present as a hemothorax, pneumothorax, or hydropneumothorax [13, 14, 19–21].

Diagnosis

Imaging

PPSS lacks specific clinical or imaging signs that are definitive; an accurate diagnosis depends on a combination of histopathologic, immunohistochemical, and molecular tests.

Initial imaging with a chest X-ray typically reveals a pleural-based mass or pleural effusion; however, it lacks specificity and often requires more advanced imaging modalities. Contrast-enhanced computed tomography (CT) scans of the chest play a vital role in assessing tumor extent and delineating its anatomical relationship with adjacent structures. In most instances, a well-circumscribed or lobulated pleural-based low-density mass is observed, exhibiting heterogeneous enhancement with hemorrhagic and necrotic foci (Fig. 15.1a, b) [9, 16, 22, 23]. The mass may originate from the visceral or parietal pleura, along the mediastinal, diaphragmatic, or costal surfaces [11, 12, 24]. In less frequent cases, CT may reveal abnormal diffuse pleural thickening [25]. Magnetic resonance imaging (MRI) is superior for detailing the nodular and internal components. Following contrast administration, rim enhancement is typically observed (Fig. 15.1c–e) [64]. Positron-emission tomography/computed tomography (PET/CT) can be used to assess the metabolic activity of the mass and detect distant metastases. Typically, there is moderate to intense FDG uptake in the mass or pleural thickening on PET/CT; however, the pleural effusion generally does not demonstrate FDG uptake (Fig. 15.1f–h) [12, 23, 25, 26].

Pathology

Tissue sampling is essential for diagnosing PPSS. This can be achieved through various methods, including percutaneous image-guided

Fig. 15.1 (continued) (**g**) PET/CT of the para-esophageal mass showing heterogeneous hypermetabolism with a large central necrotic component. Two smaller pleural nodules (white circles) exhibit mild FDG uptake
(**h**) PET/CT of the perihepatic nodular lesion showing marked FDG avidity (white circle)
Panels **a–h** represent a single patient case contributed by *Dr. Firas Ido*
(**i**) Hematoxylin- and eosin-stained section (×40) showing sheets of spindle cells with minimal intervening stroma
(**j**) Immunohistochemical staining for BCL-2 demonstrates diffuse cytoplasmic positivity
(**k**) Immunohistochemical staining for CD99 showing strong, diffuse membranous positivity

Panels **i–k** originate from a different case of primary pleural synovial sarcoma and are included for histopathologic comparison

Attribution: Panels **a–h** courtesy of *Dr. Firas Ido*; original, unpublished images reproduced with permission of the author

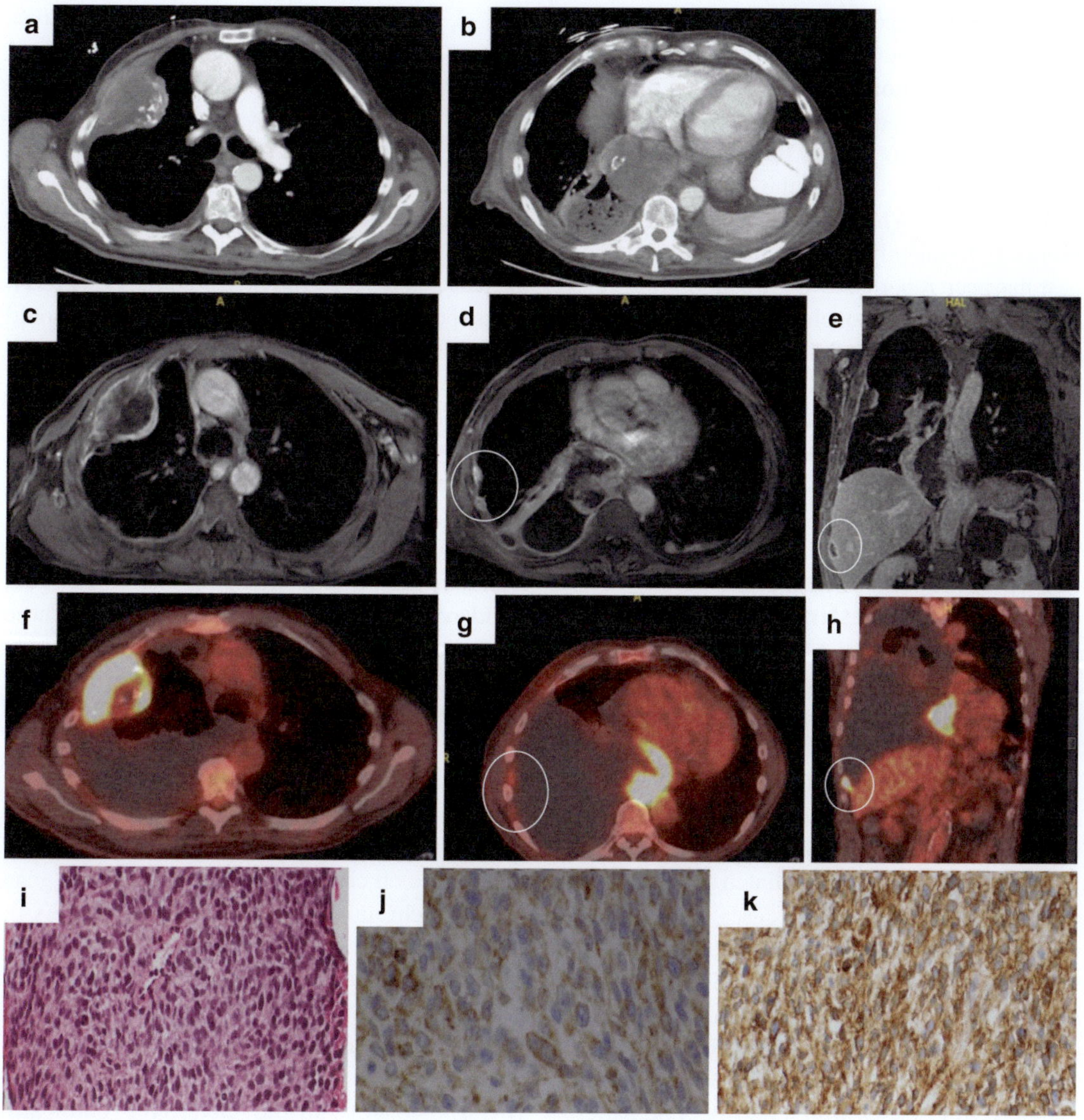

Fig. 15.1 Radiologic and histopathologic features of primary pleural synovial sarcoma

(**a**) Contrast-enhanced computed tomography of the chest showing a large, heterogeneous mass arising from the right anterior pleura at the level of the upper lobe. The lesion contains punctate calcifications and demonstrates chest-wall invasion with associated nodular circumferential pleural thickening

(**b**) Contrast-enhanced CT depicting a second large, rounded para-esophageal pleural mass with internal calcifications. An adjacent complex pleural effusion is partially drained, leaving a trapped lung. Nodular pleural thickening extends along the lateral chest wall

(**c**) Magnetic resonance angiography (MRA) of the chest wall, revealing the pleural mass from panel A, characterized by heterogeneous internal signal intensities and peripheral rim enhancement, suggestive of internal necrosis or fluid content

(**d**) MRA demonstrating a large heterogeneous para-esophageal mass with associated loculated pleural effusion and trapped lung. Two additional nodular metastatic lesions (white circles) are better visualized on MRA than on CT

(**e**) MRA image showing a nodular metastatic lesion adjacent to the liver, likely involving the peritoneum (white circle)

(**f**) Positron-emission tomography/computed tomography (PET/CT) of the pleural mass from panel A demonstrating intense hypermetabolism with non-avid regions corresponding to necrosis

(continued)

(CT or ultrasound) transthoracic core-needle biopsy, pleuroscopy with parietal pleural biopsy, or surgical resection via video-assisted thoracoscopy or thoracotomy. Among these techniques, surgical resection remains the gold standard for tissue acquisition, offering the highest diagnostic yield [27, 28]. While percutaneous core-needle biopsy is frequently utilized, its diagnostic success has been reported to vary, with multiple case reports indicating inconclusive biopsies or misdiagnoses [15, 18]. Additionally, pleural fluid cytology is often negative, exhibiting a sensitivity of only 38% in cases of malignant pleural effusion attributable to sarcoma [29, 30].

Histopathology, Immunohistochemistry, and Molecular Testing

PPSS is typically divided into four subtypes based on histological features: (1) biphasic, with both epithelial and spindle cells; (2) monophasic epithelial, made up entirely of epithelial cells; (3) monophasic fibrous, consisting solely of spindle cells (Fig. 15.1l); and (4) poorly differentiated [31, 32]. The poorly differentiated subtype occurs in approximately 20% of cases and typically indicates a less favorable prognosis [12, 27]. A review of 14 PPSS cases showed that half were biphasic [14]. Hematoxylin-eosin (H&E) staining of monophasic PPSS shows dense sheets of small, round, or oval spindle cells, sometimes arranged in fascicles with a herringbone pattern, and with minimal eosinophilic cytoplasm [14, 18, 23, 33]. Additionally, a vascular pattern resembling hemangiopericytoma has been described [12].

Immunohistochemistry (IHC) staining can further assist in diagnosing PPSS and help distinguish it from malignancies with similar morphological features. PPSS tumors have been observed to demonstrate positive expression for vimentin, epithelial membrane antigen (EMA), cytokeratin, BCL-2, and CD99, while negative for S-100, desmin, CD34, smooth muscle actin, TTF-1, chromogranin A, synaptophysin, and WT-1 (Fig. 15.1j, k) [14, 22–24, 29, 33, 34]. Positive immunohistochemical staining for CD99 and BCL2 may help differentiate PPSS from malignant mesothelioma, which is typically negative for these markers [18]. TLE1 is a highly sensitive nuclear marker for synovial sarcoma; however, it lacks specificity; therefore, a positive stain should be supported by other molecular studies when possible [35]. IHC with antibodies targeting the SS18::SSX fusion protein and the SSX C-terminus is a reliable marker of synovial sarcoma, particularly when used in combination [36, 37].

Cytogenetic testing using RT-PCR, FISH, or next-generation sequencing, remains the gold standard for diagnosing synovial sarcoma. These tests are valuable, especially if histopathology and IHC results are inconclusive. Additionally, it can aid in differentiating PPSS from other similar-appearing pleural neoplasms [32]. PPSS is characterized by the SS18::SSX fusion oncogene, which results from a balanced chromosomal translocation between the SS18 (formerly SYT) gene on chromosome 18 and an SSX gene on the X chromosome (SSX1, SSX2, or SSX4), t(X;18)(p11;q11) [38]. The precise way this translocation promotes oncogenesis is not fully understood; however, it is believed to disrupt various tumor suppressor and cellular differentiation pathways, including the displacement of the BAF47 subunit in the SNF/SWI chromatin remodeling complex, effects on the polycomb repressor complex, and the Wnt/β-catenin signaling pathway [39, 40]. The SS18:SSX fusion oncogene is diagnostic for synovial sarcoma, present in over 90% of cases overall, and detectable in 98% of primary pulmonary synovial sarcomas [41]. An immunohistochemical stain for SS18-SSX fusion detection has been developed with high sensitivity (95%) and specificity (100%) [37]. The specific SSX translocation that partners with the SS18 influences tumor epithelial differentiation; monophasic synovial sarcoma may harbor SSX1, SSX2, or both, whereas biphasic types are usually SSX2-positive, which is found in only 3% of cases. SSX4 is rare, occurring in less than 1% of tumors [40–42].

Additionally, less common genetic changes in synovial sarcoma include the heterozygous deletion of the p16INK4A (CDKN2A) gene, observed in 74% of tumors, and EZH2 overexpression. EZH2 is involved in various tumor types, including carcinomas, lymphomas, and sarcomas, and is primarily present in the poorly differentiated subtype of synovial sarcoma. Elevated EZH2 levels may serve as a marker for more aggressive disease and worse clinical outcomes [43, 44].

Staging

The most widely used staging system for soft-tissue sarcoma, including PPSS, is the tumor-node-metastasis (TNM) system developed by the American Joint Committee on Cancer (AJCC) and the Union for International Cancer Control (UICC). Unlike earlier versions, which applied a uniform staging system regardless of tumor location, the current eighth edition does not assign prognostic stage groupings (e.g., stage I-IV) for soft-tissue sarcomas of the abdomen or thorax. The current "T" criteria specify whether the tumor remains within the organ of origin (T1), extends into adjacent tissues (T2), invades another organ (T3), or shows multifocal local involvement (T4). The "N" criteria assess regional lymph node involvement; N1 indicates the presence of lymph node involvement. The "M" criterion refers to distant metastasis [45]. The majority of patients with PPSS present with localized disease confined to a hemithorax, without invasion into the lung, spread to regional lymph nodes, or to extrathoracic sites [14].

Treatment

Surgical Management

As with primary extremity soft-tissue sarcomas, complete surgical resection, whenever possible, remains the primary treatment approach. Treatment goals for synovial sarcoma of the pleura include minimizing the risk of local recurrence, perioperative morbidity, and mortality, while maximizing function and long-term survival. Currently, there are no recommendations or expert opinions on the optimal surgical approach, which can vary depending on the pleural surface involved and the extent of intrathoracic disease. Surgical techniques can include lung-sparing wedge resections for visceral PPSS, partial pleurectomy, radical resection with chest wall reconstruction, or an extrapleural pneumonectomy, among others [12, 24, 25, 33]. Complete resection of the tumor with clear margins is essential to achieve the best outcomes, as there is a greater probability of local recurrence and reduced disease-specific survival with incomplete resection [46]. However, the optimal negative margin width to achieve local control is unknown, and given the tumor's location, achieving clear margins can be challenging. Despite resection, PPSS can have a high local recurrence rate, with one case series reporting a disease-free interval of 2 to 14 months following resection [47]. A study involving 26 patients with primary pleuropulmonary and mediastinal synovial sarcoma found that 20 of them had surgical resection or lobectomy, resulting in a median survival of 14.5 months. The main factor associated with better overall survival was performing tumor resection and achieving clear margins without residual tumor [48]. Katsurada et al. described a case of recurrent metastatic primary synovial sarcoma of the pleura managed with repeated surgical resections on the same hemithorax. The patient underwent two additional surgeries following the initial resection due to tumor recurrence, ultimately achieving a survival duration exceeding 12 years [24]. It is noteworthy, however, that this is a single case report, and the patient's indolent disease course with slow, late recurrence limits the generalizability of this outcome.

Radiation Therapy

Adjuvant radiation therapy may be administered to target residual disease or to reduce the risk of local recurrence, particularly in cases where complete surgical resection has not been achieved. The potential role of radiation therapy in pleural synovial sarcoma includes neoadjuvant radiation therapy and postsurgical adjuvant radiation therapy. Neoadjuvant radiotherapy has been shown to achieve better local control in soft-tissue sarcomas [50–53]. Preoperative radiotherapy was associated with a slight increase in wound healing complications. While there is no data on its use in pleural synovial sarcoma, it may present future opportunities for ongoing research. When complete surgical removal is not feasible, radiation therapy may serve as an adjunct to lower the risk of local recurrence. AlQatari et al. reported a case in which radiotherapy was administered after surgery [19]. The patient received two rounds of radiation: a volumetric modulated arc therapy photon technique delivering 50 Gy over 25 fractions at the surgical site, followed by an additional 10 Gy over five fractions. The patient unfortunately passed away 26-month post-diagnosis. Another case involved proton beam therapy for tracheal synovial sarcoma after surgical resection [54]. An 18-month follow-up using serial CT scans and bronchoscopy showed no signs of recurrence. A retrospective review of over 100 patients who underwent definitive surgery for synovial sarcoma, with or without radiotherapy, found that those who received radiotherapy had better local recurrence-free and progression-free survival at 5 and 10 years of follow-up [55].

Chemotherapy

Due to the rarity of PPSS and limited data, chemotherapy use is mainly inferred from studies on extrathoracic soft-tissue sarcomas. It is typically reserved for metastatic or unresectable cases, or as an adjuvant in high-risk patients, given the toxicity of these drugs and their uncertain benefit on survival [56].

Pleural synovial sarcoma is generally a chemosensitive cancer treated primarily with anthracyclines like doxorubicin, with or without ifosfamide, as the first-line therapy for metastatic cases [41]. A review of 15 clinical trials involving 3330 patients with soft-tissue sarcoma, including 313 with synovial sarcoma, showed that patients with synovial sarcoma respond better to chemotherapy and have higher overall and progression-free survival rates than those with other soft-tissue sarcomas [57]. In a prospective study of 101 patients with primary extremity synovial sarcoma from two institutes, ifosfamide was associated with improved disease-specific survival and distant recurrence-free survival [56]. Additionally, neoadjuvant combination therapy with ifosfamide and doxorubicin, followed by local treatment, has demonstrated improvements in 5-year distant metastasis-free survival, disease-specific survival, and overall survival compared with local treatment alone in patients with primary soft-tissue sarcoma [58].

For patients with metastatic disease who have progressed despite anthracycline and ifosfamide treatments, options include trabectedin, pazopanib, or afamitresgene autoleucel. The selection of therapy depends on various factors, such as performance status, overall health, and the presence of tumor antigens, which may make a patient eligible for targeted immunotherapy [59].

Regorafenib is another option for second- or third-line therapy in patients who have progressed after anthracycline treatment. A phase 2 randomized controlled trial in patients with soft-tissue sarcoma, including synovial sarcoma, demonstrated modest improvements in progression-free survival [60].

Prognosis

The prognosis of pleural synovial sarcoma is generally poor due to its aggressive nature and the challenges associated with treatment. In a case series of 26 patients with PPSS, the median time until recurrence or metastasis was 8.5 months [48]. A more recent series of 20 patients reported a 2-year overall survival rate of 51%, a 5-year overall survival rate of 22%, and a median disease-free period of 8.5 months [61].

Prognosis is influenced by factors such as tumor size and stage, as defined by previous AJCC staging criteria, with larger tumors and advanced stages linked to poorer outcomes. Studies by Janssen and colleagues, as well as Nascimento and colleagues, have shown that patients with tumors larger than 4 cm and 5 cm, respectively, tend to have a worse prognosis [48, 49]. Tumor resectability is another key factor; complete surgical removal is associated with improved survival. In a study involving 15 patients with primary thoracic synovial sarcoma, negative prognostic factors included tumors larger than 10 cm, incomplete resections, and absence of adjuvant therapy [62]. Furthermore, low-grade sarcomas are typically associated with a more favorable prognosis compared to those of higher grade [63, 64].

References

1. Brand RA. 50 years ago in CORR®: synovial Sarcoma Kirk J. Anderson, MD and Orliss Wildermuth, MD CORR 1961;29:55-70. Clin Orthopaed Relat Res. 2013;471(3):1064–6. https://doi.org/10.1007/s11999-013-2792-2.
2. Blay J, von Mehren M, Jones RL, Martín-Broto J, Stacchiotti S, Bauer S, et al. Synovial sarcoma: characteristics, challenges, and evolving therapeutic strategies. ESMO Open. 2023;8(5):101618.
3. Arun RD. A rare primary synovial sarcoma of lung – case report with literature review. Res Rev J Nurs Health Sci. 2017;3(1):15–7.
4. Mrabet FZ, El Ouazzani H, Akkari LE, Hammi S, Bourkadi JE, Zouaidia F. Primary pleuropulmonary synovial sarcoma: a case. Case Rep Pulmonol. 2018 Jan 1 [cited 2025 Mar 17]; 2018:1–4.
5. Zeren H, Moran CA, Suster S, Fishback N, Koss M. Primary pulmonary sarcomas with features of monophasic synovial sarcoma: a clinicopathological, immunohistochemical, and ultrastructural study of 25 cases. Hum Pathol. 1995;26(5):474–80.
6. Gaertner E, Zeren HE, Fleming MV, Colby TV, Travis WD. Biphasic synovial sarcomas arising in the pleural cavity. Am J Surg Pathol. 1996;20(1):36–45.
7. Etienne-Mastroianni B, Falchero L, Chalabreysse L, Loire R, Ranchère D, Souquet PJ, et al. Primary sarcomas of the lung. Lung Cancer. 2002;38(3):283–9.
8. Wang W, Guo J, Bao M, Liu X, Wang H, Ye C. Primary pulmonary synovial sarcoma. JTCVS Open. 2022;10:404–14.
9. Tailor J, Roy PG, Bowker C, Lakhoo K. Primary pleural synovial sarcoma presenting as a multiloculated cyst in an adolescent. Pediatr Surg Int. 2008;24(5):597–9.
10. Begueret H, Galateau-Sallé F, Guillou L, Chetaille B, Brambilla E, Vignaud J-M, et al. Primary Intrathoracic Synovial Sarcoma. Am J Surg Pathol. 2005;29(3):339–46.
11. Sharif A, Akhtar T, Akhtar M, Zia N. Cystic pleural synovial sarcoma. J Coll Physicians Surg Pak. 2016;26(11):127–9.
12. Kang MK, Cho KH, Lee YH, Han IY, Yoon YC, Park KT, et al. Primary synovial sarcoma of the parietal pleura: a case report. Korean J Thorac Cardiovasc Surg. 2013;46(2):159–61.
13. Travis WD, Brambilla E, Burke AP, Marx A, Nicholson AG, editors. WHO classification of tumours of the lung, pleura, thymus and heart. 4th ed. International Agency for Research on Cancer: Lyon; 2015. ISBN 978-92-832-2436-5
14. Ng SB, Ahmed Q, Tien SL, Sivaswaren C, Lau LC. Primary pleural synovial sarcoma. Arch Pathol Lab Med. 2003;127(1):85–90.
15. Silva RGM, Gross JL, Silva RA, Haddad FJ, Younes RN, Cruz VM, et al. Primary monophasic synovial sarcoma of the pleura: Neoadjuvant chemotherapy followed by complete resection. Thoracic Cancer. 2010;1(3):95–101.
16. Wan JL, Lam YF, Foong KW, Abdul Ghani N, Lachmanan K. A case of primary pleural synovial sarcoma with endobronchial recurrence. Respirol Case Rep. 2020;8(3).
17. Hartel P. EC pulmonology and respiratory medicine research article primary pleural synovial sarcoma: clinicopathologic evaluation of 19 cases with focal unusual histology and diagnostic pearls [cited 2025 Mar 17].
18. Yamaki M, Yonehara S, Noriyuki T. Large primary pleural synovial sarcoma with severe dyspnea: a case report. Surg Case Rep. 2017;3(1)
19. AlQatari A, Ahmed A, AlHije F, Sabry M, Elbawab H. Primary pulmonary synovial sarcoma with hemothorax: a case report. Med Arch. 2023 [cited 2025 Jan 15];77(6):496.
20. Yin T, Liu B, Xue J, Liu X, Shang S, Wang Y. Primary pulmonary monophasic synovial sarcoma initially presenting with bloody pleural effusion: a case report and literature review. Clin Case Rep. 2024;12(5).

21. Chen S, Zhang K, Wan X, Chen Y, Ma S, Deng Q. The use of apatinib in treating primary pleural synovial sarcoma. Medicine. 2019;98(51):e18382.
22. Teng C, Li LI, Shen W, Li J, Liu Y, Jiang Q, et al. Pleural synovial sarcoma patient treated with combined chemotherapy and Endostar, plus sunitinib maintenance therapy: a case report and review of the literature. Oncol Lett. 2015;10(2):1141–4.
23. Won JH, Chin S, Park JS, Paik SH, Lee H, Cha JG, et al. Primary pleural synovial sarcoma with metastatic cardiac involvement: a case report. Iran J Radiol. 2016 Sep 7 [cited 2025 Mar 17];13(4).
24. Katsurada N, Ohnishi H, Ikeda M, Jimbo N, Hatakeyama Y, Okamura K. Primary pleural synovial sarcoma with repeated resection leading to long-term survival. Respirol Case Rep. 2019 Aug 20 [cited 2025 Mar 17];7(8):e00480.
25. Vandaele T, Van Slambrouck J, Schöffski P, Dumez H, Weynand B, Sciot R, et al. Extensive surgical resections for rare pleural neoplasms: a single-center experience with a yolk sac tumor and synovial sarcoma. World J Surg Oncol. 2024;22(1).
26. Harisankar CNB, John J, Gangadharan KV. Fluoro deoxyglucose positron emission tomography-computerized tomography in primary staging and response assessment of a rare case of primary pleural synovial sarcoma. Indian J Nucl Med. 2015;30(1):62.
27. Chabowski M, Szymańska-Chabowska A, Janczak D, Dorobisz T, Leśniak M, Jeleń M, et al. A giant pleural poorly differentiated synovial sarcoma (PDSS) in a 64-year-old woman. J Thorac Dis. 2016 Sep [cited 2025 Mar 17];8(9):E938–41.
28. Sugitani A, Asai K, Kojima K, Eguchi Y, Kawaguchi T, Ohsawa M, et al. Primary pleural synovial sarcoma treated with Pazopanib. Intern Med. 2015 [cited 2025 Mar 17];54(16):2051–5.
29. Pereira G, Pires A, Barbosa S, Cotter J. Pulmonary synovial sarcoma: an unpleasant surprise. Eur J Case Rep Intern Med. 2021;8(3):002149.
30. Grosu HB, Kazzaz F, Vakil E, Molina S, Ost D. Sensitivity of initial thoracentesis for malignant pleural effusion stratified by tumor type in patients with strong evidence of metastatic disease. Respiration. 2018 [cited 2023 Mar 17];96(4):363–9.
31. Okamoto S. Primary pulmonary synovial sarcoma: a clinicopathologic, immunohistochemical, and molecular study of 11 cases. Hum Pathol. 2004;35(7):850–6.
32. Colwell AS, D'Cunha J, Vargas SO, Parker BL, Cin PD, Maddaus MA. Synovial sarcoma of the pleura: a clinical and pathologic study of three cases. J Thorac Cardiovasc Surg. 2002;124(4):828–32.
33. Imen M, Ahmed L, Wissal R, Bechir BR, Taieb C. A case report of primary pleural synovial sarcoma, an uncommon etiology of a thoracic parietal mass. Int J Surg Case Rep. 2024;126:110663.
34. Karpathiou G, Stefanou D, Froudarakis M. Pleural neoplastic pathology. Respir Med. 2015;109(8):931–43.
35. Foo WC, Cruise MW, Wick MR, Hornick JL. Immunohistochemical staining for TLE1 distinguishes synovial sarcoma from histologic mimics. Am J Clin Pathol. 2011;135(6):839–44.
36. Zaborowski M, Vargas AC, Pulvers J, Clarkson A, Guzman D, Sioson L, et al. When used together SS18–SSX fusion-specific and SSX C-terminus immunohistochemistry are highly specific and sensitive for the diagnosis of synovial sarcoma and can replace FISH or molecular testing in most cases. Histopathology. 2020;77(4):588–600.
37. Baranov E, McBride MJ, Bellizzi AM, Ligon AH, Fletcher CDM, Kadoch C, et al. A novel SS18-SSX fusion-specific antibody for the diagnosis of synovial sarcoma. Am J Surg Pathol. 2020;44(7):922–33.
38. Törnkvist M, Brodin B, Bartolazzi A, Larsson O. A novel type of SYT/SSX fusion: methodological and biological implications. Mod Pathol. 2002;15(6):679–85.
39. McBride MJ, Pulice JL, Beird HC, Ingram DR, D'Avino AR, Shern JF, et al. The SS18-SSX fusion oncoprotein hijacks BAF complex targeting and function to drive synovial sarcoma. Cancer Cell. 2018;33(6):1128–1141.e7.
40. Nielsen TO, Poulin NM, Ladanyi M. Synovial sarcoma: recent discoveries as a roadmap to new avenues for therapy. Cancer Discov. 2015;5(2):124–34.
41. Mishra P, Panigrahi M, Pradhan G, Sahoo N, Patra S, Mohapatra P. Primary pulmonary synovial sarcoma: a reappraisal. J Cancer Res Ther. 2018;14(3):481.
42. Saito T. The SYT-SSX fusion protein and histological epithelial differentiation in synovial sarcoma: relationship with extracellular matrix remodeling. Int J Clin Exp Pathol. 2013;6(11):2272–9.
43. Subramaniam MM, Noguera R, Piqueras M, Navarro S, López-Guerrero JA, Llombart-Bosch A. p16INK4A (CDKN2A) gene deletion is a frequent genetic event in synovial sarcomas. Am J Clin Pathol. 2006 Dec;126(6):866–74.
44. Changchien Y-C, Tátrai P, Papp G, Sápi J, Fónyad L, Szendrői M, et al. Poorly differentiated synovial sarcoma is associated with high expression of enhancer of zeste homologue 2 (EZH2). J Transl Med. 2012;10(1).
45. Amin MB, Edge SB, Greene FL, et al. AJCC cancer staging manual. 8th ed. New York: Springer; 2017.
46. Suster S, Fisher C, Moran CA. Expression of bcl-2 oncoprotein in benign and malignant spindle cell tumors of soft tissue, skin, serosal surfaces, and gastrointestinal tract. Am J Surg Pathol. 1998;22(7):863–72.
47. Duran-Mendicuti A, Costello P, Vargas SO. Primary synovial sarcoma of the chest: radiographic and clinicopathologic correlation. J Thorac Imaging. 2003;18(2):87–93.
48. Lan T, Chen H, Xiong B, Ting-qing Z, Peng R, Chen M, et al. Primary pleuropulmonary and mediastinal synovial sarcoma: a clinicopathologic and molecular study of 26 genetically confirmed cases in the largest institution of southwest China. Diagn Pathol. 2016;11(1).
49. McCormack PM, Martini N. Primary sarcomas and lymphomas of the lung. In: Martini N, Vogt-Moykopf I, editors. Thoracic surgery: frontiers and uncom-

mon neoplasms, vol. 5. St. Louis: CV Mosby; 1989. p. 261–83.
50. Kobus M, Roohani S, Ehret F, Flörcken A, Striefler JK, Brandes F, et al. The role of neoadjuvant radiochemotherapy in the management of localized high-grade soft tissue sarcoma. Radiat Oncol. 2022;17(1):139.
51. Lansu J, Braam PM, van Werkhoven E, Scholten AN, Schrage Y, van Houdt WJ, et al. A moderate dose of preoperative radiotherapy may improve resectability in myxoid liposarcoma. Eur J Surg Oncol. 2021;47(10):2633–9.
52. Larrier NA, Czito BG, Kirsch DG. Radiation therapy for soft tissue sarcoma. Surg Oncol Clin N Am. 2016;25(4):841–60.
53. Kubicek GJ, LaCouture T, Kaden M, Kim TW, Lerman N, Khrizman P, et al. Preoperative radiosurgery for soft tissue sarcoma. Am J Clin Oncol. 2018;41(1):86–9.
54. Ye C, Guo J, Liu X, Jiang G, Wang W. Surgery and proton beam therapy for tracheal synovial sarcoma. Ann Thorac Surg. 2020;110(4):e265–7.
55. Song S, Park J, Kim HJ, Kim IH, Han I, Kim HS, et al. Effects of adjuvant radiotherapy in patients with synovial sarcoma. Am J Clin Oncol. 2017;40(3):306–11.
56. Eilber FC, Brennan MF, Eilber FR, Eckardt JJ, Grobmyer SR, Riedel E, et al. Chemotherapy is associated with improved survival in adult patients with primary extremity synovial sarcoma. Ann Surg. 2007;246(1):105–13.
57. Vlenterie M, Litière S, Rizzo E, Marreaud S, Judson I, Gelderblom H, et al. Outcome of chemotherapy in advanced synovial sarcoma patients: review of 15 clinical trials from the European Organisation for Research and Treatment of Cancer Soft Tissue and Bone Sarcoma Group; setting a new landmark for studies in this entity. Eur J Cancer 2016;58:62–72.
58. Goy BW, Syed SP, Padmanabhan A, Burchette RJ, Helmstedter CS. The role of Ifosfamide–doxorubicin chemotherapy in histology-specific, high grade, locally advanced soft tissue sarcoma, a 14-year experience. Radiother Oncol. 2021;(165):174–8.
59. D'Angelo SP, Araujo DM, Abdul Razak AR, Agulnik M, Attia S, Blay JY, et al. Afamitresgene autoleucel for advanced synovial sarcoma and myxoid round cell liposarcoma (SPEARHEAD-1): an international, open-label, phase 2 trial. Lancet. 2024; 403:1460–71.
60. Mir O, Brodowicz T, Italiano A, Wallet J, Blay JY, Bertucci F, et al. Safety and efficacy of regorafenib in patients with advanced soft tissue sarcoma (REGOSARC): a randomised, double-blind, placebo-controlled, phase 2 trial. Lancet Oncol. 2016;17(12):1732–42.
61. Pieropan S, Mercier O, Mitilian D, Pradère P, Fabre D, Ion DI, et al. Feasibility and long-term outcomes of surgery for primary thoracic synovial sarcoma. Interactive Cardio Vasc Thoracic Surg. 2022;35(4).
62. Galetta D, Pelosi G, Leo F, Solli P, Veronesi G, Borri A, et al. Primary thoracic synovial sarcoma: factors affecting long-term survival. J Thorac Cardiovasc Surg. 2007;134(3):808–9.
63. Dail DH, Hammar SP. Uncommon tumors. In: Pulmonary pathology. Springer; 1987. p. 928–41.
64. Burt M, Zakowski M, Pearson FG, Deslauriers J, Ginsberg RJ, McKneally NF, Urschel HC. Rare primary malignant neoplasms. Thorac Surg. 1995:808–26.

Primary Pleural Angiosarcoma

16

Meng-Shan Lin, Firas Ido, and Matthew Zheng

Introduction

Angiosarcoma is a rare, highly aggressive malignant tumor of endothelial cell origin, accounting for approximately 1–2% of all soft-tissue sarcomas [1]. Epidemiology regarding the most common primary anatomic sites varies slightly; however, cutaneous lesions of the head and neck, breast involvement, and neoplasms arising from the deep muscles of the lower extremities collectively comprise more than 50% of all angiosarcomas [1–3]. Primary visceral involvement is less common and can arise from the liver, heart, or spleen [4]. Lung involvement is typically due to metastasis from an extrapulmonary site in nearly 90% of cases. However, primary pulmonary angiosarcoma has been reported to occur in the remaining 10%, with an incidence of 0.001–0.03% [5–7]. Primary pleural angiosarcoma (PPA) is an extraordinarily rare subcategory with no reported incidence or prevalence. The disease is limited to case reports and case series. The first description of PPA is attributed to Arthur Stout, MD, in 1943; however, he referred to the neoplasm as a hemangioendothelioma [8]. Over the years, additional cases were published, and a separate category for this high-grade vascular tumor was recognized as angiosarcoma [9–13]. Further distinctions between the two vascular malignant tumors were identified based on genetic alterations and included in the World Health Organization's classification of soft-tissue tumors [14, 15].

The mean age of onset for PPA has been reported to occur during the fifth or sixth decade, with cases ranging from 17 to 87 years of age. There is a male predominance, occurring in 65%–82% of cases based on several reviews [16, 17]. The ethnicities reported were predominantly white (44%) and Asian (49%), with Black (5%) and other ethnicities (2%) much less common. The etiology and potential associated exposures of pulmonary and pleural angiosarcomas are not well defined, primarily because of their rarity. Case reports and small case series provide some data for potential risk factors. Tobacco (28%), tuberculosis (21%), and radiation (9%) exposures were among the reported potential risk factors [1, 18]. Chronic TB pyothorax, in particular, has been reported as possibly associated with PPA [19, 20]. Heavy tobacco exposure, along with other pneumoconiosis and asbestos exposures, has also been listed as a possible risk factor [21, 22]. Cases linked to postradiation have typically occurred years after the initial exposure [23, 24]. A single case with potential linkage to

M.-S. Lin · F. Ido · M. Zheng (✉)
Department of Pulmonary and Critical Care Medicine, St. Luke's University Health Network, Bethlehem, PA, USA
e-mail: Meng-Shan.Lin@sluhn.org; firas.ido@sluhn.org; Matthew.zheng@sluhn.org

F. Ido (ed.), *Rare Pleural Diseases*, https://doi.org/10.1007/978-3-032-14873-5_16

Klippel–Trenaunay syndrome (KTS), in which a PIK3CA gene mutation was detected within the tumor in a 17-year-old female, has been documented [25].

Pathophysiology

The pathogenesis of primary pleural angiosarcoma is unclear, and genomic data are limited; however, mutational analyses of angiosarcomas arising from other sites can provide insights into potential mechanisms underlying its development. Somatic mutations, such as those in PTPRB (protein tyrosine phosphatase receptor type B) and PLCG1 (phospholipase C and gamma 1), have been identified as potential driver mutations. PTPRB is expressed exclusively in endothelial cells and functions as a negative regulator of vascular endothelial growth factor (VEGF). This mutation can be commonly observed in tumors with concomitant MYC amplifications, which are often present in angiosarcoma associated with radiation exposure. PLCG1, a transducer downstream of tyrosine kinase receptors, plays a significant role in angiogenesis signaling [26]. These mutations contribute to the upregulation of receptor tyrosine kinases, such as KDR (kinase insert domain receptor), FLT1 (FMS-like tyrosine kinase 1), TIE1, and TIE2, collectively driving inappropriate angiogenesis and endothelial cell proliferation [27].

In secondary angiosarcomas, particularly those arising after radiation therapy, amplification of the oncogene c-MYC is common and plays a pivotal role in tumor progression. MYC amplification promotes transcription of genes involved in cell cycle progression and proliferation, contributing to the aggressive nature of these tumors. Approximately 25% of secondary angiosarcomas also exhibit FLT4 (FMS-like tyrosine kinase 2) amplification, which encodes VEGFR3 (vascular endothelial growth factor receptor 3), a key receptor in lymphangiogenesis and vascular development. Co-amplification of FLT4 and MYC may exert a synergistic effect, enhancing tumor vascularity, growth, and metastatic potential [28–30]. Distinct from these mechanisms, a subset of primary angiosarcomas, particularly in younger patients, harbors mutations in the CIC (Capicua transcriptional repressor) gene or gene rearrangements. The CIC gene encodes a transcriptional repressor that helps regulate cell growth and maintain differentiation. Loss-of-function mutations or oncogenic fusions involving CIC lead to transcriptional dysregulation and are associated with a round cell or epithelioid phenotype, as well as a poor prognosis. These cases represent a genetically distinct subgroup of angiosarcoma with unique biology and clinical behavior [30].

Clinical Features

Symptoms of PPA are nonspecific but may be severe at the time of presentation. The most common symptoms reported include pleuritic chest pain (47.5%), shortness of breath (35%), hemoptysis (27.5%), cough (15%), and weight loss (10%) [20]. Severe back pain has also been reported, depending on the location of the mass [31]. Diminished breath sounds, dullness to percussion, and palpable masses are all signs reflecting the presence of a pleural effusion and chest wall invasion of the neoplasm [32].

Diagnosis

The detection of PPA can be challenging due to its insidious nature, which can lead to significant diagnostic delays [33]. Additionally, PPA can mimic mesothelioma and pleural hematomas [34, 35]. A confirmatory diagnosis requires a histopathologic examination. Thoracotomy and video-assisted thoracoscopic surgery (VATS) with biopsy or tumor resection were the two most reliable modalities for tissue sampling [1]. Thoracoscopy has been used as a less invasive alternative when neither approach is available [36]. Less often, a CT-guided percutaneous pleural biopsy was performed; however, only 43% of samples yielded tumor tissue. Thoracentesis, when performed, typically demonstrates a hemorrhagic effusion in nearly all cases. However, in almost all attempts, cytology is negative for malignancy but may reveal atypical cells. A single case of positive cytopathology following thoracentesis has been documented. In cases of pulmonary involvement, bronchoscopy with bronchoalveolar lavage often reveals blood within the airways; however, cytology typically fails to demonstrate malignant cells. Transbronchial biopsy is rarely performed and usually insufficient for providing a diagnosis. Biopsy or resection of distant metastatic lesions can be diagnostic. Several cases with rapid progression led to postmortem diagnosis on autopsy [1, 11, 17, 20, 22, 25].

Radiologic imaging, although usually obtained, does not predict PPA [37]. Pleural lesions can occur as solitary nodules or multifocal nodules, both of which can be bilateral or unilateral (Fig. 16.1a, b) [1]. Depending on the size of the pleural lesions, which can range from 1 to 10 cm, multidetector computed tomography may demonstrate well-circumscribed ovoid pleural nodules or large lobulated masses with surrounding invasion (Fig. 16.1a, b). The lesions can arise from the visceral or parietal pleura and exhibit heterogeneous internal densities and variable contrast enhancement. Other CT findings include free or loculated ipsilateral or bilateral pleural effusions, which are present in approximately 70% of cases, and focal or diffuse pleural thickening may also be present. PET/CT typically shows significant uptake and hyperintensities and can also assess metastatic lesions (Fig. 16.1c) [20, 36–38]. A single case of bilateral hemothoraces, without pleural lesions, has been documented as the only presenting feature of PPA [17]. The pleural lesions may invade adjacent structures, including lung parenchyma, major vasculature, ribs, diaphragm, and the pericardium [39]. Pleural effusions, if drained, typically recur. The effusions are classically high volume, exudative, and consistent with hemorrhagic fluid [40–42].

Magnetic resonance imaging (MRI) can aid in differentiating between benign and malignant pleural lesions; however, it cannot determine the specific type of neoplasm. Using signal intensities and contrast enhancement, along with morphologic clues such as nodularity, pleural irregularities, and evidence of invasion, MRI can suggest malignancy with high diagnostic accuracy [43, 44]. T2-weighted sequences consistently demonstrate a markedly heterogeneous internal architecture, often described as "cauliflower-like" due to interspersed regions of high signal intensity set against a background of intermediate signal, features attributable to hemorrhagic, necrotic, and vascular components intrinsic to the tumor's biology. On T1-weighted imaging, lesions typically exhibit heterogeneous signal intensities, including areas of relatively high signal and scattered hypointense foci, further reflecting the mass's internal complexity. After administration of gadolinium-based contrast agents, MRI frequently reveals peripheral rim enhancement with multiple linear enhancing structures coursing inward from the periphery, indicative of prominent vascular supply and internal septation. These vascular channels enhance the recognition of the tumor's angiogenic nature and may help differentiate it from more common pleural or pulmonary neoplasms, which often lack such internal vascular complexity. Additional imaging findings may include mass effect on adjacent structures, infiltration of the mediastinum or chest wall, and associated pleural effusion. While MRI remains complementary to CT in assessing pleural masses, its superior soft-tissue contrast provides critical insights into tumor morphology, internal composition, and local extent, making it particularly valuable for the noninvasive evaluation of suspected PPA and narrowing the differential diagnosis [42, 45, 46].

Positron emission tomography (PET) with 18F-fluorodeoxyglucose (18F-FDG) is an essential tool for diagnosing, staging, restaging, and monitoring angiosarcoma. PET/CT imaging provides valuable information for assessing tumor response and detecting recurrence, making it a critical component of patient follow-up. PPA is hypermetabolic on PET/CT, with markedly elevated standardized uptake values (SUVs) that often exceed 10 [47, 48]. Lesions may appear as focal nodular masses or multifocal infiltrative pleural thickenings and, at times, demonstrate heterogeneous FDG uptake with central necrosis [49]. Unlike the

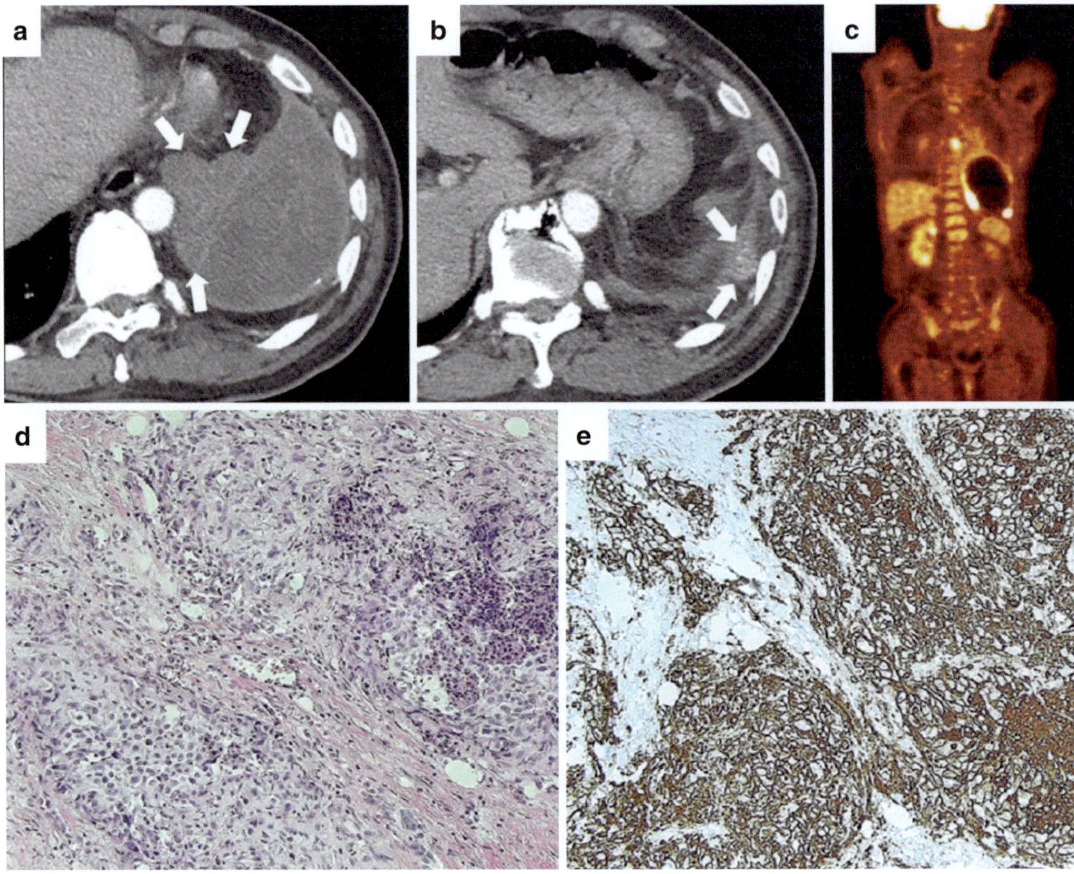

Fig. 16.1 Radiologic and histopathologic features of primary pleural epithelioid angiosarcoma
(**a**, **b**) Contrast-enhanced computed tomography demonstrates a left hemithoracic lobulated pleural-based mediastinal mass and a separate peripheral pleural nodule, both separated by a loculated pleural effusion
(**c**) F-18 fluorodeoxyglucose positron emission tomography/computed tomography showing marked hypermetabolic activity corresponding to the two pleural lesions and a hypermetabolic subcarinal lymph node. The loculated pleural effusion shows no FDG avidity
(**d**) Hematoxylin and eosin-stained section of pleural tissue revealing sheets of epithelioid tumor cells with abundant eosinophilic cytoplasm and prominent nucleoli
(**e**) Immunohistochemical staining showing strong membranous positivity for CD34, confirming endothelial differentiation

smooth, diffuse pleural thickening observed in malignant pleural mesothelioma (MPM), PPA lesions are often irregular and bulky and demonstrate intense metabolic activity [50]. Additionally, PET/CT is particularly effective in detecting early extrathoracic metastases, including those to the bone, brain, liver, and adrenal glands, which can often be present at the time of presentation [49, 50]. In contrast to pleural metastatic disease, which typically shows multiple discrete pleural nodules with variable FDG avidity, PPA tends to exhibit a more confluent and metabolically aggressive pattern [50]. Solitary fibrous tumors of the pleura, which may be confused with PPA on anatomical imaging, usually demonstrate lower SUV values and lack evidence of distant metastatic spread on PET [51]. These distinct metabolic profiles provide important diagnostic cues, and 18F-FDG PET/CT serves as a crucial modality for lesion characterization, staging, biopsy guidance, and treatment planning.

Pathology

Histologically, PPA comprises two subtypes: the classical spindle-shaped type and the epithelioid type. The epithelioid subtype is more prevalent, accounting for approximately 60–75% of reported cases, and is associated with a significantly worse prognosis compared to the spindle cell variant [52–54].

Classical Spindle Cell Variant

The classical spindle cell variant of PPA exhibits a characteristic vasoformative pattern, often resembling that of other vascular neoplasms. The histological features include irregular, anastomosing vascular channels lined by atypical and pleomorphic malignant endothelial cells. These vascular channels may vary significantly in diameter and organization. In well-differentiated regions, these channels often maintain connections to the native vasculature, mimicking typical sinusoidal structures. As the disease progresses and becomes less differentiated, these features are lost, and the tumor may appear as cellular sheets with poorly formed or absent vascular spaces [54].

Epithelioid Variant

The epithelioid subtype, which accounts for the majority of PPA cases, differs markedly from the classical morphology. It typically manifests as solid sheets or nodular aggregates of neoplastic cells (Fig. 16.1d). These tumor cells are round to polygonal, with abundant eosinophilic cytoplasm, and exhibit large, pleomorphic nuclei with vesicular chromatin and prominent nucleoli. High mitotic activity is frequently observed, along with variable degrees of necrosis and hemorrhage. A distinctive feature is the presence of intracytoplasmic lumina containing extravasated red blood cells, which supports the tumor's vascular origin. Some cases may demonstrate papillary structures with fibrovascular cores. Electron microscopy, although infrequently employed in modern diagnostic settings due to the availability of specific immunohistochemical markers, may reveal Weibel–Palade bodies and pinocytic vesicles, hallmark features of endothelial differentiation [54, 55].

Immunohistochemical Profile

Immunohistochemistry (IHC) serves as a cornerstone in the diagnosis of PPA, particularly in cases where morphological features are ambiguous. Among the available endothelial markers, CD31 is considered the most sensitive and specific, showing intense membranous staining in approximately 90% of angiosarcomas, including poorly differentiated and epithelioid variants. Nuclear transcription factors such as ERG and FLI-1 are also highly sensitive markers of endothelial lineage and provide valuable diagnostic utility. CD34, although commonly used, is supportive but less specific and can be expressed in other types of soft-tissue tumors (Fig. 16.1e). Factor VIII-related antigen is highly specific but less sensitive than CD31. Vimentin is consistently expressed in both histological subtypes, reflecting the tumor's mesenchymal origin [1, 56].

The epithelioid subtype, in particular, may express epithelial markers, including cytokeratins such as CK7, CK8, CK18, and CAM5.2. However, this expression is variable and nonspecific, as cytokeratins are also commonly observed in other pleural malignancies, including mesotheliomas and metastatic carcinomas. Therefore, cytokeratin expression should be interpreted with caution and in conjunction with endothelial markers. Cytokeratin expression in angiosarcoma can range from focal and weak to diffuse and strong, further complicating the differential diagnosis. Excluding mesothelial origin is of great importance. It is facilitated by the use of mesothelial markers such as calretinin, CK5/6, WT1, and HBME-1, which are typically negative in angiosarcoma but positive in mesothelioma. Thus, a panel of positive endothelial markers (CD31, ERG, FLI-1, CD34, and Factor VIII) and negative mesothelial markers strengthens the diagnosis of PPA [1, 5, 19, 21].

Diagnosis

The definitive diagnosis of PPA requires a comprehensive histopathological evaluation supported by a robust panel of immunohistochemical stains. CD31 and ERG are the most reliable and specific indicators of vascular differentiation and should be included in all diagnostic panels evaluating suspected PPA [20, 56]. The epithelioid variant presents unique diagnostic difficulties due to its morphological overlap with epithelial neoplasms and its potential expression of cytokeratins [19]. In contrast to other pleural malignancies, PPA is distinguished by its unique immunophenotypic profile, characterized by strong positivity for vascular markers and the absence of mesothelial antigen expression. While the epithelioid subtype may occasionally show cytokeratin positivity, this should not be relied on solely for diagnosis. Instead, it is the combination of histological architecture, immunohistochemical staining, and the exclusion of alternative diagnoses that leads to an accurate diagnosis [1, 5, 19, 21].

Treatment

General Management Approach

The management of PPA remains a significant clinical challenge due to its rarity, rapid progression, and poor prognosis. At present, there is no standardized treatment regimen for PPA. Treatment modalities reported in the literature include surgery, chemotherapy, radiotherapy, and, more recently, immunotherapy. The choice of treatment is often based on tumor resectability, histological subtype, and patient performance status. Most patients experience rapid disease progression and succumb within months of diagnosis [19]. While surgery remains the cornerstone for localized disease, the integration of chemotherapy, radiotherapy, and emerging immunotherapies offers limited but expanding therapeutic avenues. Both epithelioid and spindle cell subtypes exhibit aggressive behavior and poor responsiveness to current treatment options, underscoring the need for further research into targeted and immune-based therapies.

Surgical Intervention

Surgical resection is typically the first-line treatment for localized PPA. Procedures range from pleurectomy and pneumonectomy to debulking surgeries that may include rib excision and cauterization of bleeding foci [53, 57]. In a reported case, a patient presented with spontaneous hemothorax, which led to pleurectomy, and experienced uncontrolled postoperative bleeding. This underscores the complexity and risk associated with surgical interventions [58]. Although rare, wedge biopsy has been reported to result in hemorrhage, necessitating 99mTc-labeled red blood cell scintigraphy to localize the site of active bleeding, and subsequently embolized via endovascular techniques to achieve hemostasis [59]. While very rare, long-term survival has been reported. A single case involving a solitary tumor treated with surgical resection and adjuvant radiotherapy resulted in disease-free survival 15 years later, highlighting the possibility of curative outcomes [39].

Chemotherapy and Immunotherapy

Chemotherapy has been applied in multimodal regimens but is generally of limited efficacy. Agents used include gemcitabine, docetaxel, paclitaxel, cisplatin, ifosfamide, doxorubicin, and albumin-bound paclitaxel [52]. Partial remission has been documented after four cycles of albumin-bound paclitaxel in a patient with recurrent disease [57]. Adjuvant chemotherapy with doxorubicin and ifosfamide has shown temporary disease control in some cases, with survival extending up to 5 months posttreatment [60]. A systematic review of both epithelioid and spindle cell variants showed poor response to chemotherapy: Patients experienced either rapid progression or limited survival despite initial stabilization, highlighting the aggressive nature of both subtypes [61].

Immunotherapy has emerged as a promising avenue. Nivolumab combined with ipilimumab has shown response rates of up to 60% in cutaneous angiosarcomas and was associated with significant tumor reduction and improved hemoglobin levels in a case of PPA [62, 63]. Pembrolizumab, used postoperatively in a PDL-1-positive epithelioid PPA, stabilized disease for an extended period [64]. Tyrosine kinase inhibitors (TKIs), such as sorafenib and pazopanib, have also been employed with modest success. Sorafenib, for example, yielded a progression-free survival of 3.8 months and an overall survival of 14.9 months in patients with angiosarcoma, although this was not specifically reported in PPA [52]. Anlotinib has shown potential through its inhibition of VEGFR2 and antiangiogenic effects, although its role in PPA remains unvalidated [23]. The Taxotere–gemcitabine combination continues to show promise due to its synergistic activity and favorable toxicity profile. The effectiveness of this combination lies partly in docetaxel-mediated modulation of DNA repair and resistance pathways, enhancing gemcitabine incorporation into tumor DNA.

Radiotherapy

Radiation therapy may be used postoperatively or in cases where resection is not possible. Angiosarcomas are known to be radiosensitive, and radiotherapy has been applied to achieve local control and symptom relief [52]. A single case of an unresectable PPA treated with radiation and recombinant interleukin-2 resulted in 1-year recurrence-free survival [24]. A second case with inoperable right-sided epithelioid PPA received a total dose of 3750 cGy in 15 fractions along with multi-agent chemotherapy and remained alive 9 months following diagnosis [33].

Prognosis

The prognosis for pleural angiosarcoma remains extremely poor, with most patients experiencing rapid clinical decline and survival typically limited to less than a year [19]. Mortality frequently results from severe complications such as respiratory failure, hemorrhagic shock, or cardiac arrest [16, 40]. Prognosis is particularly poor in patients presenting with multiple pleural lesions, as multifocal disease reflects more aggressive tumor biology and confers greater resistance to therapy compared with solitary lesions. The presence of a hemothorax represents a significant adverse prognostic factor and has been consistently identified as the strongest independent predictor of increased mortality.

Other variables, such as inoperability or the lack of adjuvant radiotherapy, have been associated with poorer outcomes in some studies; however, their prognostic significance is less robust and often fails to retain statistical independence in multivariable analyses [18, 53]. Given the frequent presentation of advanced or disseminated disease and the limited effectiveness of existing therapies, there is an urgent need for further research to improve understanding and management of both primary and metastatic pleural angiosarcomas [19].

References

1. Mark RJ, Poen JC, Tran LM, Fu YS, Juillard GF. Angiosarcoma: a report of 67 patients and a review of the literature. Cancer. 1996;77(11):2400–6.
2. Fletcher CDM, Krishnan Unni K, Mertens F, International Agency for Research on Cancer. Pathology and genetics of tumours of soft tissue and bone. Lyon: International Agency For Research On Cancer (Iarc), Imp; 2006.

3. Young RJ, Brown NJ, Reed MW, Hughes D, Woll PJ. Angiosarcoma. Lancet Oncol. 2010;11(10):983–91.
4. Wilson R, Glaros S, Brown RK, Michael C, Reisman D. Complete radiographic response of primary pulmonary angiosarcomas following gemcitabine and Taxotere. Lung Cancer. 2008;61(1):131–6. https://doi.org/10.1016/j.lungcan.2007.12.006. Epub 2008 Feb 19. PMID: 18243404.
5. Rana MK, Rahman O, O'Brien A. Primary pulmonary angiosarcoma. BMJ Case Rep. 2021;14(11):e244578. https://doi.org/10.1136/bcr-2021-244578. PMID: 34753722; PMCID: PMC8578948.
6. Patel AM, Ryu JH. Angiosarcoma in the lung. Chest. 1993;103(5):1531–5.
7. Stout AP. Hemangio-Endothelioma. Ann Surg. 1943;118(3):445.
8. McCaughey WT, Dardick I, Barr JR. Angiosarcoma of serous membranes. Arch Pathol Lab Med. 1983;107(6):304–7. PMID: 6687794.
9. Tandon RK, Srivastava VK, Pandey RP. Hemangio endotheliosarcoma of chest wall and pleural cavity. Indian J Cancer. 1971;8(3):205–7. PMID: 5168901.
10. Perry KD, Al-lbraheemi A, Rubin BP, Jen J, Ren H, Jang JS, et al. Composite hemangioendothelioma with neuroendocrine marker expression: an aggressive variant. Mod Pathol. 2017;30(11):1589–602.
11. Verbeke SL, Bovée JV. Primary vascular tumors of bone: a spectrum of entities? Int J Clin Exp Pathol. 2011;4(6):541–51. Epub 2011 Jul 25. PMID: 21904630; PMCID: PMC3160606.
12. Fletcher CDM, Unni KK, Mertens F. World Health Organization classification of tumours: pathology and genetics of tumours of soft tissue and bone. IARC Press; 2002. p. 322–5.
13. Cao Y, Zou S-M, Zhang K-T, Lu N, Liu Y, Feng L, et al. Genetic alterations in pulmonary epithelioid hemangioendothelioma and epithelioid angiosarcoma. Histol Histopathol. 2011;26(4):491–6.
14. Gambarotti M. Vascular tumors: hemangioma, epithelioid Hemangioendothelioma, and Angiosarcoma. In: Picci P, Manfrini M, Fabbri N, Gambarotti M, Vanel D, editors. Atlas of musculoskeletal tumors and Tumorlike lesions. Cham: Springer; 2014.
15. Azzakhmam M, Elktaibi A, Reda M, Allaoui M, Albouzidi A, Oukabli M. Primary epitheloid angiosarcoma of the pleura: an exceptional tumor location. Pan Afr Med J. 2019;33.
16. Levi G, Orzes N, Uccelli S, Cettolo F, Arici M, Ciarfaglia M, et al. Spontaneous synchronous bilateral hemothorax as the only finding in primary pleural angiosarcoma: a case report and a literature review. Monaldi Arch Chest Dis. 2021;91(1).
17. Cabibi D, Pipitone G, Porcasi R, Ingrao S, Benza I, Porrello C, et al. Pleural epithelioid angiosarcoma with lymphatic differentiation arisen after radiometabolic therapy for thyroid carcinoma: immunohistochemical findings and review of the literature. Diagn Pathol. 2017;12(1).
18. Bruixola G, Díaz-Beveridge R, Jiménez E, Caballero J, Salavert M, Escoin C, et al. Pleuropulmonary angiosarcoma involving the liver, the jejunum and the spine, developed from chronic tuberculosis pyothorax: multidisciplinary approach and review of literature. Lung Cancer. 2014;86(1):105–11.
19. Sedhai YR, Basnyat S, Golamari R, Koirala A, Yuan M. Primary pleural angiosarcoma: case report and literature review. SAGE Open Med Case Rep. 2020 Feb;8:2050313X20904595.
20. Matsuda K, Yamaryo T, Akazawa Y, Kawakami K, Nakashima M. Primary pleural angiosarcoma associated with pneumoconiosis: an autopsy case. Pathol Int. 2015;65(11):603.
21. Wang H, Shi J, Liu H, Chen Y, Wang Y, Wang W, Zhang L. Clinical and diagnostic features of angiosarcoma with pulmonary metastases: a retrospective observational study. Medicine (Baltimore). 2017;96(36):e8033. https://doi.org/10.1097/MD.0000000000008033. PMID: 28885371; PMCID: PMC6392612.
22. Davies JD, Rees GJ, Mera SL. Angiosarcoma in irradiated post-mastectomy chest wall. Histopathology. 1983;7(6):947–56. https://doi.org/10.1111/j.1365-2559.1983.tb02309.x. PMID: 6363269.
23. Zhang PJ, Livolsi VA, Brooks JJ. Malignant epithelioid vascular tumors of the pleura: report of a series and literature review. Hum Pathol. 2000;31(1):29–34. https://doi.org/10.1016/s0046-8177(00)80194-x. PMID: 10665909.
24. Xu J, Liu M, Yuan H, Liu Z, Zhu D. Case report: primary pleural Angiosarcoma in a patient with Klippel-Trenaunay syndrome. Front Genet. 2022;28:13.
25. Nakamura M, Watanabe K, Nishimura T, Yoshida K, Fukumoto K, Hiyama N, et al. Primary pleural Angiosarcoma treated with Nivolumab and Ipilimumab: a case report. Case Rep Oncol. 2023:81–7.
26. Behjati S, Tarpey PS, Sheldon H, Martincorena I, Van Loo P, Gundem G, Wedge DC, Ramakrishna M, Cooke SL, Pillay N, Vollan HKM, Papaemmanuil E, Koss H, Bunney TD, Hardy C, Joseph OR, Martin S, Mudie L, Butler A, Teague JW, Patil M, Steers G, Cao Y, Gumbs C, Ingram D, Lazar AJ, Little L, Mahadeshwar H, Protopopov A, Al Sannaa GA, Seth S, Song X, Tang J, Zhang J, Ravi V, Torres KE, Khatri B, Halai D, Roxanis I, Baumhoer D, Tirabosco R, Amary MF, Boshoff C, McDermott U, Katan M, Stratton MR, Futreal PA, Flanagan AM, Harris A, Campbell PJ. Recurrent PTPRB and PLCG1 mutations in angiosarcoma. Nat Genet. 2014;46(4):376–9. https://doi.org/10.1038/ng.2921. Epub 2014 Mar 16. PMID: 24633157; PMCID: PMC4032873.
27. Chan JY, Lim JQ, Yeong J, Ravi V, Guan P, Boot A, Tay TKY, Selvarajan S, Md Nasir ND, Loh JH, Ong CK, Huang D, Tan J, Li Z, Ng CC, Tan TT, Masuzawa M, Sung KW, Farid M, Quek RHH, et al. Multiomic analysis and immunoprofiling reveal distinct subtypes of human angiosarcoma. J Clin Invest. 2020;130(11):5833–46.

28. Manner J, Radlwimmer B, Hohenberger P, Mössinger K, Küffer S, Sauer C, Belharazem D, Zettl A, Coindre JM, Hallermann C, Hartmann JT, Katenkamp D, Katenkamp K, Schöffski P, Sciot R, Wozniak A, Lichter P, Marx A, Ströbel P. MYC high level gene amplification is a distinctive feature of angiosarcomas after irradiation or chronic lymphedema. Am J Pathol. 2010;176(1):34–9.
29. Guo T, Zhang L, Chang NE, Singer S, Maki RG, Antonescu CR. Consistent MYC and FLT4 gene amplification in radiation-induced angiosarcoma but not in other radiation-associated atypical vascular lesions. Genes Chromosomes Cancer. 2011;50(1):25–33.
30. Cornejo KM, Deng A, Wu H, Cosar EF, Khan A, St Cyr M, Tomaszewicz K, Dresser K, O'Donnell P, Hutchinson L. The utility of MYC and FLT4 in the diagnosis and treatment of postradiation atypical vascular lesion and angiosarcoma of the breast. Hum Pathol. 2015;46(6):868–75.
31. Chang JH, Kim JH, Hong SH, Song ME, Ryu YJ, Lee JH, et al. Angiosarcoma presenting with spontaneous hydropneumothorax: report of a case and review of the literature. Open Respir Med J. 2014;8(1):48–54.
32. Antonescu CR, Yoshida A, Guo T, Chang NE, Zhang L, Agaram NP, Qin LX, Brennan MF, Singer S, Maki RG. KDR activating mutations in human angiosarcomas are sensitive to specific kinase inhibitors. Cancer Res. 2009;69(18):7175–9. https://doi.org/10.1158/0008-5472.CAN-09-2068. Epub 2009 Sep 1. PMID: 19723655; PMCID: PMC2763376.
33. Kao YC, Chow JM, Wang KM, Fang CL, Chu JS, Chen CL. Primary pleural angiosarcoma as a mimicker of mesothelioma: a case report. Diagn Pathol. 2011;6(1).
34. Chen CY, Wu YC, Chou TY, Yang KY. Pleural angiosarcoma mimicking pleural haematoma. Interact Cardiovasc Thorac Surg. 2013;17(5):886–8.
35. Chong AR, Ng KL, Huan N, Mohd Aminudin NH, Ahmad Sharifuddin M, Raja Rahaizat RNA, et al. Unveiling a rare haemorrhagic malignant pleural effusion: the role of medical thoracoscopy in diagnosing primary pleural angiosarcoma. Respirol Case Rep. 2024;12(11).
36. Gil BM, Chung MH, Lee KN, Jung JI, Yoo WJ, Kwon SS, et al. Multidetector CT findings of primary pleural angiosarcoma: a systematic review, an additional cases report. Cancer Imaging. 2022;22(1).
37. Woo JJ, Kim Y, An JK, Lee H. Primary pleural epithelioid angiosarcoma manifesting as a loculated hemothorax: a case report and literature review focusing on CT findings. Radiol Case Rep. 2021;16(10):3072–5.
38. Sinkler MA, Ullah A, Wehrle CJ, Ibrahim MA, White J. Primary pleural epithelioid Angiosarcoma with extensive and rapid metastasis to brain and bilateral adrenal glands. Cureus. 2020;12(8).
39. Alexiou C, Clelland CA, Robinson D, Morgan WE. Primary angiosarcomas of the chest wall and pleura. Eur J Cardiothorac Surg. 1998;14(5):523–6.
40. Urshila Durani, Gallo A, Beachey J, Nelson D, Robinson S, Anavekar NS. Epithelioid angiosarcoma: a rare cause of pericarditis and pleural effusion. Respir Med Case Rep. 2018;24:77–80.
41. Moriya Y, Sugawara T, Arai M, Tsuda Y, Uchida K, Noguchi T, et al. Bilateral massive bloody pleurisy Complicatedby Angiosarcoma. Intern Med. 2007;46(3):125–8.
42. Atasoy C, Fitoz S, Yiğit H, Atasoy P, Erden I, Akyar S. Radiographic, CT, and MRI findings in primary pulmonary angiosarcoma. Clin Imaging. 2001;25(5):337–40. https://doi.org/10.1016/s0899-7071(01)00302-3. PMID: 11682292.
43. Hierholzer J, Luo L, Bittner R, Stroszczynski C, Schröder R, Schoenfeld N, et al. MRI and CT in the differential diagnosis of pleural disease. Chest. 2000;118(3):604–9.
44. Grafino M, Alves P, de Almeida MM, Garrido P, Hasmucrai D, Teixeira E, Sotto-Mayor R. Angiosarcoma of the lung. J Bras Pneumol. 2016;42(1):68–70. https://doi.org/10.1590/S1806-37562016000000193. PMID: 26982044; PMCID: PMC4805390.
45. Szczyrek M, Bitkowska P, Jutrzenka M, Szudy-Szczyrek A, Drelich-Zbroja A, Milanowski J. Pleural neoplasms—what could MRI change? Cancer. 2023;15:3261. https://doi.org/10.3390/cancers15123261.
46. Piamonti D, Giannone S, D'Antoni L, Sanna A, Landini N, Pernazza A, Bassi M, Carillo C, Diso D, Venuta F, et al. Bilateral spontaneous Hemothorax: a rare case of primary pleural Angiosarcoma and literature review. J Clin Med. 2025;14:3377. https://doi.org/10.3390/jcm14103377.
47. Zhang GX, Zheng Y, Huang WS, Yang M, Xu JH. FDG PET/CT findings of unsuspected pulmonary epithelioid Angiosarcoma manifested as a brain metastasis. Clin Nucl Med. 2019;44(8):e489–91.
48. Wang J, Song Z, Zhang Y, Li J, Yu Y. Primary pleural angiosarcoma: a case report and review. Radiol Case Rep. 2022;17(1):55–9.
49. Sedhai YR, Basnyat S, Golamari R, Koirala A, Yuan M. Primary pleural angiosarcoma: Case report and literature review. SAGE Open Med Case Rep. 2020;8:2050313X20904595. https://doi.org/10.1177/2050313X20904595. PMID: 32095244; PMCID: PMC7011321.
50. Kim YK, Lee KS, Kim BT, Choi JY, Yoon YC, Kwon GY. Comparison of FDG PET/CT findings in malignant mesothelioma and metastatic pleural disease. AJR Am J Roentgenol. 2015;205(2):307–12.
51. Hodgson NC, Jackson C, Mentias M. Solitary fibrous tumor of the pleura: diagnostic challenges and imaging appearances. Cancer Imaging. 2021;21(1):17.
52. Wang X, Lu Z, Luo Y, Cai J, Wei J, Liu A, Zeng Z. Characteristics and outcomes of primary pleural angiosarcoma: a retrospective study of 43 published cases. Medicine (Baltimore). 2022;101(6):e28785. https://doi.org/10.1097/MD.0000000000028785. PMID: 35147108; PMCID: PMC8830823.
53. Lorentziadis M, Sourlas A. Primary de novo angiosarcoma of the pleura. Ann Thorac Surg.

2012;93(3):996–8. https://doi.org/10.1016/j.athoracsur.2011.07.023. PMID: 22365000.
54. Abu-Zaid A, Mohammed S. Primary pleural angiosarcoma in a 63-year-old gentleman. Case Rep Pulmonol. 2013;2013:974567. https://doi.org/10.1155/2013/974567. Epub 2013 Jun 13. PMID: 23844302; PMCID: PMC3697234.
55. Chong AR, Ng KL, Huan NC, Mohd Aminudin NH, Ahmad Sharifuddin M, Raja Rahaizat RNA, Mohamed NK. Unveiling a rare haemorrhagic malignant pleural effusion: the role of medical thoracoscopy in diagnosing primary pleural angiosarcoma. Respirol Case Rep. 2024;12(11):e70068. https://doi.org/10.1002/rcr2.70068. PMID: 39588325; PMCID: PMC11586632.
56. Kurtz JE, Serra S, Duclos B, Brolly F, Dufour P, Bergerat JP. Diffuse primary angiosarcoma of the pleura: a case report and review of the literature. Sarcoma. 2004;8(4):103–6. https://doi.org/10.1155/2004/794907. PMID: 18521403; PMCID: PMC2395614.
57. Hara N, Fujimoto N, Miyamoto Y, Yamagishi T, Asano M, Fuchimoto Y, Wada S, Ozaki S, Nishi H, Kishimoto T. Angiosarcoma of the thoracic wall responded well to nanoparticle albumin-bound paclitaxel: a case report. Drug Discov Ther. 2016;10(2):114–6. https://doi.org/10.5582/ddt.2016.01005. Epub 2016 Feb 15. PMID: 26875587.
58. Yavuz H, Ahmet Kayahan Tekneci, Tevfik Ilker Akcam, Kutsal Turhan, Taner Akalın. Pleural angiosarcoma presenting with spontaneous hemothorax. Indian J Thorac Cardiovasc Surg. 2023;39(5):543–6.
59. Provost K, Charest M. Detection of intrathoracic bleeding by 99mTc-labeled red blood cell SPECT/CT after wedge biopsy of pulmonary Angiosarcoma. J Nucl Med Technol. 2016;44(3):205–6. https://doi.org/10.2967/jnmt.116.174235. Epub 2016 Jun 30. PMID: 27363446.
60. Roh MS, Seo JY, Hong SH. Epithelioid angiosarcoma of the pleura: a case report. J Korean Med Sci. 2001;16(6):792–5. https://doi.org/10.3346/jkms.2001.16.6.792. PMID: 11748365; PMCID: PMC3054810.
61. Gil BM, Chung MH, Lee KN, Jung JI, Yoo WJ, Kwon SS, Lee H. Multidetector CT findings of primary pleural angiosarcoma: a systematic review, an additional cases report. Cancer Imaging. 2022;22(1):6. https://doi.org/10.1186/s40644-021-00435-1. PMID: 35022068; PMCID: PMC8756718.
62. Wagner MJ, Othus M, Patel SP, Ryan C, Sangal A, Powers B, Budd GT, Victor AI, Hsueh CT, Chugh R, Nair S, Leu KM, Agulnik M, Sharon E, Mayerson E, Plets M, Blanke C, Streicher H, Chae YK, Kurzrock R. Multicenter phase II trial (SWOG S1609, cohort 51) of ipilimumab and nivolumab in metastatic or unresectable angiosarcoma: a substudy of dual anti-CTLA-4 and anti-PD-1 blockade in rare tumors (DART). J Immunother Cancer. 2021;9(8):e002990. https://doi.org/10.1136/jitc-2021-002990. PMID: 34380663; PMCID: PMC8330584.
63. Nakamura M, Watanabe K, Nishimura T, Yoshida K, Fukumoto K, Hiyama N, Masuda Y, Morikawa T, Matsumoto J, Usui K. Primary pleural Angiosarcoma treated with Nivolumab and Ipilimumab: a case report. Case Rep Oncol. 2023;16(1):75–81. https://doi.org/10.1159/000529447. PMID: 36820215; PMCID: PMC9938394.
64. Wang X, Wei J, Zeng Z, Cai J, Lu Z, Liu A. Primary pleural epithelioid angiosarcoma treated successfully with anti-PD-1 therapy: a rare case report. Medicine (Baltimore). 2021;100(35):e27132. https://doi.org/10.1097/MD.0000000000027132. PMID: 34477160; PMCID: PMC8415961.

Pulmonary and Pleural Epithelioid Hemangioendothelioma

17

Matthew Bittner, Shuanzeng Wei, and Rohit Kumar

Introduction

Pulmonary epithelioid hemangioendothelioma (P-EHE), described initially as intravascular bronchioloalveolar tumor (IVBAT) by Dail and Liebow in 1975, is a rare vascular neoplasm that may involve the pleura [1, 2]. The designation "epithelioid hemangioendothelioma" was later introduced by Weiss and Enzinger in 1982, who characterized the tumor as exhibiting histological features intermediate between hemangioma and angiosarcoma [2, 3]. The authors also observed positive cytoplasmic staining for factor VIII-related antigen and the presence of Weibel–Palade bodies, both of which confirmed the vascular endothelial origin of the neoplasm.

P-EHE develops from the proliferation of malignant vascular endothelial or pre-endothelial cells and displays variable angiogenic properties [4, 5]. The clinical course of P-EHE is heterogeneous, ranging from slow progression over several decades to highly aggressive presentations that can be fatal within months [4]. Despite its rarity, P-EHE warrants consideration due to its potential aggressiveness, particularly when the pleura is involved, and should be included in the differential diagnosis under appropriate clinical circumstances.

Epidemiology and Risk Factors

Epithelioid hemangioendothelioma (EHE) is an exceedingly rare vascular tumor, with an incidence of less than 1 per 1,000,000 and representing fewer than 1% of all vascular neoplasms [1–5]. By site of origin, the tumor most frequently arises from the soft tissue and skin (30.8%), followed by the abdomen (28%), respiratory system (19%), and bone and joints (8.6%) In contrast, data from the Hemangioendothelioma, Epithelioid Hemangioendothelioma, and Related Vascular Disorders (HEARD) Support Group indicate that the most common initial presentations involve the liver alone (21%), followed by liver and lung involvement (18%), lung alone (12%), and bone alone (14%) [1, 4, 5, 7–10].

Pulmonary EHE is particularly uncommon; as of 2014, only 248 cases had been documented [1–5]. Among these, pleural involvement is observed in 10%–49% of cases [3, 7, 8]. When the pleura is affected, the disease tends to involve the right side of the chest more often [11, 12]. A review found that 28 of 32 patients with pleural

M. Bittner
Department of Thoracic Medicine and Surgery, Temple University, Philadelphia, PA, USA

S. Wei
Department of Pathology, Fox Chase Cancer Center, Philadelphia, PA, USA

R. Kumar (✉)
Department of Medicine, Section of Pulmonary, Interventional & Critical Care, Fox Chase Cancer Center, Temple University Health System, Philadelphia, PA, USA
e-mail: Rohit.Kumar@fccc.edu

F. Ido (ed.), *Rare Pleural Diseases*, https://doi.org/10.1007/978-3-032-14873-5_17

involvement also had a pleural effusion, with 72% of these occurring on the right side [12]. At diagnosis, approximately 20–30% of EHE patients present with metastatic disease [11, 12]. EHE most commonly affects individuals in their fourth or fifth decade of life, with a mean age of 36 years [1, 3, 4, 7, 8, 13–17]. Demographically, the tumor is most prevalent among Caucasians (80–83%), followed by African Americans (9%–11%) and Hispanics (11%) [18].

Females are disproportionately affected by epithelioid hemangioendothelioma, with some studies reporting a female-to-male ratio as high as 4:1 [1, 3, 4, 7, 8, 13, 16, 17]. In contrast, pleural involvement is more common in males. Instances of pulmonary epithelioid hemangioendothelioma have also been observed in both peripartum and postpartum patients [2]. The increased incidence among females of reproductive age suggests a possible role for sex hormones in the pathogenesis of the disease; however, this hypothesis remains speculative and warrants further investigation [19–21].

Additional potential risk factors for EHE include previous radiation therapy, viral hepatitis, hepatic trauma, alcohol consumption, asbestos exposure, and exposure to vinyl chloride [22–25]. However, these associations are derived from a limited number of case reports involving hepatic EHE and have not been established in P-EHE.

Genetic abnormalities have been recognized as potential factors influencing the age at diagnosis. Patients presenting with the *YAP–TFE3* fusion are generally diagnosed at a younger age than those with the more prevalent *WWTR1–CAMTA1* gene fusion [26].

Pathophysiology

Genetic studies of epithelioid hemangioendothelioma have revealed two primary fusion mutations arising from distinct chromosomal translocations. The first is characterized by a t(1;3)(p36.23;q25) translocation, which generates a fusion between *WWTR1* (WW domain-containing tr*ans*cription regulator 1, located at 3q25) and *CAMTA1* (*calm*odulin-binding transcription activator 1, situated at 1p36.23). The second genetic alteration is characterized by a fusion event between *YAP1* (Yes-associated protein 1, located at 11q22) and *TFE3* (Transcription factor E3, located at Xp11.23) [4, 7, 8, 26, 27]. The *WWTR1–CAMTA1* fusion is the predominant genetic alteration, comprising up to 90% of EHE cases, whereas the *YAP1–TFE3* fusion is observed in approximately 5% of cases [26]. Additional, less frequently observed fusion genes include *WWTR1–MAML2* (mastermind-like transcriptional coactivator 2, located at 11q21), which demonstrates a propensity for cardiac involvement, as well as *WWTR1–ACTL6A* (actin-like 6A, located at 3q26.33) [26].

Although somatic mutations are generally considered to occur spontaneously, there is a hypothesis proposing a possible association with Bartonella infection, which has been linked to other vascular neoplasms [1, 28]. The capacity of these bacteria to promote VEGF-mediated vasoproliferation and establish intra-endothelial infections offers a theoretical basis for understanding vascular tumorigenesis [1, 28].

P-EHE may disseminate contiguously through the lung parenchyma, including local alveolar spread via the pores of Kohn. This represents structured, localized alveolar infiltration rather than classic spread through air spaces (STAS) characterized by detached tumor clusters. Additionally, EHE may also disseminate hematogenously, across pleural surfaces, or through lymphatic channels [1, 16]. Primary P-EHE metastasizes in approximately 20–40% of cases, with the majority spreading to the liver (18–23%) and to bone (4–10%). Brain and intestinal metastasis are relatively rare, occurring in only 1–3% of cases [29, 30].

Clinical Features

The clinical course of EHE is highly variable [12]. Stable, asymptomatic nodules can persist for years, while others can develop rapid, widespread metastases resembling high-grade angiosarcoma. The relative frequency of indolent versus aggressive presentations remains unclear due to the rarity of the disease and limited data [4, 7, 10, 15, 17].

Over 50% of individuals diagnosed with EHE present without symptoms at the time of diagnosis [1]. Affected males report symptoms more frequently than females [16, 17]. The most frequently reported symptom is pain localized to the tumor site, which may manifest as pleuritic chest pain, right upper quadrant abdominal discomfort, or pain associated with pathological fractures [1, 31]. In instances of pulmonary involvement, patients may also present with symptoms such as cough, hemoptysis, or dyspnea [1, 2, 9, 17, 32].

Diagnosis

Imaging

The radiologic appearance of epithelioid hemangioendothelioma is variable and often nonspecific. On conventional chest radiography, bilateral pulmonary nodules are the most frequent finding, typically measuring less than 1 cm in diameter, though some may reach up to 2 cm. Approximately 60% of nodules are located in the basilar regions of the lungs [1, 5]. On computed tomography (CT), the most common pattern consists of multiple small bilateral nodules, observed in 71.4% of cases in a single-center series of 35 patients (Fig. 17.1a) [33]. In another cohort of 18 patients, 61.1% exhibited multiple perivascular lesions in both lungs, with 61.1% of nodules measuring <20 mm. Additional CT findings included ground-glass opacities (27.8%), calcification (27.8%), cavitation (16.7%), pleural thickening (27.8%), and pleural effusion (33.3%). Contrast enhancement was noted in 81.8% of cases, underscoring the utility of contrast-enhanced CT in assessing potential mediastinal or pleural involvement [29]. Pleural disease may appear as either smooth or nodular pleural thickening, and associated pleural effusions may be loculated [3, 34]. Additionally, CT may reveal multiple organ involvement, with hepatic nodules or bone sclerotic lesions (Fig. 17.1b, c) [30]. On positron emission tomography–computed tomography (PET–CT), pulmonary lesions demonstrate fluorodeoxyglucose (FDG) avidity in approximately 73% of patients, and lesion size correlated positively with SUVmax [29].

Magnetic resonance imaging (MRI) of the thorax typically reveals lesions with low-to-intermediate T1 and intermediate-to-high T2 signal intensity, along with post-contrast enhancement. MRI is beneficial for delineating pleural extent, chest-wall or mediastinal invasion, and bone marrow involvement [35]. In pleural-predominant disease, MRI typically demonstrates smooth or nodular pleural thickening, fissural extension, and a frequently associated pleural effusion, findings that may partially assist in distinguishing epithelioid hemangioendothelioma from mesothelioma or metastatic pleural disease, as the latter most commonly demonstrates circumferential involvement of the entire hemithoracic pleura [3, 35].

Magnetic resonance angiography (MRA) can further depict vascular encasement or intraluminal extension in select cases, complementing CT and PET–CT for operative planning [35]. Overall, MRI and MRA serve as valuable problem-solving tools for delineating pleural extent, vascular anatomy, and mediastinal relationships in thoracic EHE; however, these modalities do not reliably differentiate pleural EHE from MPM. Findings such as a circumferential pleural rind and marked diffusion restriction on diffusion-weighted imaging (DWI) are more characteristic of MPM and, while suggestive, are not diagnostic in the context of EHE [35–37].

Pathology

Since radiographic findings in epithelioid hemangioendothelioma are often nonspecific, definitive diagnosis relies on obtaining adequate tissue samples for histopathologic evaluation, immunohistochemical staining, and molecular testing to identify the characteristic gene fusions.

In pulmonary EHE, bronchoalveolar lavage (BAL) is essentially nondiagnostic, and transbronchial biopsy (TBBx) has a very low diagnostic yield. Most studies and reviews report negative

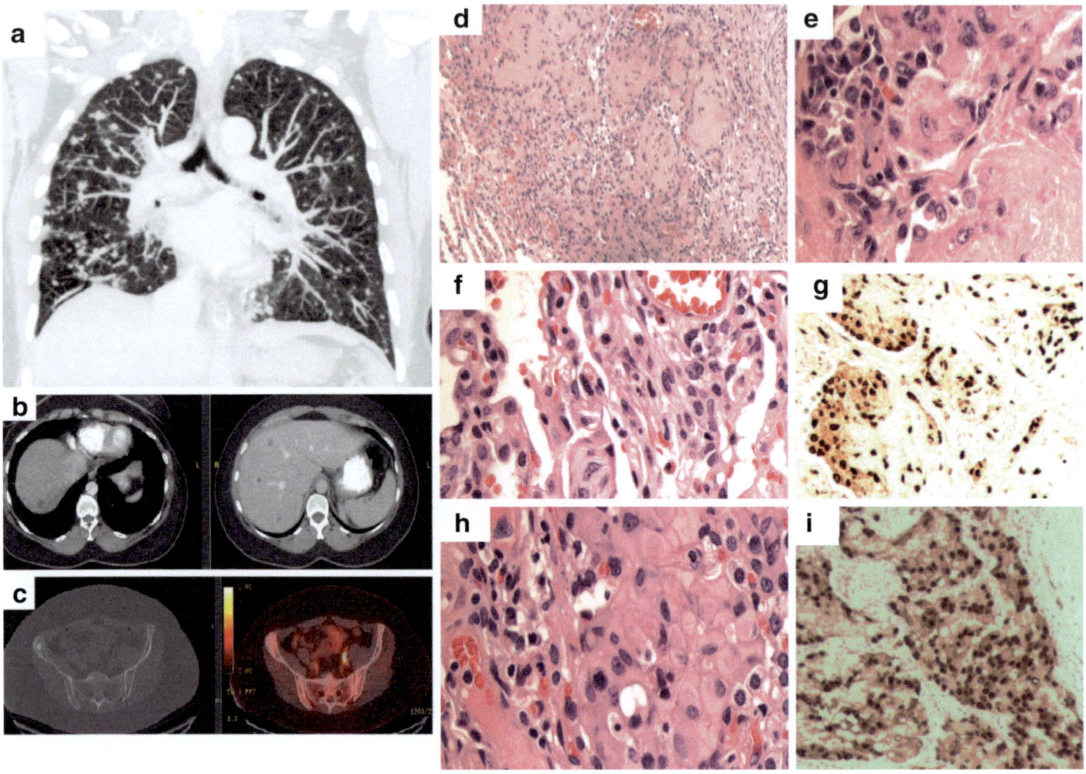

Fig. 17.1 Radiologic and histopathologic features of epithelioid hemangioendothelioma involving the pleura, lungs, liver, and bone

(**a**) Computed tomography (CT) of the chest using a maximum intensity projection (MIP) in coronal section demonstrates innumerable, bilateral, well-circumscribed pulmonary nodules of varying sizes, predominantly distributed peripherally and adjacent to pulmonary vasculature

(**b**) Abdominal CT showing multiple, well-circumscribed hypodense lesions within the liver parenchyma

(**c**) Pelvic CT in bone window (left panel) revealing a sclerotic lesion of the right iliac crest; corresponding PET/CT image (right panel) demonstrates minimal FDG uptake within the lesion

(**d**) Low-power hematoxylin and eosin (H&E)–stained section (×250) showing focal clustered proliferation of neoplastic cells within some of the pulmonary nodules. A nodular pattern of hyalinization is evident in even the smallest neoplastic cell aggregates

(**e**) Higher-power H&E section (×400) showing neoplastic clusters. Most of the cells are round, small, and bland, but a large epithelioid cell has formed at the edge of the cluster

(**f**) In non-hyalinized regions, round to oval tumor cells line newly-formed red blood cell-containing vascular spaces. (H&E, ×400)

(**g**) Immunohistochemical stains for CD31 and ERG further support the endothelial nature of these cells (×400)

(**h**) At the periphery of pulmonary nodules, clusters of larger epithelioid tumor cells with eccentric nuclei and abundant eosinophilic cytoplasm containing vacuolated or luminal spaces are evident (H&E, ×400)

(**i**) Immunohistochemistry showing strong nuclear reactivity for CAMTA1, confirming the diagnosis of epithelioid hemangioendothelioma

Attribution: Panels **a–c** courtesy of *Dr. Firas Ido*; panels **d–i** courtesy of *Dr. Santo Longo*. All images are original and unpublished, reproduced here with permission of the respective authors

BAL findings and insufficient TBBx samples, with only rare diagnostic success when the tumor directly involves a bronchus [17, 30, 35, 38, 39]. When tissue sampling is required, image-guided transthoracic core needle biopsy is the preferred approach for obtaining tissue samples. This method provides sufficient material for immunohistochemistry (including CD31, ERG, and CAMTA1) and achieves high diagnostic accuracy for pulmonary lesions overall, with reported sensitivities of approximately 90–95% and specificities of 95–100%. Several pulmonary EHE cases have been successfully diagnosed using this technique, whereas fine-needle aspiration (FNA) alone is less reliable and may yield misleading results if immunostains are limited [40–43]. When less invasive modalities fail to establish a diagnosis, surgical lung biopsy remains the gold standard for obtaining diagnostic tissue [17, 32]. In patients with pleural effusion, pleural fluid is typically exudative; however, diagnostic yield is limited, with a reported sensitivity of approximately 20% for detecting EHE [34]. If cytology is negative but clinical suspicion for malignancy remains high, a pleural biopsy should be performed to obtain diagnostic material [12].

Histologically, pulmonary EHE demonstrates an angiocentric growth pattern, tracking along small arterioles, venules, and lymphatics within the interstitium, often extending across adjacent alveolar septa with focal intra-alveolar colonization [7, 45]. The tumor is composed of infiltrative cords, strands, and nests of epithelioid cells embedded in a variably myxoid to hyalinized stroma, frequently containing intracytoplasmic vacuoles. On routine hematoxylin and eosin (H&E) staining, tumor cells exhibit moderate amounts of glassy eosinophilic cytoplasm, round to ovoid nuclei, inconspicuous nucleoli, minimal atypia, and a very low mitotic index [7, 8, 45]. Intracytoplasmic vacuoles are a common feature and may contain erythrocytes [9, 15, 45]. Well-formed vascular channels are typically absent (Fig. 17.1d–f, h) [7, 8, 15, 17, 26]. Notably, tumors harboring the *YAP1–TFE3* fusion may demonstrate greater vasoformative features and more pronounced cytologic atypia compared with those containing the *WWTR1–CAMTA1* fusion [27]. In pulmonary EHE, histologic sections often reveal multifocal infiltration of small airspaces, with tumor spread from alveolus to alveolus via the pores of Kohn [5, 7, 17].

Immunohistochemical staining is essential for confirming the diagnosis of EHE [1, 2, 9]. A panel of endothelial markers is typically employed, including CD31, ERG, and FLI-1 (Fig. 17.1g) [1, 8, 15]. Among these, CD31 is the most specific and consistently expressed marker, demonstrating near-universal positivity across published studies [8]. ERG and FLI-1, both nuclear transcription factors of the E26 - erythroblast transformation specific family (ETS), are highly sensitive indicators of endothelial differentiation. ERG has demonstrated 100% sensitivity in several large series, while FLI-1 has shown similarly high sensitivity in multiple cohorts [1, 8, 15, 26]. At the molecular level, the *WWTR1–CAMTA1* fusion gene is detected in approximately 90% of cases, while the *YAP1–TFE3* fusion gene is found in around 5%. Identification of either fusion by next-generation sequencing (NGS) or fluorescence in situ hybridization (FISH) is the most specific ancillary method for distinguishing EHE from histologic mimics [45]. Nuclear CAMTA1 immunostaining has emerged as a highly specific surrogate marker for the *WWTR1–CAMTA1* gene fusion, demonstrating positivity in approximately 86% of conventional EHEs (Fig. 17.1i) [46, 47]. Importantly, CAMTA1 staining is negative in the *YAP1–TFE3* subset. For CAMTA1-negative cases, TFE3 immunohistochemistry and confirmatory fusion testing are recommended to ensure diagnostic accuracy.

Differential Diagnosis

P-EHE may mimic other neoplasms with pleural involvement. The differential diagnosis includes epithelioid angiosarcoma, epithelioid hemangioma, pseudomyogenic hemangioendothelioma, and mesothelioma, particularly in cases with pleural involvement [7, 8, 14, 17, 26, 27, 48]. Additional mimics include metastatic signet-ring adenocarcinoma, alveolar soft part sarcoma, and Xp11 translocation-positive renal cell carcinoma, among others [14, 27]. Accurate diagnosis requires adequate tissue sampling, supplemented by immunohistochemistry and molecular genetic testing to confirm defining fusion events. Compared with epithelioid angiosarcoma, EHE typically lacks necrosis, marked cytologic atypia, a high mitotic index, and the irregular, anastomosing vascular channels characteristic of angiosarcoma. An exception is EHE harboring the *YAP1–TFE3* fusion, which may display slightly increased atypia and vascular complexity [17, 45].

Epithelioid hemangioma can be distinguished from EHE by its lobular architecture and well-formed vascular channels. Molecularly, EHE is defined by *WWTR1–CAMTA1* or *YAP1–TFE3* gene fusions, whereas epithelioid hemangioma more commonly exhibits *FOS* or *FOSB* rearrangements [26, 49].

Pseudomyogenic hemangioendothelioma shows fascicular arrangements of plump spindle cells often accompanied by a neutrophilic infiltrate. It is genetically characterized by *FOSB* fusion events, including *FOSB–ACTB*, *FOSB–SERPINE1*, or *FOSB–WWTR1* [26].

In pleural-based disease, distinguishing EHE from sarcomatoid mesothelioma is particularly challenging. Both may exhibit epithelioid to spindle-shaped cells embedded in a dense desmoplastic stroma [7, 48]. Immunohistochemistry provides important clues: Mesothelioma typically expresses pancytokeratin, whereas EHE shows strong positivity for endothelial markers such as CD31 and ERG [50]. Nonetheless, given the potential for histologic and immunophenotypic overlap, molecular testing remains the most reliable method for definitively distinguishing between these entities.

Treatment

Due to its rarity, epithelioid hemangioendothelioma lacks a standardized treatment algorithm. Management is individualized and depends on clinical presentation, disease extent, anatomic location, and the presence or absence of symptoms.

For patients with indolent or asymptomatic disease, particularly when lesions are multifocal or surgically unresectable, a strategy of active surveillance is often appropriate. In asymptomatic patients, close clinical and radiographic monitoring is preferred to allow for timely intervention should progression occur [4, 10]. When possible, surgical resection for limited disease is the preferred treatment modality. Decisions to pursue surgery in multifocal disease depend on the extent of disease burden, lesion location and size, and whether it is technically feasible [6, 16, 32]. Some patients may benefit from resection of the progressive or symptomatic lesions, while leaving other stable lesions to be monitored by surveillance [6, 16, 32]. For pulmonary EHE presenting as a solitary lesion, wedge resection offers survival outcomes comparable to those achieved with more extensive anatomic resections such as segmentectomy or lobectomy [1, 13, 51]. In one study of patients undergoing primary surgical resection for EHE, 75% remained recurrence-free at 5 years, with 71% of these patients having unifocal disease, supporting surgery as an acceptable therapeutic strategy even in select multifocal cases [4, 7].

There is currently no universally accepted systemic therapy for EHE; however, several agents have demonstrated clinical efficacy and are considered reasonable first-line or investigational options. These include pazopanib, sirolimus, paclitaxel, and trametinib, each used according to disease behavior, molecular profile, and patient tolerance. Sirolimus, an inhibitor of the mammalian target of rapamycin (mTOR) pathway, has demonstrated clinical activity in epithelioid hemangioendothelioma. In a multicenter retrospective study of 38 patients with progressive, unresectable disease, treatment with sirolimus resulted in partial responses in 11%, stable disease in 76%, and progressive disease in 13%, yielding a median progression-free survival (PFS) of 13 months [52]. Pulmonary involvement was present in approximately 68% of patients. Outcomes differed significantly based on serosal involvement. Patients without pleural or peritoneal effusions achieved a median PFS of 47.8 months. In contrast, those with serosal effusions had a markedly shorter median PFS of 4.8 months, underscoring the prognostic significance of serosal effusion as a negative marker in EHE. Sirolimus was generally well tolerated; however, ovarian dysfunction, manifesting as new-onset secondary amenorrhea or menstrual irregularity, occurred in 41% of premenopausal women [52]. Given its relative efficacy in achieving disease stabilization, particularly in patients without serosal involvement, sirolimus is frequently employed as a first-line systemic therapy in appropriate cases of unresectable or progressive EHE.

Pazopanib, a vascular endothelial growth factor receptor (VEGFR) tyrosine kinase inhibitor, has been utilized in the management of advanced epithelioid hemangioendothelioma [53–55]. The antiangiogenic mechanism of action aligns with the tumor's vascular origin, and multiple retrospective studies and case reports have reported significant disease control [53–55]. In a multicenter study conducted by the European Organisation for Research and Treatment of Cancer (EORTC) involving patients with vascular sarcomas, ten individuals with EHE received pazopanib. The overall response rate was 20%, with a median progression-free survival of 6.6 months and a median overall survival (OS) of 27.8 months [55]. Several case reports have corroborated these findings, documenting prolonged disease stability over several years in patients with metastatic pulmonary and hepatic EHE [53, 54]. Although objective response rates remain modest, pazopanib represents a noncytotoxic, orally administered therapeutic option with a favorable tolerability profile. It may be beneficial in patients with symptomatic disease, progressive lesions, or evidence of VEGF pathway activation.

Trametinib, a mitogen-activated protein kinase (MEK) inhibitor, was evaluated in a 2024 prospective phase II clinical trial involving 44 patients with advanced EHE [56]. Although the objective response rate (ORR) by *Response Evaluation Criteria in Solid Tumors (RECIST)* was modest at 3.7%, 85.7% of participants experienced some degree of tumor burden reduction [56, 57]. Among patients with TAZ–CAMTA1-positive disease, the median progression-free survival was 10.4 months; in contrast, those without this fusion, including a single case harboring YAP1–TFE3, had a median PFS of 8.25 months [56, 57]. Notably, 73% of patients reported clinically meaningful pain improvement within 4 weeks of therapy initiation, indicating potential symptomatic benefit even in the absence of significant radiographic response [56]. Serious adverse events were uncommon but included a single fatal case of pneumonitis [56, 57]. Overall, trametinib appears to provide symptom relief and disease stabilization in a subset of patients with advanced EHE, particularly those harboring MAPK pathway alterations. However, larger confirmatory studies are needed to further define its therapeutic role.

Paclitaxel, a microtubule-stabilizing chemotherapeutic agent, has demonstrated limited efficacy in the treatment of epithelioid hemangioendothelioma based on available case reports and retrospective series. In a literature review of 63 patients with pulmonary EHE, paclitaxel, either as monotherapy or in combination with platinum-based agents, was among the most frequently utilized cytotoxic regimens; however, therapeutic outcomes were variable, with some patients achieving temporary disease stabilization and others exhibiting no response or progression [13]. Similarly, in a case series of three patients with pulmonary EHE treated with combination chemotherapy, paclitaxel (administered with carboplatin and either bevacizumab or endostar) led to transient clinical and radiographic improvement. However, all patients ultimately experienced disease progression [32]. Given the rarity of EHE and the absence of prospective trials evaluating cytotoxic chemotherapy, the role of paclitaxel remains poorly defined and is generally reserved for cases in which targeted or biologic therapies are contraindicated or have failed.

The choice to use sirolimus, trametinib, and pazopanib should be individualized based on disease characteristics and patient-specific factors. For patients without serosal involvement, sirolimus offers the most reported disease control with a favorable toxicity profile [52]. Trametinib may be considered in those with symptomatic or rapidly progressive disease, particularly when cancer-related pain is prominent [56, 57]. Pazopanib represents a reasonable option across diverse clinical contexts, especially when an anti-angiogenic strategy is preferred [53–55].

Beyond these commonly utilized agents, several additional systemic therapies have shown limited or inconsistent activity in EHE and are not currently recommended as frontline treatments. These include bevacizumab, sorafenib, and PD-1 inhibitors, which may be considered only in select, refractory cases within a clinical trial or compassionate-use framework. Bevacizumab, a monoclonal antibody targeting vascular endothelial growth factor (VEGF), has demonstrated limited but measurable activity in epithelioid hemangioendothelioma. In a phase II trial including seven patients, two (29%) achieved a partial response, four (57%) had stable disease, and one (14%) experienced disease progression at the first evaluation after two treatment cycles. The median progression-free survival was 39.1 weeks, and the median overall survival reached 142.6 weeks [58].

Sorafenib, a multi-kinase inhibitor that targets both VEGF receptors and RAF kinases, has also demonstrated modest clinical activity. In a prospective phase II trial of 15 patients with progressive EHE, sorafenib achieved a 9-month non-progression rate of 31%, including two partial responses and a median PFS of 6 months [59]. Although significant tumor reduction was not observed, the drug prolonged disease stabilization in a subset of patients and may be considered a therapeutic option when other agents have failed or are contraindicated.

PD-1 inhibitors have shown variable efficacy in EHE, though evidence remains limited to isolated case reports. In one report, a patient with pulmonary endovascular EHE harboring an *MSH2* mutation achieved a marked response to paclitaxel–carboplatin chemotherapy followed by pembrolizumab maintenance [60]. Another case described prolonged stable disease lasting more than 13 months with toripalimab in a patient with retroperitoneal EHE [61]. These observations suggest a potential role for immune checkpoint inhibition, particularly in patients with microsatellite instability (MSI) or DNA mismatch repair deficiency, though larger studies are needed to confirm efficacy.

Radiation therapy is generally ineffective for pulmonary EHE due to the tumor's indolent growth and relative radioresistance. However, it may be beneficial for osseous lesions or for palliation of localized pain or mass effect [1, 13, 16, 32].

Pleural involvement in EHE is associated with more aggressive clinical behavior and reduced survival. Management often necessitates a multimodal approach. Video-assisted thoracoscopic surgery (VATS) with pleural decortication may offer both diagnostic confirmation and symptomatic relief [12, 44, 62]. Some reports have described adjunctive systemic chemotherapy to limit further pleural dissemination and alleviate effusion-related pain [44, 57]. Recurrent pleural effusions are frequently loculated and often refractory to simple thoracentesis. Placement of an indwelling pleural catheter may be considered for symptomatic management, although its efficacy in this setting has not been systematically evaluated [57]. The development of serosal effusions should prompt early initiation of systemic therapy, given the strong association with poor prognosis.

In summary, the management of advanced EHE requires a highly individualized, multidisciplinary approach. Patients with indolent disease and no serosal involvement may derive the most significant benefit from sirolimus. In contrast, those with aggressive or symptomatic disease may require MEK inhibition (e.g., trametinib) or anti-VEGF-based therapy (e.g., pazopanib or bevacizumab). Ongoing and future studies are critical for refining therapeutic algorithms, establishing biomarker-driven treatment selection, and exploring combination strategies that incorporate targeted and immunomodulatory agents for this rare vascular malignancy.

Prognosis

Overall mortality in epithelioid hemangioendothelioma varies widely depending on clinical presentation, anatomic distribution, and histopathologic features. Reported 5-year survival rates range between 70 and 80% across most studies [1, 2, 7, 10, 14, 51]. Patients with inoperable hepatic EHE exhibit a median survival of approximately 9.8 years, whereas those with pulmonary EHE have a considerably shorter median survival of 3.6 years [10].

Five-year survival for pulmonary EHE is notably poorer among patients older than 80 years, those of African American, American Indian, or Asian/Pacific Islander descent, and individuals with respiratory involvement [19–21]. While much of the survival data derive from mixed-organ EHE cohorts, pulmonary or pleural involvement appears to represent an independent predictor of worse prognosis.

Several clinical and histopathologic variables correlate with adverse outcomes. Metastatic disease remains the strongest predictor, with a reported hazard ratio of 19.8. Other independent markers of poor prognosis include tumor size greater than 3 cm, Ki-67 proliferation index >10%, symptomatic presentation, pleural effusion, lymph node involvement, and primary pulmonary localization [2, 7–9, 15, 16, 51]. The *WWTR1–CAMTA1* fusion mutation may be associated with poorer outcomes compared with *YAP1–TFE3*, although this difference has not reached statistical significance [7].

As previously noted, pleural involvement is consistently associated with unfavorable outcomes [2, 5, 6, 15, 16]. One study reported a median survival of only 1 month in patients with pleural EHE, comparable to that in patients with lymphangitic carcinomatosis [3, 7]. Another series documented a 66% 1-year mortality among three patients with pleural disease, and 5-year survival in pleural EHE has been reported as low as 22% [7, 16].

To better stratify prognosis, one study proposed a two-pattern phenotypic classification [2]. Pattern A: characterized by discrete, well-defined lesions, potentially multinodular, and limited skeletal involvement (≤2 bones or multiple lesions within a single bone). Survival rates for Pattern A were 96% at 1 year, 84% at 5 years, and 78% at 10 years. Pattern B: defined by infiltrative or poorly circumscribed lesions associated with pleural effusion, ascites, hemoptysis, or skeletal involvement of ≥3 bones. Survival rates were 62% at 1 year, 25% at 5 years, and 10% at 10 years. This classification provided superior prognostic discrimination compared with a simpler single versus multi-organ framework, which failed to demonstrate significant survival differences. Patients who transitioned from Pattern A to Pattern B during follow-up exhibited intermediate outcomes (5-year survival 62%) compared with those who remained Pattern A (89%) or initially presented as Pattern B (20%) [2].

There are currently no formal surveillance guidelines specific to pulmonary EHE. In clinical practice, most centers adopt short-interval imaging during early follow-up. Data from a contemporary sarcoma cohort, including patients with multifocal pulmonary involvement, support the use of cross-sectional imaging (CT or MRI) every 3–6 months during the initial surveillance phase, a reasonable approach for P-EHE as well, particularly when the disease is multifocal or higher risk [4]. Observation alone is a common and often appropriate strategy in P-EHE, as many patients experience indolent disease courses. In one series (median follow-up 63 months), the 5-year overall survival reached 96.3%, supporting a surveillance-first approach for stable disease; imaging intervals can be lengthened if radiographic stability is confirmed [33]. Following complete resection of a solitary lesion, some reports describe no recurrence on long-term follow-up, justifying imaging intervals of 6–12 months. Conversely, patients with multifocal ("Pattern B") disease or pleural/thoracic extension should undergo closer 3-month surveillance, given their association with markedly poorer survival outcomes [2, 33].

References

1. Sardaro A, Bardoscia L, Petruzzelli MF, Portaluri M. Epithelioid Hemangioendothelioma: an overview and update on a rare vascular tumor. Oncol Rev. 2014;8(2):259.
2. Lau K, Massad M, Pollak C, Rubin C, Yeh J, Wang J, et al. Clinical patterns and outcome in epithelioid hemangioendothelioma with or without pulmonary

involvement: insights from an internet registry in the study of a rare cancer. Chest. 2011;140(5):1312–8.
3. Woo JH, Kim TJ, Lee KS, Kim TS, Kim BT. Epithelioid hemangioendothelioma in the thorax: Clinicopathologic, CT, PET, and prognostic features. Medicine (Baltimore). 2016;95(30):e4348.
4. Tong D, Constantinidou A, Engelmann B, Chamberlain F, Thway K, Fisher C, et al. The role of local therapy in multi-focal epithelioid Haemangioendothelioma. Anticancer Res. 2019;39(9):4891–6.
5. Epelboym Y, Engelkemier DR, Thomas-Chausse F, Alomari AI, Al-Ibraheemi A, Trenor CC, et al. Imaging findings in epithelioid hemangioendothelioma. Clin Imaging. 2019;58:59–65.
6. Liu Z, He S. Epithelioid Hemangioendothelioma: incidence, mortality, prognostic factors, and survival analysis using the surveillance, epidemiology, and end results database. J Oncol. 2022;2022:2349991.
7. Rosenbaum E, Jadeja B, Xu B, Zhang L, Agaram NP, Travis W, et al. Prognostic stratification of clinical and molecular epithelioid hemangioendothelioma subsets. Mod Pathol. 2020;33(4):591–602.
8. Flucke U, Vogels RJ, de Saint Aubain Somerhausen N, Creytens DH, Riedl RG, van Gorp JM, et al. Epithelioid Hemangioendothelioma: clinicopathologic, immunhistochemical, and molecular genetic analysis of 39 cases. Diagn Pathol. 2014;9:131.
9. Shiba S, Imaoka H, Shioji K, Suzuki E, Horiguchi S, Terashima T, et al. Clinical characteristics of Japanese patients with epithelioid hemangioendothelioma: a multicenter retrospective study. BMC Cancer. 2018;18(1):993.
10. Yousaf N, Maruzzo M, Judson I, Al-Muderis O, Fisher C, Benson C. Systemic treatment options for epithelioid haemangioendothelioma: the Royal Marsden Hospital experience. Anticancer Res. 2015;35(1):473–80.
11. Crotty EJ, McAdams HP, Erasmus JJ, Sporn TA, Roggli VL. Epithelioid Hemangioendothelioma of the pleura. Am J Roentgenol. 2000;175(6):1545–9.
12. Fan Y, Wang F, Li S, Ye C, Ying Y, Mao H. Pleural epithelioid Hemangioendothelioma: a case report and literature review. J Natl Med Assoc. 2016;108(2):124–9.
13. Zheng Z, Wang H, Jiang H, Chen E, Zhang J, Xie X. Apatinib for the treatment of pulmonary epithelioid hemangioendothelioma. Medicine (Baltimore). 2017;96(45):e8507.
14. Wu X, Li B, Zheng C, Hong T, He X. Clinical characteristics of epithelioid hemangioendothelioma: a single-center retrospective study. Eur J Med Res. 2019;24:16.
15. Guo Q, Xue J, Xu L, Shi Z, Zhou B. The clinical features of epithelioid hemangioendothelioma in a Han Chinese population. Medicine (Baltimore). 2017;96(26):e7345.
16. Kitaichi M, Nagai S, Nishimura K, Itoh H, Asamoto H, Izumi T, et al. Pulmonary epithelioid haemangioendothelioma in 21 patients, including three with partial spontaneous regression. Eur Respir J. 1998;12(1):89–96.
17. Amin RMS, Hiroshima K, Kokubo T, Nishikawa M, Narita M, Kuroki M, et al. Risk factors and independent predictors of survival in patients with pulmonary epithelioid haemangioendothelioma. Review of the literature and a case report. Respirology. 2006;11(6):818–25.
18. Wehbe R, Wang X, Newhall KA, Stoner MC, Mix DS, Pitcher GS. Epithelioid hemangioendothelioma involving the superficial femoral artery and femoral vein. J Vasc Surg Cases Innov Tech. 2024;11(1):101645. https://doi.org/10.1016/j.jvscit.2024.101645.
19. Singhal S, Jain S, Singla M, Pippal RB, Gondal R, Agarwal A, et al. Multifocal epitheloid hemangioendothelioma of liver after long-term oral contraceptive use--a case report and discussion of management difficulties encountered. J Gastrointest Cancer. 2009;40(1–2):59–63.
20. Ohori NP, Yousem SA, Sonmez-Alpan E, Colby TV. Estrogen and progesterone receptors in lymphangioleiomyomatosis, epithelioid hemangioendothelioma, and sclerosing hemangioma of the lung. Am J Clin Pathol. 1991;96(4):529–35.
21. Zhao M, Yin F. Hepatic epithelioid hemangioendothelioma: clinical characteristics, diagnosis, treatment, and prognosis. World J Clin Cases. 2022;10(17):5606–19.
22. Gurung S, Fu H, Zhang WW, Gu YH. Hepatic epithelioid hemangioendothelioma metastasized to the peritoneum, omentum and mesentery: a case report. Int J Clin Exp Pathol. 2015;8(5):5883–9.
23. Atyah MM, Sun Y, Yang Z. The challenges of hepatic epithelioid hemangioendothelioma: the diagnosis and current treatments of a problematic tumor. Orphanet J Rare Dis. 2024;19(1):449.
24. Mehrabi A, Kashfi A, Fonouni H, Schemmer P, Schmied BM, Hallscheidt P, et al. Primary malignant hepatic epithelioid hemangioendothelioma. Cancer. 2006;107(9):2108–21.
25. Mo WF, Tong YL. Hepatic epithelioid hemangioendothelioma after thirteen years' follow-up: a case report and review of literature. World J Clin Cases. 2022;10(18):6119–27.
26. Suurmeijer AJH, Dickson BC, Swanson D, Sung YS, Zhang L, Antonescu CR. Variant WWTR1 gene fusions in epithelioid Hemangioendothelioma—a genetic subset associated with cardiac involvement. Genes Chromosomes Cancer. 2020;59(7):389–95.
27. Antonescu CR, Le Loarer F, Mosquera JM, Sboner A, Zhang L, Chen CL, et al. Novel YAP1-TFE3 fusion defines a distinct subset of epithelioid hemangioendothelioma. Genes Chromosomes Cancer. 2013;52(8):775–84.
28. Mascarelli PE, Iredell JR, Maggi RG, Weinberg G, Breitschwerdt EB. Bartonella species bacteremia in two patients with epithelioid Hemangioendothelioma ▿. J Clin Microbiol. 2011;49(11):4006–12.
29. Liu H, Wang J, Lang J, Zhang X. Pulmonary epithelioid Hemangioendothelioma: imaging and clinical features. J Comput Assist Tomogr. 2021;45(5):788.

30. Ye B, Li W, Liu XY, Sun KL, Yang LH, Ma K, et al. Multiple organ metastases of pulmonary epithelioid Haemangioendothelioma and a review of the literature. Med Oncol. 2010;27(1):49–54.
31. Rezvani A, Shahriarirad R, Erfani A, Ranjbar K. Primary malignant epithelioid hemangioendothelioma of the pleura: a review and report of a novel case. Clin Case Rep. 2022;10(8):e6211.
32. Ye B, Li W, Feng J, Shi JX, Chen Y, Han BH. Treatment of pulmonary epithelioid hemangioendothelioma with combination chemotherapy: report of three cases and review of the literature. Oncol Lett. 2013;5(5):1491–6.
33. Onishi Y, Kusumoto M, Goto Y, Kaku S, Motoi N. Epithelioid hemangioendothelioma of the lung: CT findings and clinical course of 35 cases. Jpn J Clin Oncol. 2020;50(10):1195–200.
34. Kim EA, Lele SM, Lackner RP. Primary pleural epithelioid Hemangioendothelioma. Ann Thorac Surg. 2011;91(1):301–2.
35. Jang JK, Thomas R, Braschi-Amirfarzan M, Jagannathan JP. A review of the spectrum of imaging manifestations of epithelioid Hemangioendothelioma. Am J Roentgenol. 2020;215(5):1290–8.
36. Coolen J, De Keyzer F, Nafteux P, De Wever W, Dooms C, Vansteenkiste J, et al. Malignant pleural mesothelioma: visual assessment by using pleural pointillism at diffusion-weighted MR imaging. Radiology. 2015;274(2):576–84.
37. Usuda K, Iwai S, Funasaki A, Sekimura A, Motono N, Matoba M, et al. Diffusion-weighted imaging can differentiate between malignant and benign pleural diseases. Cancer. 2019;11(6):811.
38. Mao X, Liang Z, Chibhabha F, Ou W, Li N, Xu P, et al. Clinico-radiological features and next generation sequencing of pulmonary epithelioid hemangioendothelioma: a case report and review of literature. Thorac Cancer. 2017;8(6):687–92.
39. Sakata KK, Klassen CL, Bollin KB, Grys TE, Slack JL, Wesselius LJ, et al. Microbiologic yield of bronchoalveolar lavage specimens from stem cell transplant recipients. Transpl Infect Dis. 2017;19(3):e12684.
40. Fjaellegaard K, Petersen JK, Stamp IM, Hoegholm A, Clementsen PF, Bodtger U. Pleural epithelioid hemangioendothelioma mimicking pleural empyema: a case report. Respir Med Case Rep. 2020;31:101194.
41. Aung TT, Chu A, Kondapi D, Markabawi D, Mirchia K, Kaul P. A case of pulmonary epithelioid Hemangioendothelioma with literature review. Case Rep Oncol Med. 2020;2020:8048056.
42. Ryu HS, Lee SS, Choi HS, Baek H, Koh JS. A case of pulmonary malignant epithelioid hemangioendothelioma misdiagnosed as adenocarcinoma by fine needle aspiration cytology. Diagn Cytopathol. 2011;39(11):801–7.
43. Sasaki A, Egashira H, Sugimoto H, Seki K, Tsukiyama T, Ichita C, et al. CT-guided biopsy for the diagnosis of pulmonary epithelioid Hemangioendothelioma mimicking metastatic lung cancer. Intern Med. 2018;57(24):3631–5.
44. Pathak V, Walker C. Pleural Epithelioid Hemangioendothelioma (EHE): a case report. Cureus. 15(7):e41308.
45. World Health Organization Classification of Tumours Editorial Board. Thoracic tumours. 5th ed. Lyon: International Agency for Research on Cancer; 2021.
46. Doyle LA, Fletcher CDM, Hornick JL. Nuclear expression of CAMTA1 distinguishes epithelioid Hemangioendothelioma from histologic mimics. Am J Surg Pathol. 2016;40(1):94–102.
47. Shibuya R, Matsuyama A, Shiba E, Harada H, Yabuki K, Hisaoka M. CAMTA1 is a useful immunohistochemical marker for diagnosing epithelioid haemangioendothelioma. Histopathology. 2015;67(6):827–35.
48. Bahrami A, Allen TC, Cagle PT. Pulmonary epithelioid hemangioendothelioma mimicking mesothelioma. Pathol Int. 2008;58(11):730–4.
49. Weiss SW. Enzinger and Weiss's soft tissue tumors. 7th ed. Elsevier; 2019.
50. Husain AN, Colby TV, Ordóñez NG, Krausz T, Borczuk A, Cagle PT, et al. Guidelines for pathologic diagnosis of malignant mesothelioma: a consensus statement from the international mesothelioma interest group. Arch Pathol Lab Med. 2009;133(8):1317–31.
51. Bagan P, Hassan M, Le Pimpec Barthes F, Peyrard S, Souilamas R, Danel C, et al. Prognostic factors and surgical indications of pulmonary epithelioid hemangioendothelioma: a review of the literature. Ann Thorac Surg. 2006;82(6):2010–3.
52. Stacchiotti S, Simeone N, Lo Vullo S, Baldi GG, Brunello A, Vincenzi B, et al. Activity of sirolimus in patients with progressive epithelioid hemangioendothelioma: a case-series analysis within the Italian rare cancer network. Cancer. 2021;127(4):569–76.
53. Bally O, Tassy L, Richioud B, Decouvelaere AV, Blay JY, Derbel O. Eight years tumor control with pazopanib for a metastatic resistant epithelioid hemangioendothelioma. Clin Sarcoma Res. 2015;5:12.
54. Semenisty V, Naroditsky I, Keidar Z, Bar-Sela G. Pazopanib for metastatic pulmonary epithelioid hemangioendothelioma—a suitable treatment option: case report and review of anti-angiogenic treatment options. BMC Cancer. 2015;15(1):402.
55. Kollár A, Jones RL, Stacchiotti S, Gelderblom H, Guida M, Grignani G, et al. Pazopanib in advanced vascular sarcomas: an EORTC soft tissue and bone sarcoma group (STBSG) retrospective analysis. Acta Oncol. 2017;56(1):88–92.
56. Schuetze SM, Ballman KV, Heise R, Ganjoo KN, Davis EJ, George S, et al. A single arm phase 2 trial of Trametinib in patients with locally advanced or metastatic epithelioid Hemangioendothelioma. Clin Cancer Res. 2024;30(20):4584–92.
57. Khreisat A, Bozyk P, Hong G, Schukow CP, et al. Pleural epithelioid hemangioendothelioma: an ultra-rare cause for recurrent pleural effusion managed with trametinib and pazopanib. Cureus. 2024;16(5):e60002. https://doi.org/10.7759/cureus.60002.

58. Agulnik M, Yarber JL, Okuno SH, von Mehren M, Jovanovic BD, Brockstein BE, et al. An open-label, multicenter, phase II study of bevacizumab for the treatment of angiosarcoma and epithelioid hemangioendotheliomas†. Ann Oncol. 2013;24(1):257–63.
59. Chevreau C, Le Cesne A, Ray-Coquard I, Italiano A, Cioffi A, Isambert N, et al. Sorafenib in patients with progressive epithelioid hemangioendothelioma. Cancer. 2013;119(14):2639–44.
60. Guo W, Zhou D, Huang H, Chen H, Wu X, Yang X, et al. Successful chemotherapy with continuous immunotherapy for primary pulmonary endovascular epithelioid hemangioendothelioma: a case report. Medicine (Baltimore). 2023;102(7):e32914.
61. Bu Y, Peng L, Liu M, He L, Wang F, Li B, et al. Epithelioid hemangioendothelioma of the retroperitoneal giant type treated with Toripalimab: a case report. Front Immunol. 2023;14:1116944.
62. Salijevska J, Watson R, Clifford A, Ritchie AI, Mauri F, Adeboyeku D. Pleural epithelioid Hemangioendothelioma: literature summary and novel case report. J Clin Med Res. 2015;7(7):566–70.

Solitary Fibrous Tumor of the Pleura

18

Luis Devia, Firas Ido, and Meredith Harrison

Introduction

Solitary fibrous tumors (SFTs) are rare neoplasms first described in 1870 by Leberecht Wagner in his publication titled "Das Tuberkelahnliche lympadenoma." In the 1930s, Klemperer and Rabin published a report providing the first histopathologic description [1]. Initially, these tumors were categorized as localized mesotheliomas and have been referred to by various names, including fibromas, fibrous mesotheliomas, pleural fibromas, subserosal fibromas, and benign fibrous tumors of the pleura; however, they are now referred to as solitary fibrous tumors of the pleura (SFTP) [1, 2]. Solitary fibrous tumors most commonly arise from the pleura. Other locations of origin include intra-abdominally, the tongue, thyroid, retroperitoneum, inguinal regions, mesentery, and upper and lower limbs [3, 4]. The malignant cells stem from submesothelial mesenchymal cells, specifically, CD34+ dendritic stromal cells that are fibroblast-like [2, 8, 10]. Solitary fibrous tumors of the pleura are rare, with an incidence of 2.8 per 100,000 [5]. The incidence for men and women is similar, although marginally higher in females, with a ratio of 1:1.2–1.35 [6]. SFTP typically occurs between the ages of 30 and 80, with a mean age of presentation between 40 and 65 years of age [4–6]. Race and ethnicity exhibit minor variations in incidence rates among Asian, White, Black, and Native American populations, with respective incidences of 4.5, 3.78, 2.75, and 2.65 per 10 million person-years [7]. Environmental exposures, including tobacco use, have not been linked to SFTP [8]. Approximately 80% of these tumors arise from the visceral pleura and 20% from the parietal pleura [9]. Up to 10–20% of SFTPs have malignant features [10]. In addition, there is a several-fold increased likelihood of malignant SFTP for those originating from the parietal pleura compared to the visceral pleura [6]. Malignant SFTP can develop from the transformation of benign tumors or de novo [6, 10]. Metastasis is typically hematogenous and occurs most frequently in the liver, central nervous system, spleen, peritoneum, adrenal glands, gastrointestinal tract, kidneys, and bone [2]. Other locations of metastasis include the contralateral hemithorax, pancreas, thyroid, and bladder [10, 42].

L. Devia
Department of General Surgery, St. Luke's University Health Network, Bethlehem, PA, USA
e-mail: luis.devia@sluhn.org

F. Ido
Department of Pulmonary and Critical Care Medicine, St. Luke's University Health Network, Bethlehem, PA, USA
e-mail: firas.ido@sluhn.org

M. Harrison (✉)
Department of Thoracic Surgery, St. Luke's University Health Network, Bethlehem, PA, USA
e-mail: Meredith.Harrison@sluhn.org

F. Ido (ed.), *Rare Pleural Diseases*, https://doi.org/10.1007/978-3-032-14873-5_18

Pathophysiology

The sequence of events leading to the development of SFTP is unclear; however, somatic genetic mutations and specific intracellular pathways have been identified and postulated to play a role in pathogenesis. The development of the tumor is associated with a chromosomal inversion at 12q13, resulting in a fusion gene between the NAB2 and STAT6 genes [11]. The fusion protein leads to activation of early growth response protein 1 (EGR-1) and subsequently alters several inhibitory pathways of the cell cycle. This leads to cellular proliferation, ultimately resulting in tumor formation [12, 13]. These tumors can also express Bcl-2, a proto-oncogene that inhibits apoptosis and facilitates the progression of these tumors [2]. Telomerase reverse transcriptase (TERT) promoter mutations have also been observed, and these mutations are associated with larger tumors and high-risk features [14, 15]. Several additional genes, including ALDH1, EGFR, FGFR1, ERBB2, and JAK2 receptors, appear overexpressed; however, their direct link to pathogenesis is unclear [13]. The development of malignant SFTP may be influenced additionally by p53 mutation, which correlates with increased mortality and recurrence [16].

Clinical Features

Benign SFTP lesions are often incidentally captured on radiographic imaging in asymptomatic patients, due to their slow, indolent growth. Presenting symptoms are usually absent but can include cough, dyspnea, chest pain, obstructive pneumonia, or hemoptysis [17]. The development of these symptoms is associated with larger tumor size, typically greater than 10 cm [17, 18]. Additionally, these symptoms are more commonly associated with malignant SFTP [19]. The presence of an ipsilateral pleural effusion is more likely in malignant SFTP than in benign lesions, with reported prevalences of 32% and 8%, respectively [19, 20]. Malignant SFTP can progress rapidly and, therefore, present with symptoms early on. Although not commonly observed, in less than 10% of total cases, paraneoplastic syndromes associated with solitary fibrous tumors can manifest with a unique clinical presentation. Pierre–Marie–Bamberg syndrome, also known as hypertrophic osteoarthropathy (HOA), can occur in 10–20% cases, resulting in finger-clubbing. This phenomenon has been associated with abnormal production of hepatocyte growth factor, hyaluronic acid, vascular endothelial growth factor, and platelet-derived growth factor from benign and malignant SFTPs. HOA typically resolves within several months following complete resection of the tumor [10, 21, 22]. Doege–Potter syndrome occurs in <5% of cases in both benign and malignant SFTPs and is characterized by overproduction of insulin-like growth factor II and low levels of insulin, growth hormone, and c-peptide, leading to refractory hypoglycemic episodes [21, 22]. Surgical resection results in the resolution of the hypoglycemic events within days [23].

Diagnosis

Radiologic imaging can provide important details regarding the tumor and suggest the presence of an SFTP. The findings vary depending on size, location, and whether the tumor is benign or malignant. Chest radiograph, although not diagnostic, can demonstrate a round, well-circumscribed opacity usually located peripherally. In cases of very large tumors, the entire hemithorax may appear opacified (Fig. 18.1a). An "incomplete border" sign may be present, indicating the visibility of one free margin of the tumor, whereas the remaining portion is obscured due to merging with the pleura [24]. On computed tomography (CT) of the chest, the tumor is typically located adjacent to the chest wall and less commonly within a lung fissure. SFTPs are well circumscribed and can be lobulated on CT. Small tumors appear homogenous, with the borders forming an obtuse angle with the pleura. Large tumors are most often heterogeneous, reflecting areas of necrosis and hemorrhage (Fig. 18.1b, c). These larger lesions more commonly form an acute angle with the pleura

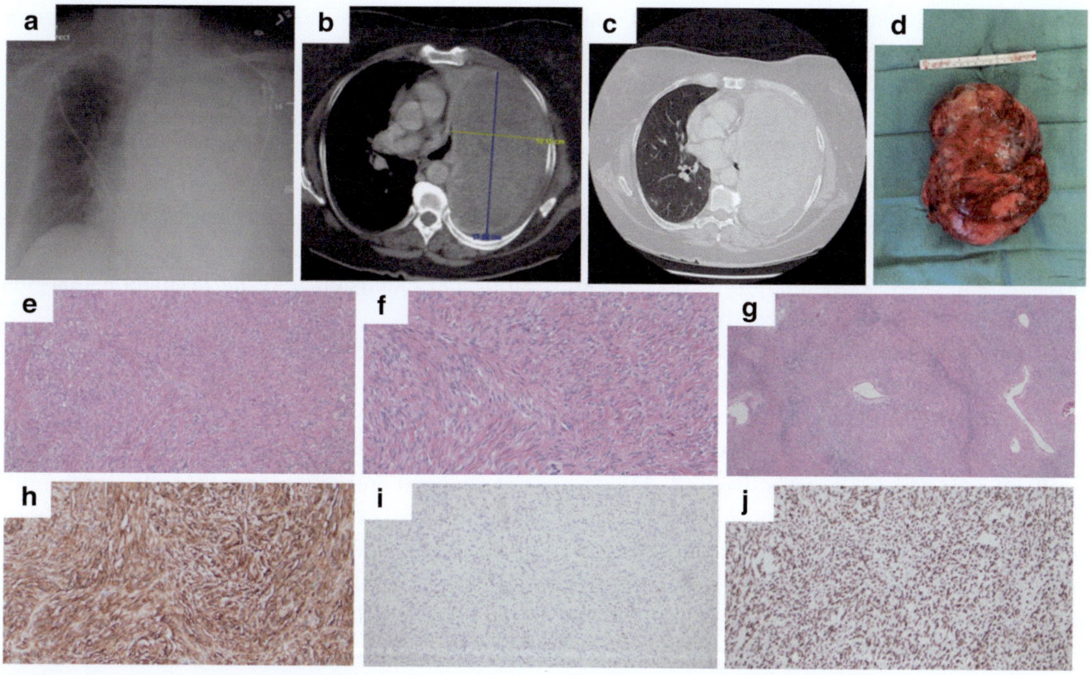

Fig. 18.1 Radiologic and histopathologic features of a solitary fibrous tumor of the pleura

(**a**) Chest radiograph demonstrating complete opacification of the left hemithorax

(**b**) Axial computed tomography (CT) of the chest (soft-tissue window) showing a large, well-circumscribed, heterogeneous soft-tissue mass occupying the entire left hemithorax with mediastinal shift toward the contralateral side

(**c**) Axial CT (lung window) showing occlusion of the left mainstem bronchus by the pleural mass

(**d**) Intraoperative gross specimen following resection, revealing a round, firm, lobulated mass measuring approximately 15 × 12 cm

(**e**) Hematoxylin and eosin (H&E) stain (×10) demonstrating ovoid to fusiform spindle cells with indistinct cell borders

(**f**) H&E stain (×20) showing haphazardly arranged ovoid to spindle cells within a hyalinized to collagenous stroma

(**g**) H&E stain (×20) highlighting dilated, branching, staghorn-like (hemangiopericytoma-like) vasculature characteristic of SFTP

(**h**) Immunohistochemistry for CD34 showing strong, diffuse cytoplasmic positivity (×20)

(**i**) Immunohistochemistry for Ki-67 demonstrating weak nuclear staining, consistent with a low proliferative index

(**j**) Immunohistochemistry for STAT6 showing strong, diffuse nuclear positivity (×20)

Attribution: Panels **a–c** courtesy of *Dr. Luis Devia*; panel **d** courtesy of *Dr. Meredith Harrison*; and panels **e–j** courtesy of *Dr. Kimberly Jaramillo*. All images are original and unpublished, reproduced here with permission of the respective authors

surface. Regardless of size, all tumors usually demonstrate soft-tissue attenuation. Peritumoral atelectasis may also be visible. A pedicle, representing a fibrous stalk, may be visible radiographically in 40% of cases [8]. SFTP usually lacks evidence of pleural seeding. Invasion of the chest wall can be present with malignant tumors, particularly neoplasms arising from the parietal pleura [25]. Other CT findings that suggest a malignant SFTP include intratumoral calcifications, hypervascularity, contrast enhancement, and an intratumoral feeding vessel [26]. Ipsilateral pleural effusions, pleural thickening, and adjacent costal destruction are findings also typically observed in malignant lesions [27]. The tumors may appear to change position on serial CTs, due to an attached stalk [28]. CT angiography can aid in visualizing the feeding artery for preoperative assessment [29]. Magnetic resonance imaging (MRI) is superior to CT for evaluating tumor-specific characteristics, extension, and invasion, as well as the relationship to surrounding structures [24]. While an MRI is not required, it may be advantageous in assessing the extent of invasion and involvement of adjacent structures preoperatively [8]. An MRI may demonstrate a hypodense solid mass with low signal intensity on T1- and T2-weighted images. Necrosis, hemorrhage, and cystic degeneration, if present, are observed as high T2 signal intensity [30]. Positron emission tomography (PET)/CT scans are often used to evaluate pulmonary neoplasms; however, both benign and malignant SFTPs have demonstrated only moderate PET avidity, with average SUVs of 3.02 and 4.89, respectively [8, 24].

Obtaining tissue samples prior to resection is not routinely performed due to its low accuracy; however, it can be considered when surgery is high risk or contraindicated. The accuracy of CT-guided fine-needle aspiration is reported to be less than 50% [8]. Core needle biopsy may provide adequate tissue; however, the success rate is highly variable, ranging from 27% to 100% [32]. Surgical biopsy is the preferred modality for obtaining tissue diagnosis, which is performed at the time of complete resection [19].

Morphologically, SFTP can appear pedunculated or sessile. Pedunculated neoplasms more often stem from the visceral pleura and are attached by a fibrovascular stalk. Rarely, sessile tumors can be inverted, with growth directed into the lung parenchyma [10]. On gross pathology, SFTPs appear as well-circumscribed, multilobulated, and encapsulated in a thin, translucent fibrous membrane (Fig. 18.1d) [31]. A pedunculated lesion may be observed with a thick fibrovascular stalk that attaches to the lung, particularly in visceral pleural tumors [32]. Upon dissection, the internal surface of the tumor reveals a white or tan, smooth, and firm texture. Areas of cystic changes and hemorrhage may be apparent. Malignant tumors often exhibit irregular borders, invasion, and areas of necrosis [31].

The most common microscopic findings with hematoxylin and eosin (H&E) staining include areas of hypo- and hypercellularity, characterized by spindle-shaped fibroblasts with minimal cytoplasm, arranged haphazardly, and surrounded by intercellular eosinophilic collagen matrix arranged in a storiform pattern (Fig. 18.1e, f). Large thin-walled blood vessels resembling a staghorn configuration are present within the stroma (Fig. 18.1g) [31, 33]. Features suggestive of malignancy include increased mitotic activity, cellular pleomorphism, nuclear atypia, presence of necrosis, evidence of stromal or vascular invasion, and extension into the peripheral margins [2, 31].

Immunohistochemical analysis is required to accurately differentiate SFTP from other soft-tissue tumors. Nearly all SFTPs are positive for CD34 and Bcl-2, which are highly sensitive markers and present in more than 90% of tumors (Fig. 18.1h) [15]. Rarely, expression of both markers can be weak or absent in malignant SFTP, specifically in high-grade or dedifferentiated tumors [10, 15]. CD34, a transmembrane glycoprotein, reflects mesenchymal cell origin and is negative in mesothelioma and many other spindle-cell neoplasms [34, 35]. In contrast to mesothelioma, SFTP is positive for vimentin and CD99, and negative for keratin, markers that help distinguish between the two pleural neoplasms [10]. SFTP is negative for S100 and SMA and is rarely positive for desmin [33]. Overexpression of Ki67, a marker of cellular proliferation, and p53 are both helpful in differentiating benign from malignant SFTP (Fig. 18.1i) [15, 36, 37]. Detection of the STAT6 molecular marker, which indicates the characteristic NAB2-STAT6 fusion gene, is highly sensitive and specific for SFTP, with reported accuracy of 95–100% (Fig. 18.1i) [33]. The NAB2-STAT6 fusion gene can be detected by gene sequencing if necessary and available [38].

Treatment

The mainstay treatment for SFTP is curative surgical resection, en bloc resection, with intraoperative negative margins. Pedunculated tumors can often be entirely resected due to the fibrovascular stalk attachment. Sessile tumors, particularly those of the parietal pleura, can be tightly adherent to adjacent structures and the chest wall, which may necessitate lobectomy, pneumonectomy, or resection of extrapleural components [10]. In <5%, the tumor may invert and grow into the lung parenchyma and therefore may require a lobectomy [10]. Preoperative CT angiography has been used to delineate the vascular supply to minimize intraoperative hemorrhage. The aberrant vascular supply has been documented to arise from the internal mammary, bronchial, inferior phrenic, or celiac trunk [8, 39]. Preoperative percutaneous arterial embolization of the feeding vessel has been documented to mitigate intraoperative hemorrhage; however, this option may be most beneficial for larger or locally aggressive tumors [8, 40]. Several surgical approaches have been utilized and include an open antero- and posterolateral thoracotomy, sternotomy, video-assisted thoracoscopic surgery (VATS), robotic-assisted thoracoscopic surgery, and mini thoracotomy [8, 39]. Caution should be taken to avoid tumor contact with the port sites during VATS to prevent contact metastasis [10, 41]. The operative approach is based on the size, location, and extent of tumor invasion into adjacent structures. SFTP <5 cm can be safely excised with VATS, although neoplasms up to 12 cm have been reportedly successfully removed with a robotic approach. For larger tumors, an open thoracotomy is necessary [8]. Regardless of the approach, the primary goal remains total resection with wide, negative margins and preservation of surrounding structures, if feasible [8]. Peritumoral adhesions and surrounding inflammatory tissue can be present in up to 60% of cases and should be resected and included in the pathological analysis to achieve negative margins [8, 18]. Since SFTP does not typically metastasize through lymphatics, lymph node dissection is usually not required, especially if a preoperative diagnosis has been achieved [8, 10, 42]. For recurrent tumors, re-resection should be performed if possible [8, 42]. Due to the variability in tumor morphology, size, and involvement of surrounding structures, intraoperative mortality varies and is reportedly 1.5–12% [8]. The 30-day postoperative mortality ranges from 0 to 3.6% [32, 40]. Perioperative morbidity rates varied between 0 and 16.7% [32]. Other postoperative complications include hemorrhage, surgical site infection, diaphragmatic paralysis, atrial fibrillation, pleural effusion, and ileus [18].

Neoadjuvant chemotherapy (anthracycline-based regimen) and radiotherapy are of limited use due to a lack of efficacy but have been employed for inoperable cases, malignant solitary fibrous tumors, and in cases of incomplete resection [8, 10]. Targeted therapy with sunitinib, temozolomide with bevacizumab, pazopanib, axitinib, and sorafenib have all been used with variable efficacy [10].

Prognosis

The overall prognosis for SFTP is favorable, particularly for benign tumors with negative microscopic histologic margins, with a reported median survival time of 14–24 years [10, 39, 42]. Hence, long-term survival is dependent on the ability to achieve complete resection. The overall SFTP 5-year and disease-free survival following resection were 83–92% and 71–87%, respectively [32]. The estimated 5-year survival rate for benign SFTP is approximately 88–100%, in contrast to malignant SFTP, which is reported to be 58–66% [10, 42]. Long-term survival, including 10- and 30-year survival rates, was estimated at 77% and 21%, respectively [43–45].

Recurrence is typically due to incomplete resection [8]. Localized recurrence usually occurs at the site of the prior resection; however, metastasis at the time of recurrence can also occur [2, 42]. Several models for predicting the risk of recurrence have been established, including Tapias, De Perrot, Demicco, and Modified Demicco scoring systems. The De Perrot scoring system uses a combination of tumor morphology and histologic features, with the remaining methods also incorporating size and age to predict recurrence [32]. Pedunculated SFTP without features of malignancy had the lowest risk of recurrence of 2%, whereas sessile SFTP with malignant features had the highest risk of recurrence, estimated at 63% [2]. Pooled data from multiple studies following complete resection showed an overall recurrent rate of 9%. Subgroup analysis of the recurrence rate for benign versus malignant SFTP showed rates of 3% and 22%, respectively [43]. Smaller studies have reported recurrence rates of up to 75% and 25% for malignant and benign SFTP, respectively. However, these studies are limited by small sample sizes. Nearly half of all recurrences occur within 5 years post-resection, with an average of 29 months to the first recurrence [46, 47]. Additionally, the reported 10-year recurrence rate is estimated to be 10–25% [10, 42]. Yet, recurrence has been documented to occur up to 20 postoperative resections along with multiple recurrences despite serial resections; therefore, long-term surveillance is necessary [8, 32]. Following complete resection, a chest CT is recommended for surveillance every 6 months for the initial 2 years, followed by annual surveillance thereafter [2, 10, 46].

Acknowledgment The authors thank *Dr. Kimberly Jaramillo*, Pathologist, St. Luke's University Health Network, for her contributions to the pathology images and corresponding figure descriptions.

References

1. Stout AP, Himadi GM. Solitary localizated mesothelioma of the pleura. Ann Surg. 1952;133(1):50–64.
2. de Perrot Mea. Solitary fibrous tumors of the pleura. Ann Thorac Surg. 2002;74(1):285–93.
3. Vallat-Decouvelaere AV, Dry SM, Fletcher CD. Atypical and malignant solitary fibrous tumors in extrathoracic locations: evidence of their comparability to intra-thoracic tumors. Am J Surg Pathol. 1998;22(12):1501–11.
4. Lee MK, Shin SD, Cho MS, Kim YM, Kim J. Extrapleural solitary fibrous tumor a clinical & pathological study of 8 cases. Korean J Pathol. 1999:108–14.
5. Khouzam MS, Khouzam N. Malignant solitary fibrous tumor of the pleura. J Cardiothorac Surg. 2022;17(1):92.
6. Chu XZL, Xue Z, Ren Z, Sun YE, Wang M, Liu M. Solitary fibrous tumor of the pleura: an analysis of forty patients. J Thorac Dis. 2012;4(2):146–54.
7. Kinslow CJ, Bruce SS, Rae AI, Sheth SA, McKhann GM, Sisti MB, Bruce JN, Sonabend AM, Wang TJC. Solitary-fibrous tumor/hemangiopericytoma of the central nervous system: a population-based study. J Neuro-Oncol. 2018;38(1):173–82.
8. Ajouz H, Sohail AH, Hashmi H, Martinez Aguilar M, Daoui S, Tembelis M, Aziz M, Zohourian T, Brathwaite CEM, Cerfolio RJ. Surgical considerations in the resection of solitary fibrous tumors of the pleura. J Cardiothorac Surg. 2023;18(1):79.
9. Briselli M, Dickersin GR. Solitary fibrous tumors of the pleura: eight new cases and review of 360 cases in the literature. Cancer. 1981;47(11):2678–89.
10. Gao X, Zhang J, Qian Z, Liu L, Wang G, Song Y, Li S. Malignant solitary fibrous tumor of the pleura: a narrative review of clinical characteristics, diagnosis and therapeutic options. Respir Med Res. 2024;86
11. Robinson DR, Wu YM, Kalyana-Sundaram S, Cao X, Lonigro RJ, Sung YS, Chen CL, Zhang L, Wang R, Su F, Iyer MK, Roychowdhury S, Siddiqui J, Pienta KJ, Kunju LP, Talpaz M, Mosquera JM, Singer S, Schuetze SM, Antonescu CR. Identification of recurrent NAB2-STAT6 gene fusions in solitary fibrous tumor by integrative sequencing. Nat Genet. 2013;45(2):180–5.
12. Demicco EGWK, Ingram D, Wagner M, Maki RG, Rizzo A, et al. TERT promoter mutations in solitary fibrous tumour. Histopathology. 2018;73(5):843–51.
13. Thway K, Ng W, Noujaim J, Jones RL, Fisher C. The current status of solitary fibrous tumor: diagnostic features, variants, and genetics. Int J Surg Pathol. 2016;24(4):281–92.
14. Bahrami ALS, Schaefer IM, Boland JM, Patton KT, Pounds S, Fletcher CD. TERT promoter mutations and prognosis in solitary fibrous tumor. Mod Pathol. 2016;29(12):1511–22.
15. Demicco EGPM, Araujo DM, Fox PS, Bassett RL, Pollock RE, Lazar AJ, Wang WL. Solitary fibrous tumor: a clinicopathological study of 110 cases and proposed risk assessment model. Mod Pathol. 2012;25:1298–306.
16. Yokoi, Tsuzuki, Yatabe, Suzuki, Kurumaya, Koshikawa, et al. Solitary fibrous tumour: significance of p53 and CD34 immunoreactivity in its malignant transformation. Histopathology. 1998;32(5):423–32.
17. Zuo Z, Zhou H, Sun Y, Mao Q, Zhang Y, Gao X. Rapidly growing solitary fibrous tumors of the pleura: a case report and review of the literature. Ann Transl Med. 2020;8(14):890.
18. Savu CMA, Pose R, Galie N, Balescu I, Diaconu C, Cretoiu D, Dima S, Filipescu A, Balalau C, Bacalbasa N. Pleural solitary fibrous tumors-a retrospective study on 45 patients. Medicina (Kaunas). 2020;56(4)
19. Lococo F, Cesario A, Cardillo G, Filosso P, Galetta D, Carbone L, Oliaro A, Spaggiari L, Cusumano G, Margaritora S, Graziano P, Granone P. Malignant solitary fibrous tumors of the pleura: retrospective review of a multicenter series. J Thorac Oncol. 2012;7(11):1698–706.
20. England DM, Hochholzer L, McCarthy MJ. Localized benign and malignant fibrous tumors of the pleura. A clinicopathologic review of 223 cases. Am J Surg Pathol. 1989;18(8):640–58.

21. Koliakos E, Chappalley D, Kalogiannis E, Sgardello S, Christodoulou M. Pierre-Marie Bamberger syndrome leading to the diagnosis and surgical treatment of a localized lung cancer. Cureus. 2023;15(11)
22. Han G, Zhang Z, Shen X, Wang K, Zhao Y, He J, Gao Y, Shan X, Xin G, Li C, Liu X. Doege-potter syndrome: a review of the literature including a new case report. Medicine (Baltimore). 2017;96(27)
23. Meng W, Zhu HH, Li H, Wang G, Wei D, Feng X. Solitary fibrous tumors of the pleura with Doege-potter syndrome: a case report and three-decade review of the literature. BMC Res Notes. 2014;7(515)
24. Chick JFCN, Madan R. Solitary fibrous tumors of the thorax: nomenclature, epidemiology, radiologic and pathologic findings, differential diagnoses, and management. AJR Am J Roentgenol. 2013;200(3):W238–48.
25. Luciano CFA, Giovanni V, Federica S, Cesare F. CT signs, patterns and differential diagnosis of solitary fibrous tumors of the pleura. J Thorac Dis. 2010;2(1):21–5.
26. Hélage SRM, Chabi ML, Audureau É, Ferretti G, Laurent F, Alifano M, Mansuet-Lupo A, Buy JN, Vadrot D. Solitary fibrous tumor of the pleura: can computed tomography features help predict malignancy? A series of 56 patients with histopathological correlates. Diagn Interv Imaging. 2016;97(3):347–53.
27. You X, Sun X, Yang C, Fang Y. CT diagnosis and differentiation of benign and malignant varieties of solitary fibrous tumor of the pleura. Medicine (Baltimore). 2017;96(49):e9058.
28. Akman CCS, Ulus S, Kaynak K, Oz B. Pedunculated localized fibrous tumor of the pleura presenting as a moving chest mass. South Med J. 2005;98(4):486–8.
29. Usami NIS, Yokoi K. Solitary fibrous tumor of the pleura: evaluation of the origin with 3D CT angiography. J Thorac Oncol. 2007;2(12):1124–5.
30. Sureka B, Thukral BB, Mittal MK, Mittal A, Sinha M. Radiological review of pleural tumors. Indian J Radiol Imaging. 2013;23(4):313–20.
31. Tariq MU, Din NU, Abdul-Ghafar J, Park YK. The many faces of solitary fibrous tumor; diversity of histological features, differential diagnosis and role of molecular studies and surrogate markers in avoiding misdiagnosis and predicting the behavior. Diagn Pathol. 2021;16(21)
32. Cieślik-Wolski BPŁ, Szlachcińska A, Walczak-Pasz G, Jesionek-Kupnicka D, Kozak J. Solitary fibrous tumor of the pleura—analysis of 18 cases. Kardiochir Torakochirurgia Pol. 2015;12(3):208–15.
33. Geramizadeh BMM, Churg A. Role of immunohistochemistry in the diagnosis of solitary fibrous tumor, a review. Iran J Pathol. 2016;11(3):195–203.
34. van LC, Rouse RV. Expression of CD34 by solitary fibrous tumors of the pleura, mediastinum, and lung. Am J Surg Pathol. 1994;18(8):814–20.
35. Sudheer Shenoy PBBI. Identification, isolation, quantification and systems approach towards CD34, a biomarker present in the progenitor/stem cells from diverse lineages. Methods. 2017;131:47–56.
36. Sun Y, Naito Z, Ishiwata T, Maeda S, Sugisaki Y, Asano G. Basic FGF and Ki-67 proteins useful for immunohistological diagnostic evaluations in malignant solitary fibrous tumor. Pathol Int. 2003;53(5):284–90.
37. Nakamori M, Oda Y, Kurihara S, Tsuneyoshi M. Clinicopathological and immunohistochemical study of extrapleural and pleural solitary fibrous tumors: a special emphasis on the comparison between ordinary tumors and their malignant variant. Mol Med Rep. 2008;1(6):797–803.
38. Chmielecki JCA, Rosenberg M, O'Connor R, Walker SR, Ambrogio L, Auclair D, McKenna A, Heinrich MC, Frank DA, Meyerson M. Whole-exome equencing identifies a recurrent NAB2-STAT6 fusion in solitary fibrous tumors. Nat Genet. 2013;45(2):131–2.
39. Guo J, Chu X, Sun YE, Zhang L, Zhou N. Giant solitary fibrous tumor of the pleura: an analysis of five patients. World J Surg. 2010;34:2553–7.
40. Weiss B, Horton DA. Preoperative embolization of a massive solitary fibrous tumor of the pleura. Ann Thorac Surg. 2002;73(3):983–5.
41. Nomori H. Contacting metastasis of a fibrous tumor of the pleura. Eur J Cardio Thorac Surg. 1997;12(6):928–30.
42. Harrison–Phipps KM, Nichols FC, Schleck CD, Deschamps C, Cassivi SD, Schipper PH, Allen MS, Wigle DA, Pairolero PC. Solitary fibrous tumors of the pleura: results of surgical treatment and long-term prognosis. J Thorac Cardiovasc Surg. 2009;138(1):19–25.
43. Zhou C, Li W, Shao J, Zhao J. Thoracic solitary fibrous tumors: an analysis of 70 patients who underwent surgical resection in a single institution. J Cancer Res Clin Oncol. 2020;146:1245–52.
44. Gold JS, Antonescu CR, Hajdu C, Ferrone CR, Hussain M, Lewis JJ, Coit DG. Clinicopathologic correlates of solitary fibrous tumors. Cancer. 2002;94(4):1057–68.
45. Cardillo G, Carbone L, Carleo F, Masala N, Graziano P, Bray A, et al. Solitary fibrous tumors of the pleura: an analysis of 110 patients treated in a single institution. Ann Thorac Surg. 2009;88(5):1632–7.
46. Mercer RM, Wigston C, Banka R, Cardillo G, Benamore R, Nicholson AG, Asciak R, Hassan M, Hallifax RJ, Wing L, Bedawi EO, Maskell NA, Harriss EK, Miller RF, Rahman NM. Management of solitary fibrous tumours of the pleura: a systematic review and meta-analysis. ERJ Open Res. 2020;6(3)
47. Lahon B, Mercier O, Fadel E, Ghigna MR, Petkova B, Mussot S, et al. Solitary fibrous tumor of the pleura: outcomes of 157 complete resections in a single center. Ann Thorac Surg. 2012;94(2):394–400.

19 Pleural Lipoma

Michael DiRico, Firas Ido, and Hiren J. Mehta

Introduction

Lipomas are benign soft-tissue tumors characterized by the presence of mature adipose tissue enclosed within a fibrous capsule. Despite the ubiquitous presence of adipose tissue throughout the body, intrathoracic lipomas are uncommon. These tumors can be classified according to their anatomical location within the thoracic cavity, which includes endobronchial, intraparenchymal, pleural, mediastinal, and cardiac [1]. Pleural lipomas are exceedingly rare and constitute less than 0.1% of all primary thoracic neoplasms [2]. Intrathoracic lipomas are often captured incidentally on imaging studies. They typically exhibit slow growth and become symptomatic primarily when compressing adjacent structures [3–6]. Although pleural lipomas rarely pose harm, their resemblance to more aggressive conditions, such as liposarcoma or metastatic disease, can lead to diagnostic challenges [3, 7, 8].

In the late 1700s, Dr. John Fothergill documented his autopsy findings on a patient who had died after reportedly experiencing angina pectoris. He observed an excessive amount of lipomatous tissue within the mediastinum, as well as surrounding the pericardium and pleura. This documented case may represent the first recorded instance of a pleural lipoma in medical literature [9]. In 1933, Dr. George Heuer published a review of over 20 cases of thoracic lipomas, since the first documented case by Dr. Fothergill, including his own case of a symptomatic 25 cm, 12.5 lbs. lipoma arising from the anterior mediastinum. He categorized thoracic lipomas into three types: dumbbell or hourglass lipomas with an intrathoracic and extrathoracic component connected by an isthmus transversing the ribs; lipomas arising from the mediastinum, often extending from the root of the neck; and purely intrathoracic lipomas with either subpleural or mediastinal origin [6].

The epidemiologic data on pleural lipomas are scarce and based on a small number of case reports. In a report of 1800 excised intrathoracic tumors, only five were consistent with the diagnosis of pleural lipoma [10]. Based on another report of over 4000 CT scans obtained, only six lesions met the criteria to be classified as pleural lipomas [11]. Existing evidence indicates that these tumors are most commonly diagnosed in individuals during the fifth to seventh decades of

M. DiRico (✉)
Department of Pulmonology, TriHealth Physician Partners, Cincinnati, OH, USA
e-mail: Michael_DiRico@TriHealth.com

F. Ido
Department of Pulmonary and Critical Care Medicine, St. Luke's University Health Network, Bethlehem, PA, USA
e-mail: firas.ido@sluhn.org

H. J. Mehta
Division of Pulmonary, Critical Care & Sleep Medicine, University of Florida, Gainesville, FL, USA
e-mail: hiren.mehta@medicine.ufl.edu

F. Ido (ed.), *Rare Pleural Diseases*, https://doi.org/10.1007/978-3-032-14873-5_19

life; however, there have been reported cases across all age groups, including within the first decade of life [6, 10–12]. The female-to-male ratio is generally equal, without a preference for any race or ethnicity. No direct link has been established between obesity and pleural lipomas, as cases have been documented in patients with both elevated and normal body mass indices [10, 11]. Tumor size at the time of presentation can vary significantly, ranging from 1 to 6 cm to gigantic lipomas that have been reported to fill the entire hemithorax [12–14]. Approximately half of these tumors arise from the parietal pleura along the costal surfaces, though neoplasms stemming from the diaphragmatic and mediastinal pleura have also been described [10]. Rarely, the tumor can grow from the visceral pleura [15].

Although lipomas are typically asymptomatic and slow-growing, their potential size and ability to mimic malignancy can cause patients to experience significant psychological stress and lead to costly diagnostic and potentially invasive evaluation [3–5].

Pathophysiology

The exact trigger and mechanism resulting in the formation of pleural lipomas is unclear. Pleural lipomas originate from well-differentiated adipocytes located in the submesothelial layer, most often from the parietal pleura [10, 12]. The focal adipocyte proliferation leads to the formation of a homogenous round tumor enclosed within a fibrous capsule [12, 14]. Chronic inflammation, genetic predisposition, obesity, or localized trauma have been postulated as contributing factors but are not strongly supported by evidence [4, 6, 10, 11, 14, 16].

Cytogenetic abnormalities are well documented in soft-tissue lipomas in general, including the translocation of 12q13-15, 13q deletions, and the 6p21-23 rearrangement; however, they have not been investigated in pleural lipomas specifically [17, 18]. It may be reasonable to assume that similar mutations contribute to the development of pleural lipomas, despite the lack of conclusive evidence.

Clinical Features

Due to the indolent growth of pleural lipomas, most are asymptomatic and detected incidentally on radiological examination [6, 18, 19]. Symptoms are estimated to be present in only 20% of cases and, when present, are due to a mass effect that the tumor imparts on surrounding anatomic structures [10, 14]. The presenting symptoms include chest pain, dyspnea, cough, or dysphagia. The tumor may compress nerves coursing from the spine or brachial plexus, resulting in back or limb pain or weakness in relation to the related nerve distribution [1, 6, 10, 13, 14, 18, 20]. Very rare systemic symptoms, such as fever, have been reported [10]. Additional compressive features, such as arrhythmias, vascular collapse, or rib lysis, have been documented in case reports [21, 22]. Pleural lipomas with an extrathoracic component may be palpable on examination [18, 20, 21].

Diagnosis

These tumors are often incidental findings but may also present with nonspecific symptoms. Clinical context guides diagnostic testing and the need for tissue sampling. Regardless of presentation, the goal of evaluation is to confirm the benign nature of the lesion and exclude malignancy, particularly liposarcoma [8, 23].

Spirometry measurements are often normal. When sufficiently large, pleural lipomas may cause compression of the small or large airways, resulting in a proportional decrease in FEV1 and FVC [23]. Although the effects of pleural lipomas on lung volumes and diffusion capacity are not well reported, such compression reduces lung volumes in proportion, while minimally affecting diffusion when adjusting for the volume loss [24].

Thoracic ultrasound can be used to visualize pleural lipomas when they are found peripherally or protrude from the chest. However, they may be mistaken for pleural effusions or other solid masses with this modality [1, 21]. On ultrasound, pleural lipomas appear as homogenous, hypoechoic areas that do not typically demonstrate any significant vascularity or calcifications [12].

Although chest radiography lacks sensitivity and specificity for pleural lipomas, it is frequently the initial modality by which these lesions are identified, either incidentally or when pursuing nonspecific symptoms [3, 4, 13, 15]. When apparent, pleural lipomas manifest as dense, well-circumscribed, round opacities located in the periphery and contiguous with the pleura, typically forming an obtuse pleural angle (Fig. 19.1a) [4]. They may simulate pleural effusions or malignant foci and, less commonly, occur in alternative locations such as the hilum or within the lung parenchyma [6, 7, 9, 25].

Computed tomography (CT) is the standard imaging modality for diagnosing pleural lipomas [7]. These lesions are typically homogeneous, well-circumscribed, and encapsulated, demonstrating characteristic fat attenuation values ranging from −50 to −150 Hounsfield units (Fig. 19.1b) [3–5, 11, 19]. They do not enhance with intravenous contrast and lack invasive features, which distinguishes them from malignancies such as liposarcomas [10, 26]. Lesions tend to arise in the periphery of the thorax, particularly on the lateral chest wall. As they enlarge, pleural lipomas may displace adjacent anatomic structures, such as the lung, great vessels, or mediastinum [11, 19]. The tumors appear to protrude from the chest wall into the pleural space at obtuse angles, a feature that supports their extrapulmonary origin [4, 12, 19].

Homogeneous fat attenuation is considered a hallmark diagnostic feature. If septations, calcifications, or heterogeneous components are present, the diagnosis can become less apparent, raising suspicion for a malignant pleural tumor such as liposarcoma [10, 11, 19, 27]. Although CT findings are generally diagnostic for pleural lipomas, additional diagnostic evaluation is frequently undertaken, particularly in the absence of prior imaging, evidence of interval growth, or even in asymptomatic patients [3, 10, 19, 28].

MRI is not required for diagnostic evaluation but can be obtained when CT tissue attenuation and features are not characteristic of pleural lipoma [7, 15, 29]. Adipose tissue appears as hyperintense signals on T1- and T2-weighted sequences [7]. MRI provides superior detail regarding soft-tissue components and may indicate attachments to the pleura. Functional MRI with diffusion-weighted imaging may provide additional value for differentiating lipomas and liposarcomas [29–32]. CT and MRI features that suggest malignancy rather than a benign lipoma include lesion size >10 cm, presence of thickened septa, globular or nodular nonadipose areas, and lesions comprised of less than 75% fat composition [8].

18-Fluorodeoxyglucose Positron Emission Tomography (18-FDG-PET) may be obtained. Even large pleural lipomas are unlikely to appear FDG avid, in contrast to liposarcomas [6, 7]. Pleural lipomas generally have an SUV maximum of 0.8 ± 0.2 [33].

Although imaging can often be definitive, a biopsy may be warranted when malignancy cannot be excluded or when a more definitive diagnosis is preferred [10, 34]. Transthoracic fine-needle aspiration or core biopsy, typically performed under ultrasound or CT guidance, is the preferred method for obtaining tissue when a biopsy is pursued [35]. CT- or US-guided transthoracic biopsies frequently yield inconclusive results and often lead to surgical excision regardless of histological findings [1, 3, 5, 11, 12, 19, 28, 35].

Although advancements in bronchoscopic techniques have achieved accuracy comparable to transthoracic core biopsies for peripheral pulmonary nodules, this has not been specifically evaluated for extraparenchymal disease or pleural lipomas [36].

Thoracoscopic biopsy not only offers an alternative means of obtaining diagnostic tissue but also has a suboptimal yield; therefore, early resection is sometimes advocated as both a diagnostic and a therapeutic strategy [3, 37].

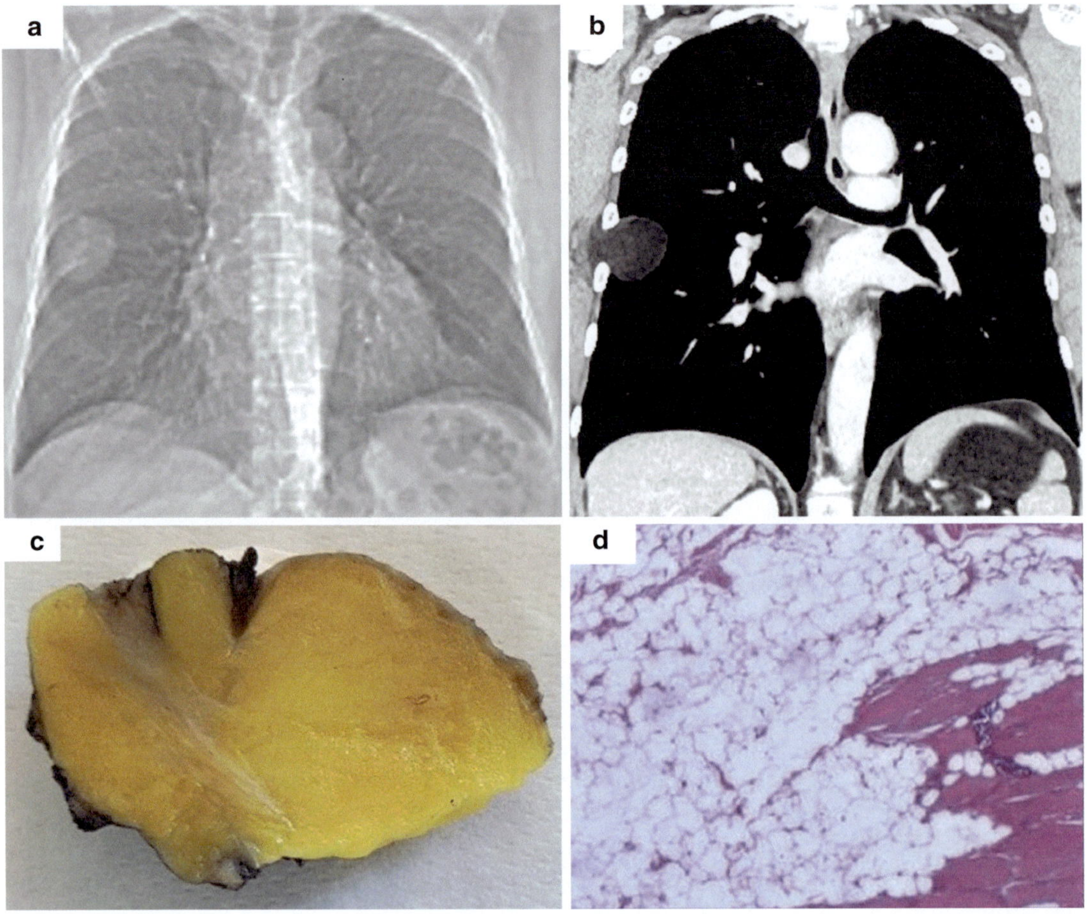

Fig. 19.1 Radiologic and pathologic features of pleural lipoma
(**a**) Chest radiograph showing a well-defined, rounded opacity in the peripheral right middle lung field
(**b**) Coronal computed tomography image demonstrating a homogeneous, fat-attenuated, encapsulated lesion situated between two ribs in the right mid-lung zone
(**c**) Gross pathological specimen revealing a lobulated, yellow, soft-tissue mass with a smooth capsule, characteristic of a lipoma
(**d**) Hematoxylin and eosin-stained section displaying uniform, mature adipocytes without cellular atypia, consistent with benign lipomatous tissue

On gross pathology, in particular, following surgical resection, the tumor appears well circumscribed, with a uniform, tan-yellow appearance when sectioned (Fig. 19.1c). Upon histopathologic analysis, abundant mature adipose tissue arranged into lobules is observed (Fig. 19.1d). The cells may vary in shape and appear larger than normal adipocytes. A thin, fibrous capsule usually surrounds the lipoma. Scattered lymphocytes and histiocytes, along with hyperchromatic stromal cells, may be present. There may be fibrous septa with or without vascular structures. The absence of cytologic atypia or mitotic figures is a key distinguishing feature that differentiates lipomas from liposarcomas. Additionally, in contrast to liposarcomas, pleural lipomas lack invasive growth or necrotic areas and tend to exhibit a low degree of vascularity [10, 12]. Areas of calcification should raise more concern for liposarcoma [10, 27]. Fat necrosis or hemorrhage may be visualized in lipomas depending on the sampling method used [10].

Treatment

Small, asymptomatic lipomas confirmed on imaging do not require interventions. Periodic imaging may be utilized to monitor for changes in size or other features. Although no formal guidelines exist for surveillance, some reported cases begin with follow-up imaging at 6 months [5, 10]. More frequent surveillance or intervention may be appropriate when concerning features are present, such as large size, proximity to vulnerable structures, or imaging characteristics atypical of benign lipomas [10, 34].

Symptomatic, enlarging, or diagnostically uncertain lipomas necessitate surgical excision. Some authors advocate for resection of all pleural lipomas, as delayed intervention may allow for growth or adhesion development, which can make future surgery more challenging [10, 12]. These lesions may have attachments to various thoracic structures; most often, a single vascular pedicle to the parietal or mediastinal pleura is reported. When lung involvement is present, wedge resections of a small portion of the lung parenchyma have been described [23].

Video-assisted thoracoscopic surgery (VATS), where available, has become the preferred approach due to its minimally invasive nature and reduced recovery time. This is especially advantageous for small, uncomplicated lesions. Thoracotomy is generally reserved for larger or more complicated lesions [14, 38, 39]. When surgery is elected, specimens should undergo histopathological evaluation for diagnostic confirmation and assessment of surgical margins, particularly if local tissue adhesion is present [10, 12, 23].

There are no recommendations on the period or frequency of surveillance of pleural lipomas once they are identified. Even among groups who advocate for early surgical resection, an observation strategy with periodic imaging has been suggested for elderly or high-risk patients, especially when lesions are asymptomatic [13, 14]. Given that lipomas may grow or mimic malignancy, some reports recommend a surveillance period of 2–3 years with CT imaging intervals of 6–12 months. If surgical resection is performed and margins are clear, a single postoperative CT scan at 3–6 months is often considered sufficient [34, 40].

Prognosis

The prognosis of pleural lipomas is excellent. Most remain asymptomatic and are believed to go undetected throughout a person's lifetime. When resected, recurrence is rare, and complete excision is typically curative. There is no reported or validated definition of an adequate surgical margin for pleural lipomas. Complications such as misdiagnosis or incomplete excision have been reported but are uncommon [6, 13, 14].

Recurrence rarely occurs and is believed to result from incomplete resection. Incomplete resection is most likely when lesions are in surgically challenging regions, such as on the diaphragm or near critical structures like the brachial plexus. In these instances, residual lipomatous tissue has been reported to remain stable, increase, or even decrease in size, making long-term outcomes in this small subset less predictable [4, 14].

References

1. Politis J, Funahashi A, Gehlsen JA, DeCock D, Stengel BF, Choi H. Intrathoracic lipomas: report of three cases and review of the literature with emphasis on endobronchial lipoma. J Thorac Cardiovasc Surg. 1979;77(4):550–6.
2. Jensen MS, Petersen AH. Bronchial lipoma. Scand J Thorac Cardiovasc Surg. 1970;4(2):131–4.
3. Gaffney H, Klebe S. Symptomatic pleural lipoma: a case report and literature review. Ann Case Rep. 2023;8:1122. https://doi.org/10.29011/2574-7754.101122.

4. Rahman SMT, Rahim A, Kibria AA. Unusual cause of large intrathoracic mass in a young male of Bangladesh: a case report of giant intrathoracic lipoma & literature review. Int J Surg Case Rep. 2020;76:73–6.
5. Malik B, Abdelazeem B, Ghatol A. Pleural lipoma: when to intervene. BMJ Case Rep. 2021;14(4):e243175.
6. Heuer GJ. The thoracic lipomas. Ann Surg. 1933;98(5):801–19.
7. Molinari F, Bankier AA, Eisenberg RL. Fat-containing lesions in adult thoracic imaging. Am J Roentgenol. 2011;197(5):W795–813.
8. Kransdorf MJ, Bancroft LW, Peterson JJ, Murphey MD, Foster WC, Temple HT. Imaging of fatty tumors: distinction of lipoma and well-differentiated Liposarcoma. Radiology. 2002;224(1):99–104.
9. Fothergil J. Wellcome Collection. [cited 2025 Jul 10]. A complete collection of the medical and philosophical works of John Fothergill, M. D. F. R. S. and S. A. member of the Royal Colleges of Physicians at London and Edinburgh; of the Royal Medical Society at Paris; and of the American Philosophical Society : with an account of his life; and occasional notes / by John Elliot, M.D. Available from: https://wellcomecollection.org/works/ugtus2gc/items
10. Jayle C, Hajj-Chahine J, Allain G, Milin S, Soubiron L, Corbi P. Pleural lipoma: a non-surgical lesion? Interact Cardiovasc Thorac Surg. 2012;14(6):735–8.
11. Epler GR, McLoud TC, Munn CS, Colby TV. Pleural lipoma: diagnosis by computed tomography. Chest. 1986;90(2):265–8.
12. Sudhakaran D, Chandrashekhara SH, Kumar S, Sulaiman M. Unusual giant pleural lipomas: imaging features. BMJ Case Rep. 2021;14(6):e238870.
13. Chen M, Yang J, Zhu L, Zhao H. Intrathoracic giant pleural lipoma: case report and review of the literature. J Cardiothorac Surg. 2013;8(1):196.
14. Sakurai H, Kaji M, Yamazaki K, Suemasu K. Intrathoracic lipomas: their clinicopathological behaviors are not as straightforward as expected. Ann Thorac Surg. 2008;86(1):261–5.
15. Nakajima E, Takahashi H, Kajiwara N, Furukawa K, Ishizumi T, Kataba H, et al. Intrathoracic lipoma in the horizontal fissure of the right lung: a case report. J Surg Case Rep. 2021;2021(9):rjab385.
16. Gaerte SC, Meyer CA, Winer-Muram HT, Tarver RD, Conces DJ. Fat-containing lesions of the chest. Radiographics. 2002 Oct;22(Suppl_1):S61–78.
17. Vaughan CJ, Weremowicz S, Goldstein MM, Casey M, Hart M, Hahn RT, et al. A t(2;19)(p13;p13.2) in a giant invasive cardiac lipoma from a patient with multiple lipomatosis. Genes Chromosomes Cancer. 2000;28(2):133–7.
18. Vougiouklakis T, Mitselou A, Agnantis NJ. Giant lipoma: an unusual cause of intrathoracic mass. Pathol Res Pract. 2006;202(1):47–9.
19. Salahudeen HM, Hoey ETD, Robertson RJ, Darby MJ. CT appearances of pleural tumours. Clin Radiol. 2009;64(9):918–30.
20. Abbott AC, Webb EGS. A case of intrathoracic lipoma. Can Med Assoc J. 1935;33(6):660.
21. Jack AI, Blohm ME, Lye M. An intrathoracic lipoma impairing left ventricular function. Br Heart J. 1995;74(1):95.
22. Buxton RC, Tan CS, Khine NM, Cuasay NS, Shor MJ, Spigos DG. Atypical transmural thoracic lipoma: CT diagnosis. J Comput Assist Tomogr. 1988;12(2):196–8.
23. Aldahmashi M, Elmadawy A, Mahdy M, Alaa M. The largest reported intrathoracic lipoma: a case report and current perspectives review. J Cardiothorac Surg. 2019;14(1):215.
24. Gold WM, Koth LL. Pulmonary function testing. In: Broaddus VC, Mason RJ, Ernst JD, King TE Jr, Lazarus SC, Murray JF, et al., editors. Murray and Nadel's textbook of respiratory medicine. 6. Philadelphia: W.B. Saunders; 2016. p. 407–435.e18.
25. Kaur N, Singh J, Haq S, Garg S, Bhatnagar S. Pleural and mediastinal lipomatosis with subpleural fat as a mimicker of pleural effusion- a rare case report. J Clin Diagn Res. 2017;11(7):TD03.
26. Sureka B, Thukral BB, Mittal MK, Mittal A, Sinha M. Radiological review of pleural tumors. Indian J Radiol Imaging. 2013;23(4):313–20.
27. Chen M, Yang J, Zhu L, Zhou C, Zhao H. Primary intrathoracic liposarcoma: a clinicopathologic study and prognostic analysis of 23 cases. J Cardiothorac Surg. 2014;9:119.
28. Crutcher TRR, Plott CL. MEDIASTINAL LIPOMA: the successful removal of an eight pound, one ounce (3,657 grams). J Thorac Surg. 1954;27(3):261–5.
29. Worden CP, Svoboda SA, Garcia EM. Pleural lipomatosis: an often-forgotten intrathoracic tumor. Radiol Case Rep. 2020;15(7):854.
30. Pessôa FMC, de Melo ASA, Souza AS, de Souza LS, Hochhegger B, Zanetti G, et al. Applications of magnetic resonance imaging of the thorax in pleural diseases: a state-of-the-art review. Lung. 2016;194(4):501–9.
31. Santos MK, Elias Júnior J, Mauad FM, Muglia VF, Trad CS. Ressonância magnética do tórax: aplicações tradicionais e novas, com ênfase em pneumologia. J Bras Pneumol. 2011;37:242–58.
32. Arcuri PP, Aiello V, Severo C, Cascini GL, Gallucci S, Laganà D. A case of pleural lipoma evaluated with multi-imaging methods. Radiol Case Rep. 2024;19(1):97–102.
33. Baffour FI, Wenger DE, Broski SM. 18F-FDG PET/CT imaging features of lipomatous tumors. Am J Nucl Med Mol Imaging. 2020;10(1):74–82.
34. Sakellaridis T, Panagiotou I, Gaitanakis S, Katsenos S. Subpleural lipoma: management of a rare intrathoracic tumor. Int J Surg Case Rep. 2013;4(5):463–5.
35. Millward S, Escott N, Masood K. The diagnosis of a pleural lipoma by CT and fine-needle biopsy to avoid thoracotomy. Can Assoc Radiol J J Assoc Can Radiol. 1988;39(1):57–8.
36. Lentz RJ, Frederick-Dyer K, Planz VB, Koyama T, Aboudara MC, Swanner B, et al. Navigational

bronchoscopy versus computed tomography-guided transthoracic needle biopsy for the diagnosis of indeterminate lung nodules: protocol and rationale for the VERITAS multicenter randomized trial. medRxiv. 2023:2023.11.22.23298915.
37. Takayama T, Hirai S, Ishihara T, Kumazaki S, Sano K, Mishima H, et al. Pleural lipoma: report of a case. Surg Today. 1994;24(2):173–5.
38. Prasad S, Ramachandra L, Agarwal S, Sharma D. Successful management of pleural lipoma by video-assisted thoracoscopic surgery. J Minimal Access Surg. 2012;8(1):19.
39. Kummari M, Narahari NK, Kapoor A, Avala RC, Paramjyothi GK. A rare case of giant mediastino-pleural lipoma. Asian Cardiovasc Thorac Ann. 2023;31(8):739–42.
40. Menon A, Marchand C, Medford ARL. Intrapleural lipoma mimicking a lung cancer. QJM Int J Med. 2015;108(8):649–50.

Primary Pleural Liposarcoma

20

William J. Moore III and Michael J. Morris

Introduction

Liposarcoma (LPS) is one of the most common soft-tissue sarcomas in adults, accounting for approximately 20% of reported mesenchymal malignancies [1]. The mesenchymal neoplasm arises from an abnormal differentiation of lipocytic cells, including adipocytes and lipoblasts [2]. The majority of liposarcomas arise from the extremities or retroperitoneum [3, 4]. Intrathoracic LPS is exceedingly rare, comprising only about 1% of all mediastinal tumors [5]. Of all intrathoracic liposarcomas, the most comprehensive review identified 198 cases; 17% originated from the pleura, while the remainder originated from the mediastinum (75%) and lung (7%) [2]. The incidence and prevalence of primary pleural liposarcoma (PPLS) are unknown due to its rarity. In 2014, only 16 PPLS cases had been documented, with a mean age of 50 years (range 19–80 years) and a 69% male predominance [6]. By 2023, a comprehensive review compiled 45 cases of primary pleural liposarcoma with reported outcomes [11]. No environmental or occupational risk factors have been identified, and most cases are believed to result from well-documented sporadic genetic mutations [7].

The first reported case of PPLS was published in 1942 by Ackermann and Wheeler. They described a 50-year-old with progressive dyspnea with a PPLS occupying the entire left hemithorax diagnosed at autopsy [12]. Following this case, Gupta documented a large right-sided PPLS with an associated pleural effusion in 1966 [13]. Additional published case reports led to the first case series, comprising only four patients, in 2000 [8]. Three larger case series have since provided additional information on PPLS histology and treatment course [9–11]. By 2020, the World Health Organization (WHO) recognized five histologic subtypes, which include atypical lipomatous tumor/well-differentiated liposarcoma (ALT/WDLPS), dedifferentiated liposarcoma

The views expressed in this chapter do not necessarily reflect the official policy or position of the Department of the Army, Defense Health Agency, the Department of Defense, or any other government agencies.

The authors have no financial conflicts of interest.

W. J. Moore III · M. J. Morris (✉)
Pulmonary/Critical Care Service, Department of Medicine, Brooke Army Medical Center, JBSA Fort Sam, Houston, TX, USA
e-mail: William.j.moore479.mil@health.mil; michael.j.morris34.civ@health.mil

F. Ido (ed.), *Rare Pleural Diseases*, https://doi.org/10.1007/978-3-032-14873-5_20

(DDLPS), myxoid/round-cell liposarcoma (MLPS/RCLPS), pleomorphic liposarcoma (PLPS), and myxoid pleomorphic liposarcoma [15]. Among all extrathoracic liposarcomas, WDLPS is the most common subtype, accounting for about 40–45% [2, 7]. Myxoid LPS is the second most common subtype overall, accounting for 30–35% of all LPS [14]. The DDLPS subtype accounts for 5% of all liposarcomas but constitutes approximately 21% of intrathoracic liposarcomas [2, 4]. In contrast, primary pleural liposarcoma has been most frequently documented among the myxoid liposarcoma (MLPS) subtype, followed by the well-differentiated subtype [8, 11, 48]. Dedifferentiated liposarcoma possesses the highest potential for metastasis and has been documented to disseminate to the bone and adrenal glands [48].

Pathophysiology

The development of most LPS has been consistently linked to several genetic abnormalities that vary by subtype [16]. Both the well-differentiated and dedifferentiated LPS subtypes are associated with a shared genetic amplification involving the chromosome 12q13-15 segment, resulting in the overexpression of MDM2 and CDK4 [7]. MDM2 is an oncogene that negatively regulates the p53 tumor suppressor protein. It binds to the p53 domain, effectively preventing transcription from occurring [17, 18]. CDK4 encodes a protein that binds to the Cyclin D family proteins and enables the transition from the G1 to the S phase of the cell cycle [7]. Coamplification of both genes is present in more than 90% of well-differentiated and dedifferentiated subtypes [32]. However, MDM2 and CDK4 have also been shown to be overexpressed in other benign and malignant mesenchymal tumors [19]. The addition of a p53 mutation has been observed in DDLPS, suggesting a role in the dedifferentiation process during the transition from the WDLPS to the DDLPS subtype [20]. These genes may also serve as adjunct immunohistochemical markers to differentiate WDLPS and DDLPS from adipose tumors [2, 16, 31–33].

Myxoid liposarcoma (MLPS) is associated with a characteristic genetic translocation involving the t(12;16)(q13;p11) chromosomal rearrangement. This results in the fusion between the DDIT3 gene (previously referred to as CHOP) and the FUS gene (FUS-DDIT3), which is present in nearly 95% of MLPS. Rarely, the translocation can involve the t(12;22)(q13;q12) genes in the remaining 5% of cases, which replace FUS with the EWS gene (EWS-DDIT3) [7, 21]. DDIT3 or CHOP is a nuclear protein that interferes with appropriate adipocyte differentiation and influences cell death in response to stress [6, 14]. The FUS and EWS proteins function in both the nucleus and the cytoplasm, binding to RNA and thereby affecting transcription and nucleocytoplasmic shuttling [7]. Genetic abnormalities involving the phosphoinositide 3-kinase (PI3k) pathway have also been documented in approximately 20% of MLPS [21].

The oncogenesis of pleomorphic liposarcoma (PLPS) is complex, involving numerous gains and losses of gene segments that span multiple chromosomes and genomic locations [7]. A common deletion involves 13q14.2-q14.3 in nearly 60%, which includes the RB1 tumor suppressor protein within that region [22]. Other genetic changes identified include an increased copy number of MAD2, which is involved in DNA replication, as well as deletions of TP53 and NF1, occurring in 17% and 8% of PLPS, respectively [7, 23, 43].

Myxoid pleomorphic liposarcoma (MPLS), named for its histologic resemblance to both PLPS and MLPS, has been associated with numerous genetic gains and deletions [24]. Most notable were genetic mutations that resulted in the deletion of the tumor suppressor protein RB1 [34].

Clinical Features

Symptoms of intrathoracic LPS, when present, are typically due to compression of surrounding structures by the mass effect. In 16% of cases involving intrathoracic LPS, the tumor was detected incidentally on radiologic imaging, without any symptoms. Whether symptoms develop may be related to tumor size, as nearly 23% were less than 10 cm. Reported symptoms of intrathoracic liposarcoma include dyspnea (nearly 50% of patients), chest pain (29%), cough (26%), dysphagia (13%), weight loss (7%), and fatigue (6%) [2]. Symptoms of PPLS are similar, such as cough, dyspnea, shortness of breath, and chest pain [9, 11]. Very large LPS in close proximity to the mediastinal structures can result in superior vena cava syndrome, Horner's syndrome, dysphagia, and cardiac symptoms [35].

Diagnosis

On chest X-ray, intrathoracic liposarcomas typically demonstrate a well-demarcated opacity; however, depending on the tumor size, complete opacification of an entire hemithorax has also been documented (Fig. 20.1a) [39]. Findings on computed tomography (CT) of the chest can vary but most commonly exhibit a heterogeneous, well-circumscribed mass with nodules or septations. Hounsfield units (HUs) can identify the fatty components of the tumor, with values well below −30 HU (Fig. 20.1b) [40]. Radiographically, WDLPS, in particular, may appear similar to benign lipomas, highlighting the diagnostic difficulties in the absence of tissue sampling [35]. Pleural liposarcomas can vary in size and have been documented to range between 3 and 29 cm. Large liposarcomas, in particular, can cause mediastinal deviation and, rarely, may occupy the entire hemithorax. Contrast imaging typically does not result in significant enhancement of the neoplasm. The tumor can arise from both the left and right hemithorax [11, 42]. Less commonly, calcifications, areas of necrosis, and ipsilateral pleural effusions may be present; however, mediastinal lymphadenopathy is typically absent [10]. In PET/CT, tumors exhibit an average SUV of 4.3 [2]. Magnetic resonance imaging (MRI), although not always performed, can reveal varying findings, depending on the LPS subtype. WDLPS can be seen as an encapsulated, homogeneous mass with internal septations, appearing as high-intensity signals on both T1- and T2-weighted imaging. A diminished T1 signal with nodules >1 cm is more suggestive of DDLPS [4]. Transthoracic ultrasound can depict a heterogeneous, hypoechoic mass [40].

Definitive diagnosis requires histopathologic analysis. Ultrasound-guided core needle biopsy and fine-needle aspiration of the mass have been performed infrequently [40, 41]. Rarely, the diagnosis has been achieved based on pleural fluid cytology [36, 37]. Given that large tumors require surgical removal, and since nearly 75% of intrathoracic liposarcomas are >10 cm, diagnosis is more often confirmed following complete resection [2, 10, 38]. Due to the rarity and limited cases regarding primary pleural liposarcoma, no formal staging criteria have been proposed.

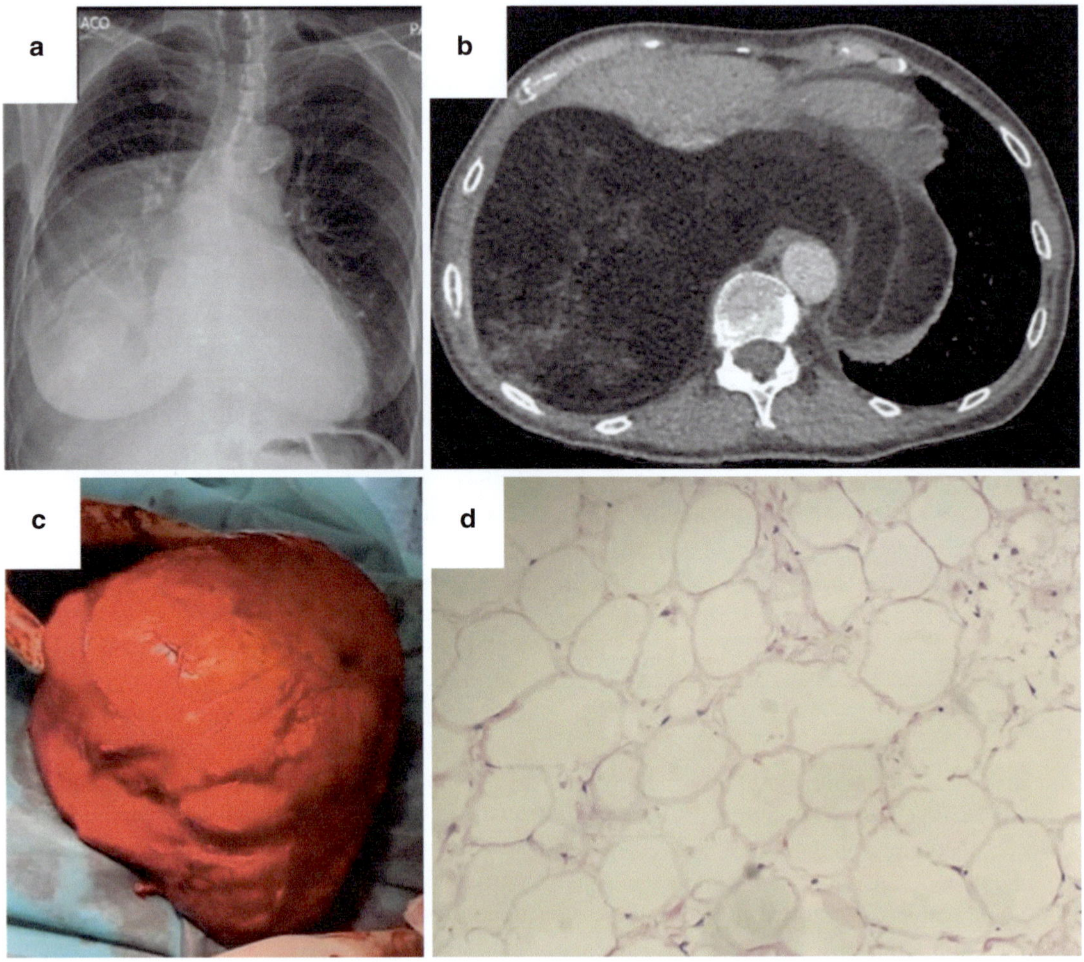

Fig. 20.1 Radiologic and histopathologic features of an intrathoracic well-differentiated liposarcoma

(**a**) Chest radiograph showing a large, well-defined opacity occupying approximately half of the right hemithorax

(**b**) Axial computed tomography (CT) image demonstrating a massive right intrathoracic, fat-attenuating lesion measuring 15.1 × 22.9 × 21.9 cm

(**c**) Intraoperative photograph following resection of the giant intrathoracic liposarcoma, revealing a well-circumscribed, lobulated mass

(**d**) Atypical lipomatous tumor (ALT)/well-differentiated liposarcoma (WDL). Microscopic section showing predominantly mature adipocytes with rare scattered spindle stromal cells exhibiting hyperchromatic nuclei (hematoxylin and eosin stain; ×400)

Pathology

On gross pathology, tumors can weigh more than 3000 g, depending on size [2]. Pleural liposarcomas are encapsulated, with a lobulated and nodular contour (Fig. 20.1c). The consistency is described as solid, rubbery, with occasional scattered myxomatous or gelatinous areas. Cut sectioning exhibits a deep yellow, ivory, or gray color. Focal areas of hemorrhage and necrosis may be visible [8, 11]. A pedicle, attaching to the pleura, can be identified intraoperatively if present [42].

Microscopically, WDLPS is further divided into lipoma-like, sclerosing, and inflammatory variants, which can be distinguished histologically [25]. Most reported cases of mediastinal or pleural WDLPS have not been further classified into subcategories; however, several have described the lipoma-like and sclerosing variants [8, 11, 26]. The term atypical lipomatous tumor, which is also used synonymously with WDLPS, is reserved for tumors arising in the extremities or soft tissue, owing to the high success rate of achieving wide clear margins during resection and the low recurrence rate [4]. WDLPS is a low-grade neoplasm without metastatic potential; however, 10% of WDLPS can transform into DDLPS, which is an aggressive, high-grade subtype of liposarcoma that can metastasize [2, 5].

Histologically, on hematoxylin and eosin (H&E) staining, WDLPS is composed of mature adipocytes of varying sizes, interspersed with fibrous tissue composed of collagen (Fig. 20.1d). Hyperchromatic atypical spindle cells are observed within the fibrous or vascular component of the stroma. The presence of lipoblasts, characterized by well-defined cytoplasmic vacuoles compressing and distorting the hyperchromatic nucleoli, is occasionally observed but not required for the diagnosis of WDLPS [8, 11, 25]. For histologic samples without classic features of WDLPS, ancillary diagnostic tests can be utilized. Immunohistochemistry for the overexpression of MDM2 and CDK4 can demonstrate nuclear reactivity in atypical spindle cells; however, despite a specificity greater than 90%, the sensitivities were only 45% and 41%, respectively [30]. Karyotype analysis can reveal supernumerary ringed or giant chromosomes, indicating the amplification of several genes. Fluorescence in situ hybridization (FISH) can be used in cases of uncertainty, as it detects MDM2 amplification with sensitivity greater than 90% [5, 27–29].

Dedifferentiated liposarcoma shares a similar immunohistochemical profile and cytogenetic features with WDLPS. However, microscopic findings of DDLPS demonstrate a lack of mature adipocytes within the neoplasm. Instead, the tumor is comprised mainly of sheets of undifferentiated pleomorphic or atypical spindle cells in a patternless arrangement (Fig. 20.2a). Mature atypical adipocytes, consistent with WDLPS, are observed at the periphery, bordering the tumor, hinting at the presence of a liposarcoma. The tumor is highly cellular with a significant mitotic count. Areas of necrosis within the neoplasm may be observed [25]. In addition to MDM2 and CDK4, other immunostains positive in pleural DDLPS include S100 and p16, with variable expression of CD99 and adipophilin (Fig. 20.2b–d) [11].

Myxoid liposarcoma of the pleura is characterized by low-to-moderate cellularity, comprised of small round or spindle-shaped tumor cells within a background of myxoid stroma containing significant mucopolysaccharide material. Most notable are scattered, very thin-walled, branching blood vessels described as "chicken-wire" vasculature. Scattered lipoblasts can also be visible (Fig. 20.2e, f) [1, 7, 44]. Immunohistochemistry for DDIT3 is typically positive in all cases containing the associated genetic abnormality [45]. The diagnosis can be confirmed using FISH to detect the DDIT3 rearrangement [44].

Pleomorphic liposarcoma is a high-grade, aggressive neoplasm that demonstrates highly cellular pleomorphic spindle cells with variable amounts of lipoblasts that vary in size (Fig. 20.2g) [7, 46]. Immunohistochemistry shows variable staining for S100, actin, desmin, and CD34 [4].

Myxoid pleomorphic liposarcoma contains features of both myxoid and pleomorphic liposarcoma. The tumor exhibits an area of low-grade

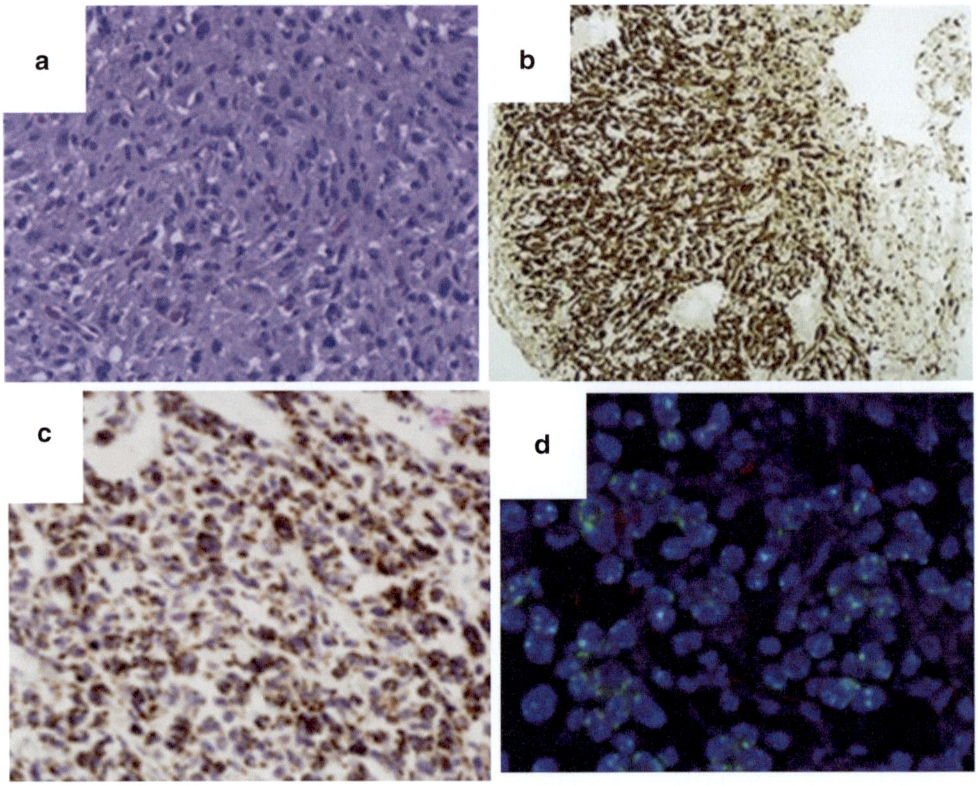

Fig. 20.2 Histopathologic spectrum of liposarcoma subtypes

(**a**) Dedifferentiated liposarcoma (×200). Hematoxylin and eosin stain demonstrating high-grade spindle and pleomorphic sarcomatous components composed of moderately atypical spindle cells with scattered mitoses and minimal adipocytic differentiation

(**b**) Immunohistochemistry showing diffuse and strong CDK4 positivity, typically coamplified with MDM2 in well- and dedifferentiated liposarcomas (×40)

(**c**) Immunohistochemistry for adipophilin showing cytoplasmic positivity in tumor cells of dedifferentiated liposarcoma

(**d**) Fluorescence in situ hybridization (FISH) for MDM2 (green signals) and centromere 12 (red signals) demonstrating MDM2 gene amplification

(**e**) Myxoid liposarcoma (×200). Characterized by bland ovoid or spindle cells dispersed in abundant myxoid stroma with a plexiform network of curvilinear thin-walled blood vessels and scattered lipoblasts with vacuolated cytoplasm (arrows)

(**f**) Pleomorphic liposarcoma (×200). Large, atypical, multivacuolated lipoblasts with indented hyperchromatic nuclei within a background of atypical spindle cells

(G) Round-cell variant of myxoid liposarcoma (×40). Marked cellular proliferation of round and ovoid cells with hyperchromatic nuclei and scant amphophilic cytoplasm

(**h**) Intermediate-power field (×100) showing juxtaposition of a myxoid liposarcoma-like area with myxoid stroma and plexiform vasculature adjacent to a more pleomorphic, lipogenic cellular region

Attribution:

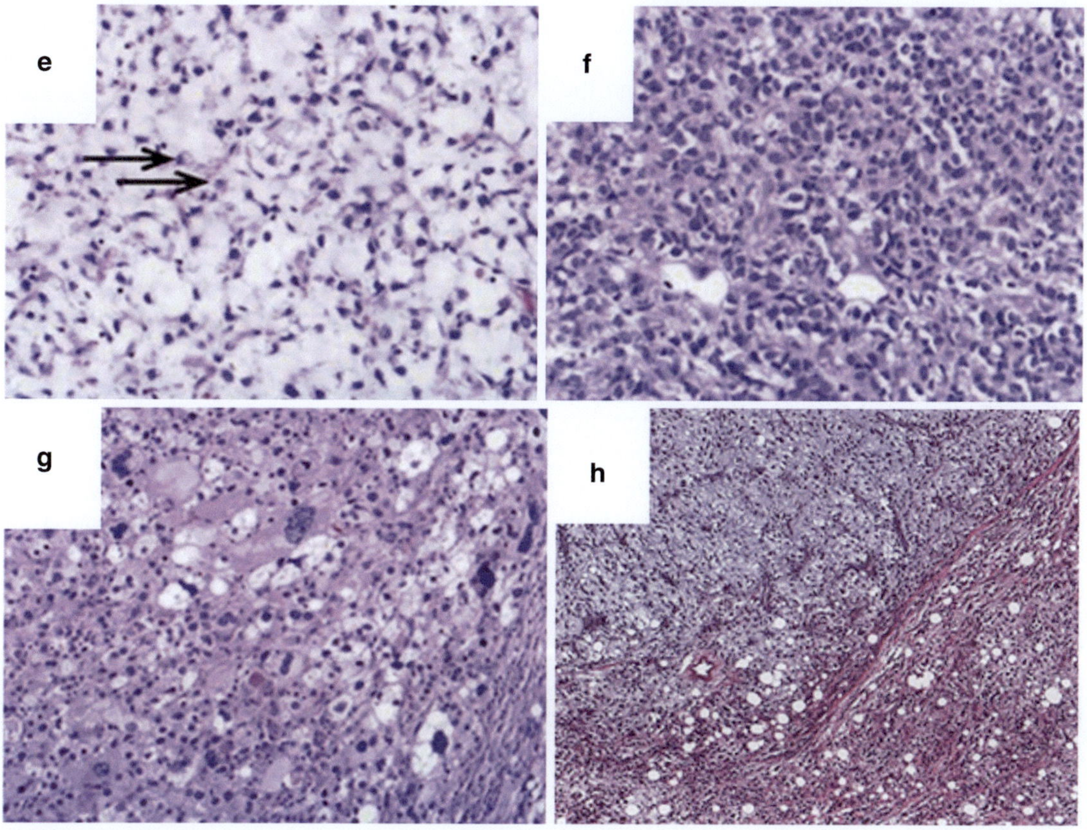

Fig. 20.2 (continued)

spindle cells within a myxomatous background stroma, accompanied by a network of thin blood vessels that transition into sheets of pleomorphic spindle cells, along with lipoblasts and multinucleated giant cells (Fig. 20.2h). Immunostaining for RB1 can exhibit a loss of nuclear reactivity [24].

Treatment

Surgical resection is the most common and preferred treatment for PLS. In a series of intrathoracic LPS, surgical resection was performed in 96% of cases [2]. Surgical success with curative intent is dependent on achieving negative pathologic margins. The presence of residual tumor increases the risk of recurrence [8]. The surgical approach to resection depends on the size and location of the tumor. Thoracotomy and video-assisted thoracoscopic surgery (VATS) have both been performed [2]. Aggressive subtypes, such as DDLPS, may exhibit evidence of surrounding pulmonary parenchymal invasion, necessitating lobectomy [48]. In some cases, adjuvant radiation therapy has been implemented in combination with surgery, with a tendency to increase survival, particularly in myxoid liposarcoma [8]. Chemotherapy has also been reported, although details of the specific regimens are often unavailable [47]. In a single case, the reported regimen included Adriamycin, vincristine, and etoposide [8]. Other chemotherapeutic agents reported to be used in liposarcomas originating from other sites, such as the retroperitoneum, include ifosfamide, doxorubicin, docetaxel, pazopanib, and eribulin, with varying results [2].

Prognosis

Prognosis is influenced by tumor type and the ability to resect the neoplasm with negative margins on pathology [9]. Data compiled from all intrathoracic liposarcomas show an overall 5-year survival of 62%. When analyzing particular subtypes of liposarcoma, the 5-year survival rates were as follows: WDLPS, 80%; DDLPS, 64%; MLPS, 31%; and PLPS, 41% [2, 10]. The overall recurrence rate for intrathoracic liposarcomas was estimated at 37% [2]. Myxoid liposarcoma demonstrates the highest mortality and recurrence rate, often progressing to death within several months. Dedifferentiated liposarcoma has also shown rapid growth with high mortality rates following incomplete resection [48]. MLPS and DDLPS may both metastasize and are associated with rapid growth [7]. WDLPS was most favorable, especially if amenable to resection with negative margins [11]. Local recurrence following resection has been documented to occur several months to years after the initial procedure [2, 8]. Management of local recurrence depends on the feasibility of performing repeat surgical resection [8, 11]. Since most cases proceed to surgery following detection, no standard imaging surveillance interval has been established for monitoring pleural liposarcoma.

References

1. Dei TA. Liposarcoma: new entities and evolving concepts. Ann Diagn Pathol. 2000;4(4):252–66.
2. Kiełbowski K, Ruszel N, Skrzyniarz SA, Wojtyś ME, Becht R, Ptaszyński K, et al. Clinicopathological features of intrathoracic liposarcoma: a systematic review with an illustrative case. J Clin Med. 2022;11(24):7353.
3. Gadgeel SM, Harlan LC, Zeruto CA, Osswald M, Schwartz AG. Patterns of care in a population-based sample of soft tissue sarcoma patients in the United States. Cancer. 2009;115(12):2744–54.
4. Henze J, Bauer S. Liposarcomas. Hematol Oncol Clin North Am. 2013;27(5):939–55.
5. Thway K, Jordan S, Fisher C, Nicholson AG. Updates in the approach to intrathoracic sarcomas. Histopathology. 2015;67(6):755–70.
6. Alberto J, Navarrete C, López A, Peláez M. Primary pleural liposarcoma, pleomorphic variant. J Thorac Dis. 2014;6(9):E166.
7. Conyers R, Young S, Thomas DM. Liposarcoma: molecular genetics and therapeutics. Sarcoma. 2011;2011:483154.
8. Okby NT, Travis WD. Liposarcoma of the pleural cavity: clinical and pathologic features of 4 cases with a review of the literature. Arch Pathol Lab Med. 2000;124(5):699–703.
9. Chen M, Yang J, Zhu L, Zhou C, Zhao H. Primary intrathoracic liposarcoma: a clinicopathologic study and prognostic analysis of 23 cases. J Cardiothorac Surg. 2014;9(1):1–8.
10. Xie Y, Jing W, Zhao W, et al. Primary intrathoracic liposarcomas: a clinicopathologic and molecular study of 43 cases in one of the largest medical centers in China. Front Oncologia. 2022;12:949962.
11. Kawai T, Nakashima H, Washimi K, Yokose T, Matsuo T, Nakayama M, et al. Liposarcoma of the pleural cavity. Hum Pathol. 2023;136:105–13.
12. Ackerman LV, Wheeler P. Liposarcoma. South Med J. 1942;35(156):12.
13. Gupta RK, Paolini FA. Liposarcoma of the pleura: report of a case with a review of literature and views on histogenesis. Am Rev Respir Dis. 1967;95(2):298–304.
14. Batchvarova N, Wang XZ, Ron D. Inhibition of adipogenesis by the stress-induced protein CHOP (Gadd153). EMBO J. 1995;14(19):4654–61.
15. Sbaraglia M, Bellan E, Dei Tos AP. The 2020 WHO classification of soft tissue tumours: news and perspectives. Pathologica. 2020;113(2):1–15.
16. Schaefer IM, Gronchi A. WHO pathology: highlights of the 2020 sarcoma update. Surg Oncol Clin N Am. 2022;31(3):321–40.
17. Mendrysa SM, McElwee MK, Michalowski J, O'Leary KA, Young KM, Perry ME. mdm2 is critical for inhibition of p53 during lymphopoiesis and the response to ionizing irradiation. Mol Cell Biol. 2003;23(2):462–73.
18. Oliner JD, Pietenpol JA, Thiagalingam S, Gyuris J, Kinzler KW, Vogelstein B. Oncoprotein MDM2 conceals the activation domain of tumour suppressor p53. Nature. 1993;362(6423):857–60.
19. Aleixo PB, Hartmann AA, Menezes IC, Meurer RT, Oliveira AM. Can MDM2 and CDK4 make the diagnosis of well differentiated/dedifferentiated liposarcoma? An immunohistochemical study on 129 soft tissue tumours. J Clin Pathol. 2009;62(12):1127–35.
20. Pilotti S, Torre GD, Lavarino C, Palma SD, Sozzi G, Minoletti F, et al. Distinct mdm2/p53 expression patterns in liposarcoma subgroups: implications for different pathogenetic mechanisms. J Pathol. 1997;181(1):14–24.
21. Trautmann M, Cyra M, Isfort I, Jeiler B, Krüger A, Grünewald I, et al. Phosphatidylinositol-3-kinase (PI3K)/Akt signaling is functionally essen-

tial in myxoid liposarcoma. Mol Cancer Ther. 2019;18(4):834–44.
22. Taylor BS, Barretina J, Socci ND, DeCarolis P, Ladanyi M, Meyerson M, et al. Functional copy-number alterations in cancer. PLoS One. 2008;3(9):e3179.
23. Barretina J, Taylor BS, Banerji S, Ramos AH, Lagos-Quintana M, DeCarolis PL, et al. Subtype-specific genomic alterations define new targets for soft-tissue sarcoma therapy. Nat Genet. 2010;42(8):715–21.
24. Fadaei S, Cordier F, Ferdinande L, Van Dorpe J, Creytens D. Myxoid pleomorphic liposarcoma. Histol Histopathol. 2024;39(9):1101–8.
25. Thway K. Well-differentiated liposarcoma and dedifferentiated liposarcoma: an updated review. Semin Diagn Pathol. 2019;36(2):112–21.
26. Iwamoto N, Matsuura Y, Ninomiya H, Ichinose J, Nakao M, Ishikawa Y, et al. An extremely rare case of rapidly growing mediastinal well-differentiated liposarcoma with a sclerosing variant: a case report. Surg Case Rep. 2020;6(1):158.
27. Thway K, Wang J, Swansbury J, Min T, Fisher C. Fluorescence in situ hybridization for MDM2 amplification as a routine ancillary diagnostic tool for suspected well-differentiated and dedifferentiated liposarcomas: experience at a tertiary center. Sarcoma. 2015;2015:1–10.
28. Gambella A, Bertero L, Rondón-Lagos M, Verdun Di Cantogno L, Rangel N, Pitino C, et al. FISH diagnostic assessment of MDM2 amplification in liposarcoma: potential pitfalls and troubleshooting recommendations. Int J Mol Sci 2023;24(2):1342.
29. Kashima T, Halai D, Ye H, Hing SN, Delaney D, Pollock R, et al. Sensitivity of MDM2 amplification and unexpected multiple faint alphoid 12 (alpha 12 satellite sequences) signals in atypical lipomatous tumor. Mod Pathol. 2012;25(10):1384–96.
30. Clay MR, Martinez A, Weiss SM, Edgar MA. MDM2 and CDK4 immunohistochemistry: should it be used in problematic differentiated lipomatous tumors? Am J Surg Pathol. 2016;40(12):1647–52.
31. Boland JM, Colby TV, Folpe AL. Liposarcomas of the mediastinum and thorax: a clinicopathologic and molecular cytogenetic study of 24 cases, emphasizing unusual and diverse histologic features. Am J Surg Pathol. 2012;36(9):1395–403.
32. Binh MBN, Sastre-Garau X, Guillou L, de Pinieux G, Terrier P, Lagacé R, et al. MDM2 and CDK4 immunostaining are useful adjuncts in diagnosing well-differentiated and dedifferentiated liposarcoma subtypes: a comparative analysis of 559 soft tissue neoplasms with genetic data. Am J Surg Pathol. 2005;29(10):1340–7.
33. Henricks WH, Chu YC, Goldblum JR, Weiss SW. Dedifferentiated liposarcoma: clinicopathological analysis of 155 cases with a proposal for an expanded definition of dedifferentiation. Am J Surg Pathol. 1997;31(3):271–81.
34. Creytens D, Folpe AL, Koelsche C, Mentzel T, Ferdinande L, van Gorp JM, et al. Myxoid pleomorphic liposarcoma: a clinicopathologic, immunohistochemical, molecular genetic and epigenetic study of 12 cases, suggesting a possible relationship with conventional pleomorphic liposarcoma. Mod Pathol. 2021;34:2043.
35. Leivaditis V, Dahm M, Papatriantafyllou A, Keul HG, Kohl L, Schafers HJ. Recurrent intrathoracic liposarcoma: a case report and a comprehensive literature review of a rare clinical entity. Cureus. 2024;16(9)
36. AbdullGaffar B, Keloth T. Pleomorphic liposarcoma cytologically detected in hemosiderotic pleural effusion: pitfalls mitigated by cytologic clues and cell-block immunocytochemistry. Diagn Cytopathol. 2024;52(12):E279–85.
37. Ng JKM, Li JJX. Liposarcoma involving serous fluid cavities: a case series illustrating clinical implications and the diagnostic role of exfoliative cytology. Int J Surg Pathol. 2024;32(5):913–9.
38. McGregor DH, Dixon AY, Moral L, Kanabe S. Liposarcoma of pleural cavity with recurrence as malignant fibrous histiocytoma. Ann Clin Lab Sci. 1987;17(2):83–92.
39. Gökçe M. Giant liposarcoma in hemithorax. Turk J Thorac Cardiovasc Surg. 2012;20(4):938–40.
40. Prabhakar N, Vaiphei K, Vishwajeet V, Ramamoorthy E, Gorsi U, Dhooria S, et al. Primary pleural liposarcoma: a rare entity. Lung India. 2019;36(5):438–40.
41. Skiranth U, Pai RR, Bukelo MM, Rao RVC. Primary pleural liposarcoma: a case report and review of the literature. Int J Med Appl Sci. 2014;3(3):98–101.
42. Wang F, Kiryu S, Li L, Wang Q, Li D, Zhang L. Resectable primary pleural myxoid liposarcoma with a pedicle: report of a rare case and literature review. J Thorac Dis. 2017;9(3):E183–7.
43. Hisaoka M, Matsuyama A, Hashimoto H. Aberrant MAD2 expression in soft tissue sarcoma. Pathol Int. 2008;58(6):329–33.
44. Fritchie KJ, Goldblum JR, Tubbs RR, Sun Y, Carver P, Billings SD, et al. The expanded histologic spectrum of myxoid liposarcoma with an emphasis on newly described patterns. Am J Clin Pathol. 2012;137(2):229–39.
45. Scapa JV, Cloutier JM, Raghavan SS, Peters-Schulze G, Varma S, Charville GW. DDIT3 immunohistochemistry is a useful tool for diagnosing myxoid liposarcoma. Am J Surg Pathol. 2020;45(2):230–9.
46. Hornick JL, Bosenberg MW, Mentzel T, McMenamin ME, Oliveira AM, Fletcher CD. Pleomorphic liposarcoma. Am J Surg Pathol. 2004;28(10):1257–67.
47. Goldsmith P, Papagiannopoulos K. Pleural myxoid liposarcoma: features of 2 cases and associated literature review. J Cardiothorac Surg. 2007;2(1):70.
48. Matsukuma S, Oshika Y, Utsumi Y, Obara K, Tanimoto T, Katsurada Y, et al. Pleural dedifferentiated liposarcoma: a case report. Mol Clin Oncol. 2018;10(1):132–6.

21 Primary Pleural Lymphoma

Kyle Admire and Joshua M. Sill

Introduction

Primary pleural lymphoma (PPL) is defined as a lymphomatous neoplasm confined to the pleura, without evidence of lymphatic or extranodal disease elsewhere at the time of diagnosis [1]. This entity is exceedingly rare, representing approximately 2.4% of all primary chest wall tumors and 0.5–7% of all lymphomas reported in the literature [2–5]. The true incidence of isolated pleural-based lymphoma may, however, be underestimated, owing to diagnostic challenges and overlap with secondary pleural involvement by systemic lymphoma.

It is important to emphasize that pleural involvement in lymphoma is more commonly a secondary manifestation of disease. Such secondary pleural lymphomas may result from hematogenous dissemination, lymphatic spread, or direct contiguous extension from adjacent mediastinal or pulmonary foci. Indeed, secondary pleural involvement has been reported in up to 30% of patients with lymphoma [6].

The pleura represents an exceptionally rare site of primary oncogenesis, accounting for less than 0.5% of all non-Hodgkin lymphomas (NHLs) [5]. Precise epidemiologic characterization of PPL remains difficult, as current understanding is largely based on isolated case reports and small case series. While many reported cases do not exhibit traditional risk factors associated with primary effusion lymphoma (PEL) or pyothorax-associated lymphoma (PAL), several demonstrate evidence of chronic inflammatory stimulation, most notably asbestos or silica exposure [7–10]. Among patients without occupational or environmental inhalational exposure, there is often an association with autoimmune or autoinflammatory disorders, including chronic lymphocytic thyroiditis, dermatomyositis, rheumatoid arthritis, Sjögren's syndrome, systemic vasculitides, and human immunodeficiency virus (HIV) [8, 11–14]. Additional predisposing factors that have been implicated in the pathogenesis of PPL include prior chest trauma, chronic heart failure with recurrent pleural effusions, cigarette smoking, and states of immunosuppression, each of which may contribute to persistent local inflammation and lymphoproliferative transformation within the pleural microenvironment [15–18].

Pathophysiology

The pathogenesis of PPL remains incompletely understood. The most widely accepted hypothesis centers on chronic B-cell stimulation within the pleural lymphatic network, triggered by persistent irritation or inflammation arising from

K. Admire · J. M. Sill (✉)
Department of Medicine, Pulmonary & Critical Care Division, Macon & Joan Brock Virginia Health Sciences, Eastern Virginia Medical School at Old Dominion University, Norfolk, VA, USA
e-mail: admirek@odu.edu; silljm@odu.edu

F. Ido (ed.), *Rare Pleural Diseases*, https://doi.org/10.1007/978-3-032-14873-5_21

inhalational exposures or autoimmune diseases [8, 13]. This sustained antigenic drive may promote clonal expansion and eventual malignant transformation of B lymphocytes residing in pleural-associated lymphoid tissue. Several case reports and series have demonstrated high levels of Epstein–Barr virus (EBV) gene expression within the neoplastic cells of PPL, suggesting a pathogenic role for EBV infection in at least a subset of cases [7, 8, 18]. EBV-associated cytokine dysregulation, particularly the overexpression of interleukins IL-6 and IL-10, contributes to enhanced in vitro proliferation of EBV-infected B cells and to the suppression of cytotoxic immune surveillance. The resultant uncontrolled lymphoid proliferation predisposes patients with chronic or latent EBV infection to the development of PPL [18–21]. Another proposed mechanism involves relative T-lymphocyte depletion secondary to chronic B-cell hyperactivation, leading to impaired immune regulation. This imbalance fosters lymphoid and plasmacytic hyperplasia within the pleural tissue, creating a microenvironment conducive to neoplastic transformation [7].

Clinical Features

Patients with PPL do not exhibit a distinctive clinical phenotype, and presenting symptoms are often nonspecific. Many individuals experience constitutional or "B-symptoms," including fever, night sweats, and unintentional weight loss [22, 23]. Owing to the anatomic involvement of the pleura and chest wall, patients may also present with pleuritic chest pain, dyspnea, or a nonproductive cough, symptoms typically associated with a pleural effusion or local pleural inflammation [23]. Neuropathic manifestations have been reported in some cases and may serve as initial or concurrent presentations. These are usually secondary either to direct tumor extension, resulting in mononeuropathy, or to paraneoplastic vasculitic processes, leading to polyneuropathy [24].

Diagnosis

The radiologic appearance of PPL is variable, reflecting the heterogeneous nature of the disease. Plain chest radiography is typically the initial imaging modality in patients presenting with dyspnea, cough, or pleuritic chest pain and may demonstrate findings suggestive of PPL. Two series have reported a 4–14% prevalence of peripheral or pleural-based nodules among patients with lymphoma; however, both acknowledged that small subpleural lesions are easily overlooked on conventional radiographs [25, 26]. Pleural effusions may also be observed, but remain a nonspecific finding and cannot, in isolation, suggest lymphoma.

With the widespread use of computed tomography (CT), the radiographic spectrum of PPL has been more clearly delineated. Reported findings include pleural thickening, focal or diffuse pleural nodularity, and recurrent or heterogeneous pleural effusions [7, 27–31]. These imaging variations are thought to correlate with the anatomic heterogeneity of pleural lymphatic drainage within the thoracic cavity [25]. An increase in Hounsfield units (HU) on CT can help distinguish malignant from benign pleural lesions; however, due to variability in standardized uptake values (SUVs) and overlapping radiodensities, differentiating lymphoma from other malignant pleural processes based solely on enhancement characteristics remains challenging [17, 25, 32]. When diagnostic uncertainty exists, particularly in the presence of adjacent pleural effusion, the use of intravenous contrast may enhance pleural surface definition and help delineate otherwise obscured lesions [14]. A distinctive CT feature, described by one group as the "pleural sandwich sign," refers to the preservation of intact intercostal arteries coursing through a confluent pleural mass (Fig. 21.1a) [33]. This finding is notable because, unlike metastatic pleural tumors, mesothelioma, or other secondary pleural neoplasms, PPL does not typically invade or erode the intercostal vasculature.

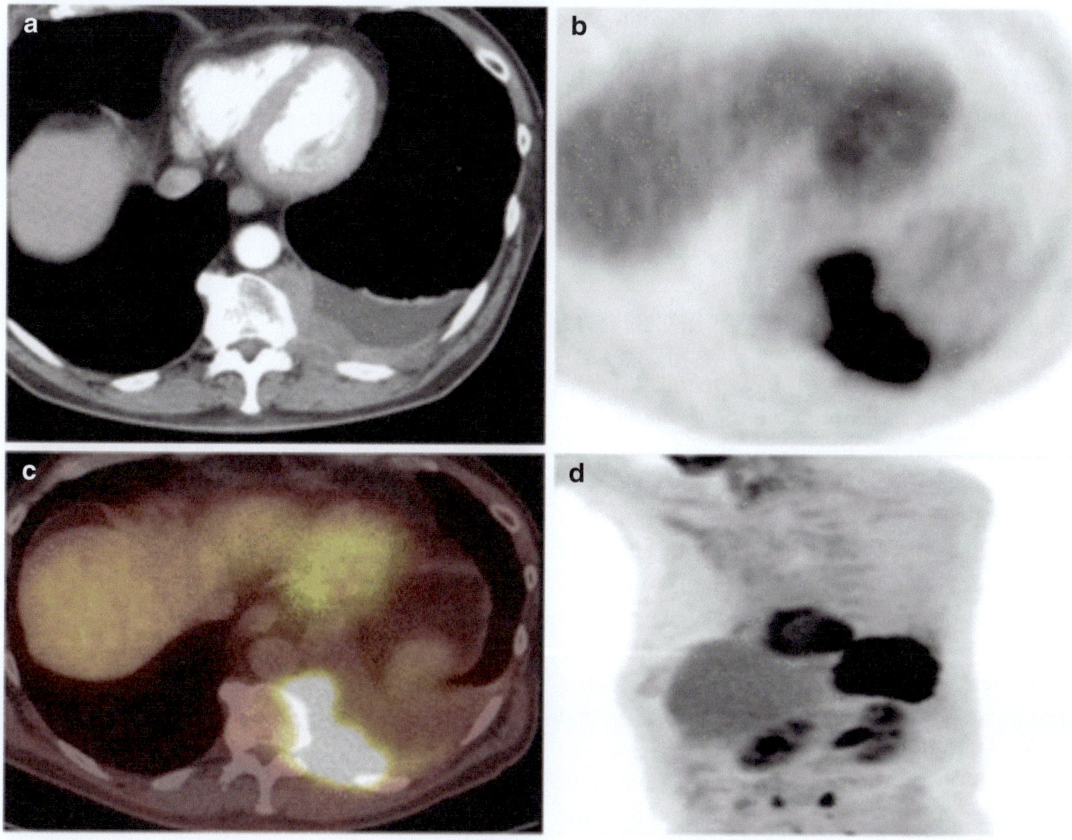

Fig. 21.1 Radiologic features of primary pleural lymphoma. (**a**) Axial computed tomography showing left pleural nodular thickening with an associated pleural effusion. An intercostal vessel is encased within the pleural thickening—characteristic of the pleural "*sandwich sign*." (**b**) Positron emission tomography/computed tomography (PET/CT) showing intense fluorodeoxyglucose (FDG) uptake with a standardized uptake value (SUV) of 14. (**c**) PET/CT fused image showing avid FDG uptake in the paravertebral nodular thickening; note the associated pleural effusion is PET negative. (**d**) Oblique maximum-intensity projection demonstrating isolated FDG uptake from the pleural thickening without associated lymphadenopathy. (Attribution: Reprinted from *Journal of Clinical Oncology*, Vol 29(14), Giardino A., O'Regan K.N., Hargreaves J., Jagannathan J., et al., "Primary Pleural Lymphoma Without Associated Pyothorax," 2011, Copyright © 2011 Wolters Kluwer Health, Inc. Reproduced by permission of Wolters Kluwer Health, Inc. through RightsLink License No. **6136860259390** for *Rare Pleural Disease* (Springer Nature, 2026). All rights reserved. No further reproduction or distribution is permitted without permission from Wolters Kluwer Health, Inc.)

Positron emission tomography (PET) plays a crucial role in the diagnostic evaluation of suspected PPL. Detection of extrapleural involvement on PET helps differentiate PPL from secondary pleural lymphoma, the latter being far more common (Fig. 21.1b–d). Furthermore, PET is valuable for disease staging, response assessment, and surveillance for recurrence or dissemination following treatment [12].

Magnetic resonance imaging (MRI) of the chest, although rarely utilized, can provide complementary soft-tissue characterization. In a reported case of PPL, MRI demonstrated hypointense signal on T1-weighted sequences, hyperintense signal on T2-weighted sequences, and no signal loss on fat-suppressed T2-weighted sequences, consistent with a cellular, non-fat-containing lesion [34].

When pleural effusion is present, the diagnostic yield of pleural fluid cytology in PPL is generally low. Moreover, misdiagnosis as tuberculous pleuritis may occur due to elevated adenosine deaminase (ADA) levels, which are commonly seen in both conditions [35, 36]. This overlap arises because ADA, a key enzyme in the purine metabolism pathway, is actively utilized by T lymphocytes during immune activation, whether in tuberculous infection or lymphomatous oncogenesis [37, 38]. Importantly, ADA concentrations are typically higher in PPL than in tuberculosis, and an ADA level exceeding 250 U/L should raise suspicion for lymphoma or empyema rather than a tuberculous effusion [39].

Definitive diagnosis of PPL requires histologic confirmation through pleural tissue biopsy, which also informs treatment planning [8, 13, 14]. This can be achieved by video-assisted thoracoscopic surgery (VATS) or image-guided pleural biopsy, both of which provide sufficient tissue for immunophenotypic analysis. Thoracoscopic visualization often reveals macular, papular, nodular, plaque-like, or mass-like pleural lesions [13, 14, 26, 40–43]. Once tissue samples are obtained, cytologic examination and immunostaining are employed to narrow the diagnosis and ultimately guide treatment. Histological findings vary depending on the type of lymphoma.

Following tissue acquisition, cytologic examination and immunohistochemical staining are used to classify the lymphoma subtype and guide therapy. The histologic features vary depending on the specific lymphoma type. Diffuse large B-cell lymphoma (DLBCL) demonstrates lymphoproliferation with large, mononuclear, and polylobulated neoplastic cells [13]. Marginal zone lymphoma shows reactive germinal centers surrounded by a mantle and marginal zone configuration [40]. Small B-cell lymphoma is characterized by diffuse proliferation of small, round lymphocytes with mature chromatin [2, 44]. Mucosa-associated lymphoid tissue (MALT) lymphoma, or MALToma, typically shows polymorphic, medium-sized lymphoid cells with basophilic cytoplasm and possible light-chain clonality [34, 45].

Immunophenotypic profiling is typically necessary for diagnostic confirmation. In B-cell lymphomas, immunostains commonly demonstrate positivity for CD19, CD20, CD45, and CD79a, consistent with a B-cell phenotype [46]. Since DLBCL is the predominant PPL subtype, additional markers such as CD10, BCL6, and MUM-1 should be assessed to aid prognostic stratification [47, 48]. T-lymphoblastic lymphomas, in contrast, exhibit positivity for T-cell markers such as CD2, CD3, CD4, CD7, CD8, and CD45 [49, 50]. In cases with diagnostic ambiguity, polymerase chain reaction (PCR) may be used to detect clonality when cytology and immunohistochemistry are inconclusive [34].

It is important to note that no specific histologic or immunohistochemical profile distinguishes PPL from secondary pleural involvement by systemic lymphoma. The differentiation between the two relies primarily on clinical context and radiographic findings, including the absence of extrapleural disease.

Treatment

The management of PPL is guided by the histologic subtype, immunophenotypic findings, and individual patient factors, with treatment tailored accordingly. For patients with diffuse large B-cell lymphoma (DLBCL) or mantle cell lymphoma, the standard of care involves systemic polychemotherapy with CHOP-based regimens (cyclophosphamide, doxorubicin, vincristine, and prednisone), administered with or without rituximab (R-CHOP) [12, 14, 30, 35, 42, 51–54]. Alternative multi-agent regimens such as cyclophosphamide, doxorubicin, vincristine, and cytarabine, or etoposide, vincristine, methotrexate, ifosfamide, and mesna, have been used with varying success in refractory or relapsed settings [55]. Adjuvant radiotherapy may be considered in patients with bulky pleural disease or those who develop chylothorax secondary to lymphatic obstruction [56, 57]. Although exceedingly rare, spontaneous remission has been documented in isolated cases of DLBCL-type PPL [27, 58]. The proposed mechanism involves a post-biopsy inflammatory response that enhances immune recognition and cytotoxic clearance of malignant B cells [27, 58].

For indolent lymphomas, including small B-cell lymphoma, follicular lymphoma, and mucosa-associated lymphoid tissue lymphoma (MALToma), a conservative approach is often appropriate. These subtypes typically follow a slow clinical course, and treatment may be deferred unless patients develop symptomatic disease or evidence of progression [2, 14, 45]. Cases of T-cell lymphoma are managed with more intensive chemotherapy protocols, such as LMT-89 or LSA2-L2, although responses are inconsistent and long-term outcomes remain suboptimal [49, 50, 59, 60]. In the relapsed or high-risk DLBCL setting, autologous hematopoietic stem cell transplantation (HSCT) may be considered following an initial response to induction therapy. HSCT has been shown to improve progression-free survival, though its impact on overall survival appears limited [61].

Prognosis

Prognostication in PPL remains difficult due to the rarity of the disease and the broad histologic spectrum of lymphomas that may originate within the pleura. Reported outcomes vary widely across studies. In pooled analyses, overall survival (OS) among patients with diffuse large B-cell lymphoma has shown considerable variability; one cohort reported a median survival of 29 months and a 2-year survival rate of 47% [62, 63]. These discrepancies likely reflect underlying heterogeneity in performance status, therapeutic responsiveness, and tumor biology, as well as small sample sizes inherent to published case series [43, 64]. Owing to the scarcity of cases, no large-scale systematic reviews or prospective studies have yet established definitive data on the long-term prognosis or the curative potential of therapy in PPL.

When extrapolating from outcomes in extranodal lymphomas at other sites, there appears to be no significant difference in overall survival between patients treated with R-CHOP versus CHOP regimens [65]. Among patients with DLBCL-type PPL, complete remission rates following polychemotherapy are reported between 35% and 50%, underscoring the poor prognosis associated with invasive or extranodal disease [51, 66]. Furthermore, treatment-related toxicity represents a significant source of morbidity and mortality. Myelosuppression is the most common adverse effect, and one study reported a treatment-related mortality rate of approximately 25% in DLBCL patients receiving systemic chemotherapy [63].

References

1. Pereira LJ, Mohrbacher S, Neves PDM d M, Zacchi FFS, Medeiros IUD, Sato VAH, et al. Primary effusion lymphoma: a rare and challenging diagnosis for recurrent pleural effusion. Diagnostics. 2023;13(3):370.
2. Ru X, Ge M, Li L, Lin Y, Liu L. Primary pleural lymphoma: a rare case and a synopsis of the literature. J Thorac Dis. 2013;5(4):E121–3.
3. King RM, Pairolero PC, Trastek VF, Piehler JM, Payne WS, Bernatz PE. Primary chest wall tumors: factors affecting survival. Ann Thorac Surg. 1986;41(6):597–601.
4. Piñel Jiménez L, Martín AR, Garza Graves M, Mesa AM. Linfoma pleural primario asociado a piotórax. Revista española de patología torácica. 2018;30:196–9.
5. Bligh MP, Borgaonkar JN, Burrell SC, MacDonald DA, Manos D. Spectrum of CT findings in thoracic extranodal non-Hodgkin lymphoma. Radiographics. 2017;37(2):439–61.
6. Alexandrakis MG, Passam FH, Kyriakou DS, Bouros D. Pleural effusions in hematologic malignancies. Chest. 2004;125(4):1546–55.
7. Ahmad H. Primary pleural lymphomas. Thorax. 2003;58(10):908–9.
8. Hirai S, Hamanaka Y, Mitsui N, Morifuji K, Sutoh M. Primary malignant lymphoma arising in the pleura without preceding long-standing pyothorax. Ann Thorac Cardiovasc Surg. 2004;10(5):297–300.
9. Pain A. Asbestos exposure and primary pleural lymphoma. Int Clin Pathol J. 2015;1(2):38–40.
10. Matano Y, Okazaki A, Iwasaki K. Primary pleural lymphoma accompanied by silicosis. Clin Case Reports. 2023;11(1):e6826.
11. Zhang Q, Ju Y, Qu T, Wang T, Liu X. Primary diffuse large B-cell lymphoma as a chest-wall mass. Medicine. 2018;97(47):e13291.
12. Lee SM, Kim YK, Lee JJ, Lee JW, Lee YJ, Kim HR, et al. 18F-FDG PET demonstration of cancer recurrence presenting as dermatomyositis in a rare case of primary pleural lymphoma. Nucl Med Mol Imaging. 2011;45(1):79–82.
13. Gastesi A, Kapadia D. Primary pleural lymphoma. Respir Med Case Rep. 2024;50:102046.
14. Oikonomou A, Giatromanolaki A, Margaritis D, Froudarakis M, Prassopoulos P. Primary pleural lymphoma: plaque-like thickening of the pleura. Jpn J Radiol. 2010;28(1):62–5.

15. Atoini F, Ouarssani A, Hachimi MA, Aitlhou F, Guenoun FZ, Elmejereb C, et al. Diffuse large B-cell lymphoma presenting as a large anterior chest wall mass involving pleura and lung: a possible result of post-traumatic chronic inflammation. Thorac Cancer. 2012;3(1):79–83.
16. Rabadão T, Naia L, Ferreira F, Teixeira M, Aveiro M, Eulálio M, et al. Not always (and only) heart failure—a case report of primary pleural lymphoma in an elderly patient. Clin Pract. 2021;11(1):32–6.
17. Jahanshahi A, Hiradfar A, Zarrintan A, Mirza-Aghazadeh-Attari M. Primary pleural lymphoma of T cell origin in a paediatric patient with a focus on radiological findings – a case report and review of literature. Pol J Radiol. 2019;84:e353–9.
18. Martin A, Capron F, Liguory-Brunaud MD, De Frejacques C, Pluot M, Diebold J. Epstein-Barr virus-associated primary malignant lymphomas of the pleural cavity occurring in longstanding pleural chronic inflammation. Hum Pathol. 1994;25(12):1314–8.
19. Kishimoto T. The biology of interleukin-6. Blood. 1989;74(1):1–10.
20. Tanner J, Tosato G. Impairment of natural killer functions by interleukin 6 increases lymphoblastoid cell tumorigenicity in athymic mice. J Clin Invest. 1991;88(1):239–47.
21. Kanno H, Naka N, Yasunaga Y, Iuchi K, Yamauchi S, Hashimoto M, et al. Production of the immunosuppressive cytokine interleukin-10 by Epstein-Barr-virus-expressing pyothorax-associated lymphoma: possible role in the development of overt lymphoma in immunocompetent hosts. Am J Pathol. 1997;150(1):349–57.
22. Carbone PP, Kaplan HS, Musshoff K, Smithers DW, Tubiana M. Report of the committee on Hodgkin's disease staging classification. Cancer Res. 1971;31(11):1860–1.
23. Truong GTD, Creech ZA, Shaffer KV, Merrill M. Diffuse large B-cell lymphoma presenting as a primary pleural mass: a case report and literature review. Cureus. 2022;14:e22765.
24. Fajraoui N, Ben Hamida K, Hadj Kacem A, Amouri R, Ben Ghars K, Khiari I, et al. Neuropathie axonale révélant un lymphome pleural primitif sur séquelles de collapsothérapie. Rev Med Interne. 2010;31(8):e3–6.
25. Shuman L, Libshitz H. Solid pleural manifestations of lymphoma. Am J Roentgenol. 1984;142(2):269–73.
26. Burgener F, Hamlin D. Intrathoracic histiocytic lymphoma. Am J Roentgenol. 1981;136(3):499–504.
27. Guerra SS, Coutinho S, Abrantes T, Rocha P, Silva HM. Primary pleural lymphoma—a rare diagnosis. Pulmonology. 2023;29(1):94–6.
28. Paredes CS, Lauretta J, Semprun M, Rivera-Porras D, Viloria ME, Bermúdez V. Primary pleural lymphoma in an immune-competent patient: a diagnostic and therapeutic challenge. J Pers Med. 2025;15(5):162.
29. Malatskey A, Fields S, Libson E. CT appearance of primary pleural lymphoma. Comput Med Imaging Graph. 1989;13(2):165–7.
30. Sun M, Shang B, Gao J, Jiang S. Rare case of primary pleural lymphoma presenting with pleural effusion. Thorac Cancer. 2016;7(1):145–50.
31. Balikian JP, Herman PG. Non-Hodgkin lymphoma of the lungs. Radiology. 1979;132(3):569–76.
32. Chaber R, Łasecki M, Kuczyński K, Cebryk R, Kwaśnicka J, Olchowy C, et al. Hounsfield units and fractal dimension (test HUFRA) for determining PET positive/negative lymph nodes in pediatric Hodgkin's lymphoma patients. PLoS One. 2020;15(3):e0229859.
33. Kim Y, Lee M, Ryu YJ, Cho MS. The pleural sandwich sign in two cases of primary pleural lymphoma. Korean J Radiol. 2015;16(1):213.
34. Barahona ML, Dueñas VP, Sánchez MT, Plaza BV. Primary mucosa-associated lymphoid tissue lymphoma as a pleural mass. Br J Radiol. 2011;84(1008):e229–31.
35. Yang X, Xu X, Song B, Zhou Q, Zheng Y. Misdiagnosis of primary pleural DLBCL as tuberculosis: a case report and literature review. Mol Clin Oncol. 2018;8:729.
36. Sun J, Li G, Zhang N, Li S, Chen R. Analysis of lymphoma presenting with pulmonary symptoms: report of 79 cases. Zhonghua Jie He He Hu Xi Za Zhi. 2014;37(8):597–600.
37. Krenke R, Korczyński P. Use of pleural fluid levels of adenosine deaminase and interferon gamma in the diagnosis of tuberculous pleuritis. Curr Opin Pulm Med. 2010;16(4):367–75.
38. Yao CW, Wu BR, Huang KY, Chen HJ. Adenosine deaminase activity in pleural effusions of lymphoma patients. QJM. 2014;107(11):887–93.
39. Porcel JM, Esquerda A, Bielsa S. Diagnostic performance of adenosine deaminase activity in pleural fluid: a single-center experience with over 2100 consecutive patients. Eur J Intern Med. 2010;21(5):419–23.
40. Fernandes FR, Oliveira RC, Rodrigues LV. Primary pleural lymphoma. Arch Bronconeumol. 2018;54(8):430.
41. Steiropoulos P, Kouliatsis G, Karpathiou G, Popidou M, Froudarakis ME. Rare cases of primary pleural Hodgkin and non-Hodgkin lymphomas. Respiration. 2009;77(4):459–63.
42. Durieux P, Ravez P. Pleural effusion revealing non-Hodgkin lymphoma. diagnose performed by videothoracoscopy. Acta Clin Belg. 2005;60(6):383–7.
43. Jardin F, Stamatoullas A, Buchonnet G, Duval C, Dujon A, Picquenot JM, et al. Lymphomes pleuraux primitifs après collapsothérapie: aspects modernes d'une maladie historique. Rev Med Interne. 1999;20(11):985–91.
44. Sander B, Campo E, Hsi ED. Chronic lymphocytic leukaemia/small lymphocytic lymphoma and mantle

cell lymphoma: from early lesions to transformation. Virchows Arch. 2023;482(1):131–45.
45. Mitchell A, Meunier C, Ouellette D, Colby T. Extranodal marginal zone lymphoma of mucosa-associated lymphoid tissue with initial presentation in the pleura. Chest. 2006;129(3):791–4.
46. Nakatsuka SI, Yao M, Hoshida Y, Yamamoto S, Iuchi K, Aozasa K. Pyothorax-associated lymphoma: a review of 106 cases. J Clin Oncol. 2002;20(20):4255–60.
47. Ahmed AM, Abdel-Hakeem SS, Amine MA, Yassin EH, Badary FAM. Prognostic value of CD10, BCL6 and MUM1 in diffuse large B-cell lymphoma. SVU-Int. J. Medi. Sci. 2021;4(2):128–40.
48. Vega F, Padula A, Valbuena JR, Stancu M, Jones D, Medeiros LJ. Lymphomas involving the pleura: a clinicopathologic study of 34 cases diagnosed by pleural biopsy. Arch Pathol Lab Med. 2006;130(10):1497–502.
49. Akbayram S, Dogan M, Akgun C, Erbey F, Taşkin GA, Peker E, et al. Report of a non-Hodgkin lymphoma case presenting with pleural effusion. J Pediatr Hematol Oncol. 2011;33(5):e192–4.
50. Karadeniz C, Güven MA, Ruacan Ş, Demirbilek S, Sağbil Ş, Akhan O. Primary pleural lymphoma: an unusual presentation of childhood non-Hodgkin lymphoma. Pediatr Hematol Oncol. 2000;17(8):695–9.
51. Farissi Y, Kouevidjin-Eppou G, Mazieres J, Abakarim O. Primary pleural lymphoma: a case report. PAMJ Clin Med. 2024;14. https://doi.org/10.11604/pamj-cm.2024.14.45.43145.
52. Sun M, Liu X, Jiang S, Yan D. Primary pleural diffuse large B cell lymphoma: a case report and review of literature. Zhonghua Jie He He Hu Xi Za Zhi. 2014;37(11):835–9.
53. Giardino A, O'Regan KN, Hargreaves J, Jagannathan J, Park D, Ramaiya N, et al. Primary pleural lymphoma without associated pyothorax. J Clin Oncol. 2011;29(14):e413–5.
54. Basuthakur S, Sarkar A, Burman S, Dandale R. A rare case of pleural lymphoma. Lung India. 2008;25(4):160.
55. Ravikumar G, Tirumalae R, Das K. Primary pleural non-Hodgkin lymphoma in a child—an exceedingly rare disease. J Pediatr Surg. 2012;47(3):e29–31.
56. Xaubet A, Diumenjo MC, Marín A, Montserrat E, Estopá R, Llebaría C, et al. Characteristics and prognostic value of pleural effusions in non-Hodgkin's lymphomas. Eur J Respir Dis. 1985;66(2):135–40.
57. American Thoracic Society. Management of malignant pleural effusions. Am J Respir Crit Care Med. 2000;162(5):1987–2001. https://doi.org/10.1164/ajrccm.162.5.ats8-00.
58. Snijder J, Mihyawi N, Frolov A, Ewton A, Rivero G. Spontaneous remission in diffuse large cell lymphoma: a case report. J Med Case Rep. 2019;13(1):28.
59. Jabbour E, Koscielny S, Sebban C, Peslin N, Patte C, Gargi T, et al. High survival rate with the LMT-89 regimen in lymphoblastic lymphoma (LL), but not in T-cell acute lymphoblastic leukemia (T-ALL). Leukemia. 2006;20(5):814–9.
60. Mora J, Filippa DA, Qin J, Wollner N. Lymphoblastic lymphoma of childhood and the LSA 2 -L 2 protocol. Cancer. 2003;98(6):1283–91.
61. Stiff PJ, Unger JM, Cook JR, Constine LS, Couban S, Stewart DA, et al. Autologous transplantation as consolidation for aggressive non-Hodgkin's lymphoma. N Engl J Med. 2013;369(18):1681–90.
62. Shao C, Guo Y, Xu X, Pan D, Wang B, Tang Y, et al. Non-pyothorax-associated primary pleural lymphoma without pleural effusion in an immunocompetent patient: a case report and literature review. J Thorac Dis. 2018;10(5):E368–71.
63. Peyrade F, Jardin F, Thieblemont C, Thyss A, Emile JF, Castaigne S, et al. Attenuated immunochemotherapy regimen (R-miniCHOP) in elderly patients older than 80 years with diffuse large B-cell lymphoma: a multicentre, single-arm, phase 2 trial. Lancet Oncol. 2011;12(5):460–8.
64. Aozasa K, Ohsawa M, Iuchi K, Mori T, Komatsu H, Tajima K, et al. Prognostic factors for pleural lymphoma patients. Jpn J Clin Oncol. 1991;21(6):417–21.
65. Gutiérrez-García G, Colomo L, Villamor N, Arenillas L, Martínez A, Cardesa T, et al. Clinico-biological characterization and outcome of primary nodal and extranodal diffuse large B-cell lymphoma in the rituximab era. Leuk Lymphoma. 2010;51(7):1225–32.
66. Bonnet C, De Prijck B, Lejeune M, Fassotte MF, Van Den Neste E, Beguin Y. Diffuse large B cell lymphoma: management in 2012. Rev Med Suisse. 2012;8(351):1582–4, 1586–90.

22 Pleuropulmonary Blastoma

Ahmad Ghabsha and Christos Deamont

Introduction

Pleuropulmonary blastoma (PPB) is a rare mesenchymal neoplasm that primarily affects the pediatric population [8]. In 1988, Manivel et al. described 11 cases of a distinctive intrathoracic tumor composed of blastematous cells, which were pathologically distinct from adult pulmonary blastoma, thereby leading to the classification of this entity as "pleuropulmonary blastoma" [2]. Pediatric lung tumors represent only 0.5–1.0% of all primary pulmonary malignancies, with PPB being the most common, accounting for an estimated 25–50 new cases annually, or nearly 8% of pediatric lung masses identified postnatally [12, 18]. Most cases are diagnosed before age 6, with a mean age at diagnosis of 2 years. Only about 10% of cases are identified after age 5 [4, 8]. A small number of adult cases have been documented [5, 20]. PPB occurs in males and females at nearly equal frequencies. Most cases are reported among Caucasians (83.4%), followed by Black individuals (11.8%), with other racial groups comprising the remainder. Approximately 15.3% of cases occur in Hispanic individuals, with the remaining cases in non-Hispanics [18, 20].

PPB is classified into three subtypes based on gross morphology: type I, a purely cystic lesion; type II, which contains both cystic and solid components; and type III, a purely solid tumor. About 70% of PPB cases are associated with a germline heterozygous mutation in the *DICER1* gene, with nearly 80% of these resulting from inherited mutations [15]. Up to 30% of PPB cases with DICER1 mutations are also linked to cystic nephroma. Other neoplasms associated with DICER1 mutations that may occur alongside PPB include Wilms tumor, sex cord-stromal tumors, and pituitary blastoma [8, 19]. Among patients who had resection for congenital cystic adenomatoid malformation (CCAM), 4% were found to have PPB, indicating a possible relation or cystic precursor lesion [17]. The three PPB subtypes are believed to exist on a spectrum, with type I regarded as a more benign tumor but potentially progressing into the more aggressive types II and III [8, 18]. Type I accounts for 15–20% of all PPB cases, while types II and III make up the remaining 80–85% [15]. At diagnosis, nearly 50% of cases are localized, about 30% exhibit regional extension, and roughly 15% show distant extension or metastasis [18]. Types II and III can metastasize, with the most common sites being the brain, followed by the liver, bones, and kidneys [12, 15].

Clinical Features

Most cases of cystic pulmonary disease are asymptomatic. When symptoms do occur, they often include nonspecific respiratory issues, such

A. Ghabsha (✉) · C. Deamont
Department of Pulmonary and Critical Care, McLaren Oakland Hospital, Pontiac, MI, USA

F. Ido (ed.), *Rare Pleural Diseases*, https://doi.org/10.1007/978-3-032-14873-5_22

as dyspnea, shortness of breath, chest or abdominal discomfort, fever, cough, hemoptysis, or respiratory distress, which may worsen as the lesion enlarges. Common associated clinical findings are spontaneous pneumothorax, pleural effusion, and recurrent pneumonia [5, 6, 8, 10]. While it is rare for purely cystic lesions to become malignant, about 10% of these lesions diagnosed in the neonatal period may eventually transform to a more aggressive and malignant subtype, particularly those linked to the DICER 1 mutation [3, 6, 8, 10, 13].

Diagnosis

The definitive diagnosis of PPB required tissue sampling with histopathologic analysis. Usually, a chest X-ray is performed initially. However, computed tomography (CT) or magnetic resonance imaging (MRI) is used to better characterize mediastinal abnormalities, which are then monitored and evaluated for malignancy (Fig. 22.1a). CT has limited diagnostic accuracy in distinguishing benign cystic pulmonary lesions from PPB, with preoperative chest CT sensitivity for detecting malignancy at only 33.3% (95% CI 15.2–58.3) [7, 8, 14]. Specifically, the sensitivity and specificity of CT for detecting PPB are approximately 58% and 83%, respectively [7, 8, 11, 14]. Lesions that cause symptoms in infancy are generally managed with surgical resection due to a higher risk of complications. In contrast, asymptomatic lesions, whose natural history is unclear, are more often followed with serial imaging and close clinical monitoring [7, 8, 14]. In 30% of types I and Ir PPB cases, pneumothorax was present at initial presentation. Most cysts across all PPB subtypes were unilateral (74%), and most exceeded 5 cm in size [13]. For patients with type II or III PPB, tumor sizes were over 10 cm in 123 cases and under 10 cm in 73 cases. Metastatic lesions were detected at diagnosis in 20 cases. While the status of mediastinal and hilar lymph node involvement was often unreported, nine cases had confirmed regional nodal metastases. Pleural effusion was observed in 77% of patients, and pneumothorax was more

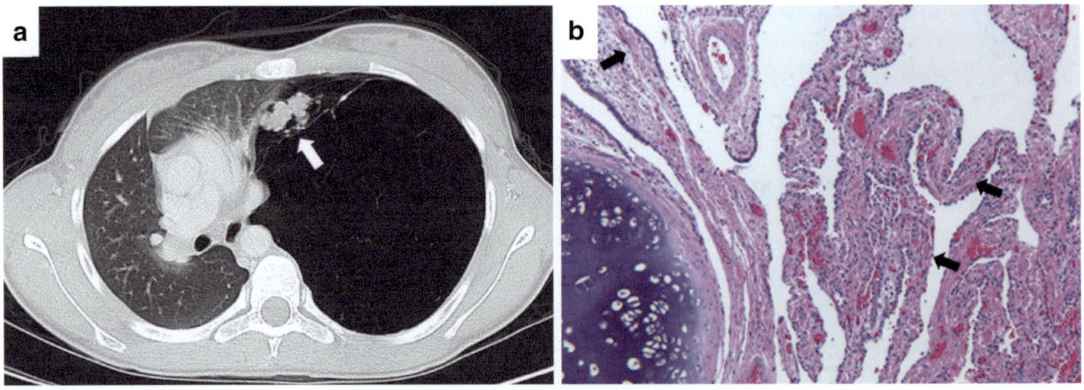

Fig. 22.1 Radiologic and histopathologic features of pulmonary and pleuropulmonary blastoma. (**a**) Axial contrast-enhanced CT of the chest showing a large pleuropulmonary mass with both a cystic lesion with thin internal septations and solid components occupying the hemithorax, resulting in rightward mediastinal shift. The combination of multiloculated cystic regions and solid nodularity is characteristic of a mixed cystic–solid lesion consistent with type II pleuropulmonary blastoma. (**b**) Histopathologic section from the same case showing primitive malignant mesenchymal proliferation with focal rhabdomyoblastic differentiation and residual cystic spaces lined by benign epithelium. Although originally reported by the authors as type Ir, the presence of solid malignant stroma supports reclassification as type II pleuropulmonary blastoma according to the current DICER1-associated classification. (Attribution: Reprinted from *Journal of Pediatric Surgery Case Reports*, Vol 59, Bownes L.V., Hutchins S.C., Cardenas A.M., Kelly D.R., Beierle E.A., "Pleuropulmonary blastoma in an adolescent," Article 101482, Copyright © 2020 Elsevier Inc. Reproduced by permission of Elsevier through RightsLink License No. 6130561092085 for *Rare Pleural Disease* (Springer Nature, 2026). All rights reserved. No further reproduction or distribution is permitted without permission from Elsevier)

common in type II patients (65%) than in type III patients [10–13, 21].

Pathology

PPB is divided into three subtypes, which are also pathologically distinct [3, 4, 6, 8]. Type I represents a purely cystic form with scattered malignant cells and entails the best prognosis if treated early. Type II exhibits both cystic and solid tumor components, reflecting a more aggressive form and the potential of disease progression (Fig. 22.1b). Type III is an exclusively solid tumor and is the most aggressive of all three subtypes, indicating a poor prognosis [3, 6, 8, 11]. Not all cases of type I cystic PPB progress to a malignant stage; some remain cystic, regress, and never metastasize, a subtype referred to as type I regressed (type Ir) PPB. Microscopically, PPB features highly mitotically active blastematous and spindle-cell areas at various stages of malignancy, resembling rhabdomyosarcoma, chondrosarcoma, or liposarcoma [1, 2, 4, 5, 8].

Pathologic specimens of type I PPB feature cystic lesions that are clearly separated from the surrounding normal lung tissue, distal airspaces, and alveoli. Within the pulmonary septa, cellular proliferation of embryonal rhabdomyosarcoma, spindle cell, or fibrosarcoma-like areas is also believed to represent a single entity of type I PPB. The exact cellular arrangement characterizes another variant of type I PPB, but the septa lack rhabdomyoblasts or other primitive cells [21–23]. Cystic tumors without a cellular component are classified as type Ir PPB, suggesting regression or nonprogression. Types II and III PPB share similar histologic features, with solid areas composed of sarcomatous patterns, embryonal rhabdomyosarcoma, spindle cell or fibrosarcoma-like regions, clusters of undifferentiated cells surrounded by primitive mesenchyme, cartilaginous nodules, and atypical anaplastic cells [21–23]. In cases of types I and Ir PPB, a pathological review confirmed cystic pathology in 115 of 350 cases (33%), with 77% type I and 23% type Ir. Males were more frequently affected than females in both subtypes, 57% vs. 43% in type I and 73% vs. 27% in type Ir.

Treatment

Surgery

The primary treatment for PPB is surgical removal. As previously noted, diagnosis often occurs after resection of high-risk cystic lesions suspected to be PPB. All cystic lesions in infants and children should initially be classified as either symptomatic or asymptomatic, with symptomatic cases given priority for prompt advanced imaging, such as MRI or CT, and early surgical intervention, especially if they carry high-risk genetic markers, such as a *DICER1* gene mutation [9, 12, 14]. Due to this link and the increased risk of multiple cancers, all PPB patients should undergo genetic counseling and *DICER1* gene screening as detailed below. Conversely, asymptomatic lesions can usually be monitored with a simple chest X-ray at birth and later categorized as low or high risk based on specific features. Low-risk features include small lesions or the absence of lesions, as well as the absence of PPB risk factors. High-risk features involve large lesions covering 20% or more of the hemithorax or significant risk factors such as bilateral or multifocal cysts, pneumothorax, DICER1 mutations, or a family history of DICER1 syndrome [8, 9, 12–14]. As noted earlier, radiographic imaging alone cannot confirm the diagnosis; thus, surgery is primarily performed to eliminate the risk of malignant transformation and to prevent complications like recurrent pneumonia or respiratory failure caused by cystic lung disease [6, 8, 14].

Chemotherapy/Radiation

In cases of type I PPB, the data regarding the use of chemotherapy is less definitive. Few case reports detail the treatment of type I PPB with surgery alone, as well as cases involving surgical intervention combined with chemotherapy. Examples of chemotherapeutic regimens include ifosfamide, vincristine, D-actinomycin, and cyclophosphamide. Conversely, for type II-III PPB, chemotherapy is universally recommended due to the more aggressive nature of the disease [8, 9, 14]. A typical regimen includes IVA (ifosfamide, vincristine, and actinomycin), or IVA in conjunction with doxorubicin, or a combination of vincristine, actinomycin, and cyclophosphamide (VAC). Currently, there is no standardized treatment protocol or data defining the optimal duration of therapy; however, it has been described to range from 21 to 45 weeks [8, 9, 13]. Radiation therapy remains an option for patients only following initial surgical resection with residual tumor tissue or after the completion of chemotherapy with persistent viable tumor tissue. Generally, radiation therapy is not recommended for type I PPB. The optimal radiation dose has not been established; however, it is recommended to deliver a total of 45–54 Gy in daily fractions of 1.8 Gy [8, 9, 13, 14].

Prognosis

Survival in PPB heavily depends on the extent of disease progression at the time of diagnosis. For type I/Ir, the overall survival rate after resection is 91%. In contrast, survival rates are 71% for type II and 53% for type III, influenced by the presence of metastatic disease. Out of 71 cases, 16 (22.5%) resulted in death. Most of these fatalities occurred in cases with distant disease, underscoring the importance of early diagnosis and quick treatment. Involvement of the pleura or mediastinum, or metastatic disease at diagnosis, is associated with significantly poorer outcomes compared to cases without such involvement. The 5-year survival rate is 83% for type I, but drops to 42% for types II and III, respectively [18].

Genetics

As previously noted, mutations in the *DICER1* gene are strongly linked to PPB. A common genetic feature in the mesenchymal cells of PPB is the presence of specific alterations in the DICER1 RNase IIIb domain, which are also observed in several other conditions. At the cellular level, these mutations lead to the dysregulation of oncofetal genes and unchecked cell proliferation. One mechanism for DICER1 dysfunction is heterozygous loss-of-function mutations, which cause the described changes. Additionally, a study of 47 PPB tumors suggests that DICER1 mutations involve only partial loss of function, with a two-hit somatic mutation mechanism. Notably, 34% of patients develop PPB without a germline DICER1 mutation, and this pathway remains under investigation [3–5, 9–11, 13, 16, 21–23].

Screening

All PPB cases require referral for genetic counseling and screening for DICER1 mutations. If positive, patients should join active surveillance programs to monitor for other DICER1-related conditions. Specifically, screening for cystic nephroma and ovarian tumors is of great importance, typically using abdominal ultrasound [8]. Infants with parents known to carry the DICER1 mutation should undergo a third-trimester ultrasound and screening chest CTs between 3 and 6 months and again at 2 to 3 years of age to detect PPB subclinically. Prenatal ultrasounds have identified lung cysts in 7 of 115 cases at 31 to 35 weeks of gestation [8, 13]. It is recommended to perform chest X-rays every 6 months from birth until age 7, then annually until age 12, with continued screening beyond age 12 based on individual cases. This screening approach aims to detect PPB early in most patients. Testing siblings of PPB patients is generally unnecessary, as their risk is similar to that of the general population, considering the low probability of germline mosaicism [6, 9, 14, 19].

Conclusion

In summary, PPB is a rare pleuroparenchymal disease predominantly seen in children. Treatment options include surgical resection, chemotherapy, radiation therapy, as well as genetic counseling and supportive care. The prognosis for PPB has improved with multimodal treatments, significantly increasing survival. Overall, the survival rate exceeds 90% for type I/Ir PPB, over 70% for type II, and more than 50% for type III [8, 9, 14]. However, the literature lacks sufficient data to establish definitive treatment protocols for all PPB cases, highlighting the need for further research to clarify these approaches.

References

1. Dehner LP. Pleuropulmonary blastoma is the pulmonary blastoma of childhood. Semin Diagn Pathol. 1994;11(2):144–51. PMID: 7809508.
2. Hill DA, Sadeghi S, Schultz MZ, Burr JS, Dehner LP. Pleuropulmonary blastoma in an adult: an initial case report. Cancer. 1999;85(11):2368–74. PMID: 10357407.
3. Walker RI, Suvarna K, Matthews S. Case report: pulmonary blastoma—presentation of two atypical cases and review of the literature. Br J Radiol. 2005;78(929):437–40. https://doi.org/10.1259/bjr/45172814. PMID: 15845939.
4. Magistrelli P, D'Ambra L, Berti S, Bonfante P, Francone E, Vigani A, Falco E. Adult pulmonary blastoma: report of an unusual malignant lung tumor. World J Clin Oncol. 2014;5(5):1113–6. https://doi.org/10.5306/wjco.v5.i5.1113. PMID: 25493248; PMCID: PMC4259939.
5. Manivel JC, Priest JR, Watterson J, Steiner M, Woods WG, Wick MR, Dehner LP. Pleuropulmonary blastoma: the so-called pulmonary blastoma of childhood. Cancer. 1988;62(8):1516–26. https://doi.org/10.1002/1097-0142(19881015)62:8<1516::aid-cncr2820620812>3.0.co;2-3. PMID: 3048630.
6. Kunisaki SM, Lal DR, Saito JM, Fallat ME, St Peter SD, Fox ZD, Heider A, Chan SS, Boyd KP, Burns RC, Deans KJ, Gadepalli SK, Hirschl RB, Kabre R, Landman MP, Leys CM, Mak GZ, Minneci PC, Wright TN, Helmrath MA, Midwest Pediatric Surgery Consortium. Pleuropulmonary blastoma in pediatric lung lesions. Pediatrics. 2021;147(4):e2020028357. https://doi.org/10.1542/peds.2020-028357. Epub 2021 Mar 24. PMID: 33762310.
7. Engwall-Gill AJ, Chan SS, Boyd KP, Saito JM, Fallat ME, St Peter SD, Bolger-Theut S, Crotty EJ, Green JR, Bowling RLH, Kumbhar SS, Rattan MS, Young CM, Canner JK, Deans KJ, Gadepalli SK, Helmrath MA, Hirschl RB, Kabre R, Lal DR, Landman MP, Leys CM, Mak GZ, Minneci PC, Wright TN, Kunisaki SM, Midwest Pediatric Surgery Consortium. Accuracy of chest computed tomography in distinguishing cystic pleuropulmonary blastoma from benign congenital lung malformations in children. JAMA Netw Open. 2022;5(6):e2219814. https://doi.org/10.1001/jamanetworkopen.2022.19814. PMID: 35771571; PMCID: PMC9247735.
8. Bisogno G, Sarnacki S, Stachowicz-Stencel T, Minard Colin V, Ferrari A, Godzinski J, et al. Pleuropulmonary blastoma in children and adolescents: the EXPeRT/PARTNER diagnostic and therapeutic recommendations. Pediatr Blood Cancer. 2021;68(S4):e29041. https://doi.org/10.1002/pbc.29041.
9. Fita AM, Llinares-Riestra E, Doménech-Abellán E, Bermúdez-Cortés M, Galera-Miñarro AM, Bas-Bernal A, Fuster-Soler JL. Type III pleuropulmonary blastoma in a DICER1 germline mutation carrier: management of residual lung cystic lesions. Pediatr Blood Cancer. 2017;64(8):e26438. https://doi.org/10.1002/pbc.26438. Epub 2017 Jan 18. PMID: 28097783.
10. Dehner LP, Messinger YH, Williams GM, Stewart DR, Harney LA, Schultz KA, Hill DA. Type I pleuropulmonary blastoma versus congenital pulmonary airway malformation type IV. Neonatology. 2017;111(1):76–81. https://doi.org/10.1159/000447992. Epub 2016 Aug 26. PMID: 27562209.
11. Priest JR, Hill DA, Williams GM, Moertel CL, Messinger Y, Finkelstein MJ, Dehner LP, International Pleuropulmonary Blastoma Registry. Type I pleuropulmonary blastoma: a report from the International Pleuropulmonary Blastoma Registry. J Clin Oncol. 2006;24(27):4492–8. https://doi.org/10.1200/JCO.2005.05.3595. PMID: 16983119.
12. Priest JR, McDermott MB, Bhatia S, Watterson J, Manivel JC, Dehner LP. Pleuropulmonary blastoma: a clinicopathologic study of 50 cases. Cancer. 1997;80(1):147–61. PMID: 9210721.
13. Messinger YH, Stewart DR, Priest JR, Williams GM, Harris AK, Schultz KA, Yang J, Doros L, Rosenberg PS, Hill DA, Dehner LP. Pleuropulmonary blastoma: a report on 350 central pathology-confirmed cases by the International Pleuropulmonary Blastoma Registry. Cancer. 2015;121(2):276–85. https://doi.org/10.1002/cncr.29032. PMID: 25209242.
14. Zhang N, Zeng Q, Ma X, Chen C, Yu J, Zhang X, Yan D, Xu C, Liu D, Zhang Q. Diagnosis and treatment of pleuropulmonary blastoma in children: a single-center report of 41 cases. J Pediatr Surg. 2020;55(7):1351–5. https://doi.org/10.1016/j.jpedsurg.2019.06.009. Epub 2019 June 27. PMID: 31277979.
15. AbuAyyash RI, Aqel W, Bannoura S, Asbeh YA. Pleuropulmonary blastoma type I presenting as a tension pneumothorax: a case report and review of the literature. Ann Med Surg. 2023;85:2024. https://doi.org/10.1016/j.amsu.2023.102024.
16. Dehner LP, Schultz KA, Hill DA. Pleuropulmonary blastoma: more than a lung neoplasm of childhood. Am J Clin Pathol. 2019;152(3):206–10. https://doi.org/10.1093/ajcp/aqz071. PMID: 31504785.

17. Nasr A, Himidan S, Pastor AC, Taylor G, Kim PS. Is congenital cystic adenomatoid malformation a premalignant lesion for pleuropulmonary blastoma? J Pediatr Surg. 2010;45(6):1086–9. https://doi.org/10.1016/j.jpedsurg.2010.02.031. PMID: 20537313.
18. Borad A, Deianni E, Burjonrappa S. Predictive factors of mortality in pediatric pleuropulmonary blastoma: a Surveillance Epidemiology and End Results database analysis. J Indian Assoc Pediatr Surg. 2024;29(3):245–50. https://doi.org/10.4103/jiaps.jiaps_28_24.
19. Abbo O, Pinnagoda K, Brouchet L, Leobon B, Savagner F, Oliver I, et al. Wilms tumor, pleuropulmonary blastoma, and DICER1: case report and literature review. World J Surg Oncol. 2018;16(1):158. https://doi.org/10.1186/s12957-018-1447-5. PMID: 30089472.
20. Chidiac C, Sferra SR, Kunisaki SM, Rhee DS. Patient characteristics, treatment, and survival in pleuropulmonary blastoma: an analysis from the National Cancer Database. Children (Basel). 2024;11(4):424. https://doi.org/10.3390/children11040424. PMID: 38638469.
21. Brenneman M, Field A, Yang J, Williams G, Doros L, Rossi C, Schultz KA, Rosenberg A, Ivanovich J, Turner J, Gordish-Dressman H, Stewart D, Yu W, Harris A, Schoettler P, Goodfellow P, Dehner L, Messinger Y, Hill DA. Temporal order of RNase IIIb and loss-of-function mutations during development determines phenotype in pleuropulmonary blastoma/DICER1 syndrome: a unique variant of the two-hit tumor suppression model. F1000Res. 2015;4:214. https://doi.org/10.12688/f1000research.6746.2. PMID: 26925222; PMCID: PMC4712775.
22. Foulkes WD, Priest JR, Duchaine TF. DICER1: mutations, microRNAs and mechanisms. Nat Rev Cancer. 2014;14(10):662–72. https://doi.org/10.1038/nrc3802. Epub 2014 Sep 1. PMID: 25176334.
23. Hong B, Chen Z, Coffin CM, Lemons R, Issa B, Brothman A, Zhou H. Molecular cytogenetic analysis of a pleuropulmonary blastoma. Cancer Genet Cytogenet. 2003;142(1):65–9. https://doi.org/10.1016/S0165-4608(02)00731-8. PMID: 12660036.

23 Desmoplastic Small Round Cell Tumor of the Pleura

Razi Even Dar and Yaniv Dotan

Introduction

Desmoplastic small round cell tumor (DSRCT) of the pleura is a rare malignant and highly aggressive soft tissue sarcoma of mesenchymal origin. The first case, documented in 1989 by Gerald and Rosai, involved an 8-year-old female with a 16 cm intra-abdominal solid mass noted to arise from the omentum during surgery. Histologically, the mass demonstrated features resembling those of epithelial, neuroendocrine, and skeletal muscle [1]. As the name implies, the tumor is composed of small polyphenotypic cells surrounded by a dense, reactive connective tissue stroma, reflecting the desmoplastic process responsible for the characteristic hard, solid appearance. Population-based registries from the United States and France have estimated its incidence at approximately 0.2 per million individuals, with a peak frequency between 20 and 24 years of age [2, 3]. Incidence rates are higher among Black Americans, reaching 0.5 per million, with a peak between 25 and 29 years [3]. The disease predominantly affects young males between 10 and 39 years of age, with a male-to-female incidence ratio of 4:1 [3]. No lifestyle or environmental risk factors have been identified, and smoking and asbestos exposure are not associated with its development [3, 4]. Instead, the tumor is associated with a unique somatic chromosomal translocation t(11;22)(p13;q12), resulting in the *EWSR1-WT1* fusion gene, which upregulates several oncogenic proteins [10]. DSRCT most frequently arises from the peritoneum, although it has been described in the ovaries, liver, lungs, and bones. Pleural DSRCT is exceedingly rare, with the medical literature limited to isolated case reports and small case series [4–9]. It may present as a primary pleural neoplasm or as secondary involvement due to metastases from extra-pleural sites. In a review of primary pleural cases, the left hemithorax was affected more frequently (46%) than the right (26%), while bilateral involvement was reported in 20% of patients. The tumor has been described in peripheral, mediastinal, and paravertebral pleural locations. In two reported cases, the origin was the parietal pleura, whereas the site of origin was not specified in other reports [10, 11]. In 70% of cases, the lung parenchyma was spared, but in the remaining cases, there was direct invasion of the lung and mediastinum. Adjacent vertebral involvement occurred in 33% of patients. Importantly, none of the documented cases of primary pleural DSRCT has reported distant metastases [4].

R. E. Dar · Y. Dotan (✉)
Pulmonary Institute, Rambam Health Care Campus, Ruth and Bruce Rappaport Faculty of Medicine, The Technion—Israel Institute of Technology, Haifa, Israel
e-mail: R_evendar@rmc.gov.il; y_dotan@rmc.gov.il

F. Ido (ed.), *Rare Pleural Diseases*, https://doi.org/10.1007/978-3-032-14873-5_23

Genetics and Molecular Mechanism

Desmoplastic small round cell tumor is defined by the chromosomal translocation t(11;22)(p13;q12), which fuses the N-terminal domain of the *Ewing sarcoma* gene (*EWS*) with the C-terminal domain of the *Wilms tumor* suppressor gene (*WT1*) [12, 13]. The resulting chimeric protein functions as a transcriptional activator for several growth factors, including PDGFRα, IGF1R, IL-2, MYC, and PAX2, among others [14–17]. The oncogenic potential of the EWS–WT1 fusion protein is extensive, encompassing the induction of fibroblast and endothelial cell proliferation through PDGFRα, IGF2, and EGFR signaling, in addition to immune system evasion and impairment of DNA repair via inhibition of p53 [18]. The EWS–WT1 rearrangement is believed to represent the predominant, and nearly exclusive, genetic abnormality associated with DSRCT. This conclusion is supported by a study that performed broad sequencing of 29 oncogenes and tumor suppressor genes in 24 patients with DSRCT, identifying no other consistent genetic alterations [19]. The low somatic mutation burden observed in DSRCT is similar to that of other pediatric-onset sarcomas, including Ewing sarcoma and rhabdomyosarcoma. However, several case reports have described additional genetic alterations, including single-nucleotide polymorphisms and copy number variations in more than ten genes, such as *AURKB*, *MCL1*, and *ARID1A* [20–22]. However, the lack of reproducibility, combined with their coexistence alongside the t(11;22)(p13;q12) rearrangement, raises uncertainty about their clinical significance. The predominance of the EWS–WT1 translocation suggests potential applications as a biomarker, such as quantification of circulating tumor DNA for disease monitoring, or as a target for individualized biologic therapies. However, neither approach is currently employed in clinical practice [20].

Clinical Features

The most common clinical presentation of isolated pleural DSRCT is acute, sharp chest pain. Back and neck pain, resulting from tumor invasion into adjacent ribs and soft tissues, has been reported either as accompanying symptoms or as the sole manifestation [23, 24]. Dyspnea is observed in approximately 50% of patients. Dry cough and unintentional weight loss have been described in up to 25% of cases [4, 10]. Fever is rare, documented in only one case involving a child with DSRCT [23]. The disease typically follows an aggressive course, with the interval from symptom onset to diagnosis being short, most often ranging from several days to 1–2 months [11, 23, 25]. A notable exception is a report of an elderly woman who presented with a 6-month history of indolent symptoms and in whom the pathological diagnosis remained uncertain [26]. The tumor is generally confined to a single hemithorax, either right or left, although bilateral pleural effusion has been reported in a single case [27]. Both the mediastinal and peripheral aspects of the pleura may be involved, and simultaneous involvement of both has also been described [11, 25]. Less common thoracic presentations include a primarily intraparenchymal tumor with secondary pleural extension, as well as abdominal disease with subsequent pulmonary parenchymal metastases [8, 28].

Diagnosis

Computed tomography (CT) remains the primary and most important imaging modality for evaluating DSRCT. However, only a limited number of case reports have described the radiographic appearance of pleural DSRCT, and the reported findings are heterogeneous. Several reports describe the pleural mass as nodular or irregular, while a single case characterized it as round-edged (Fig. 23.1a) [30, 32, 33]. Late (venous)-

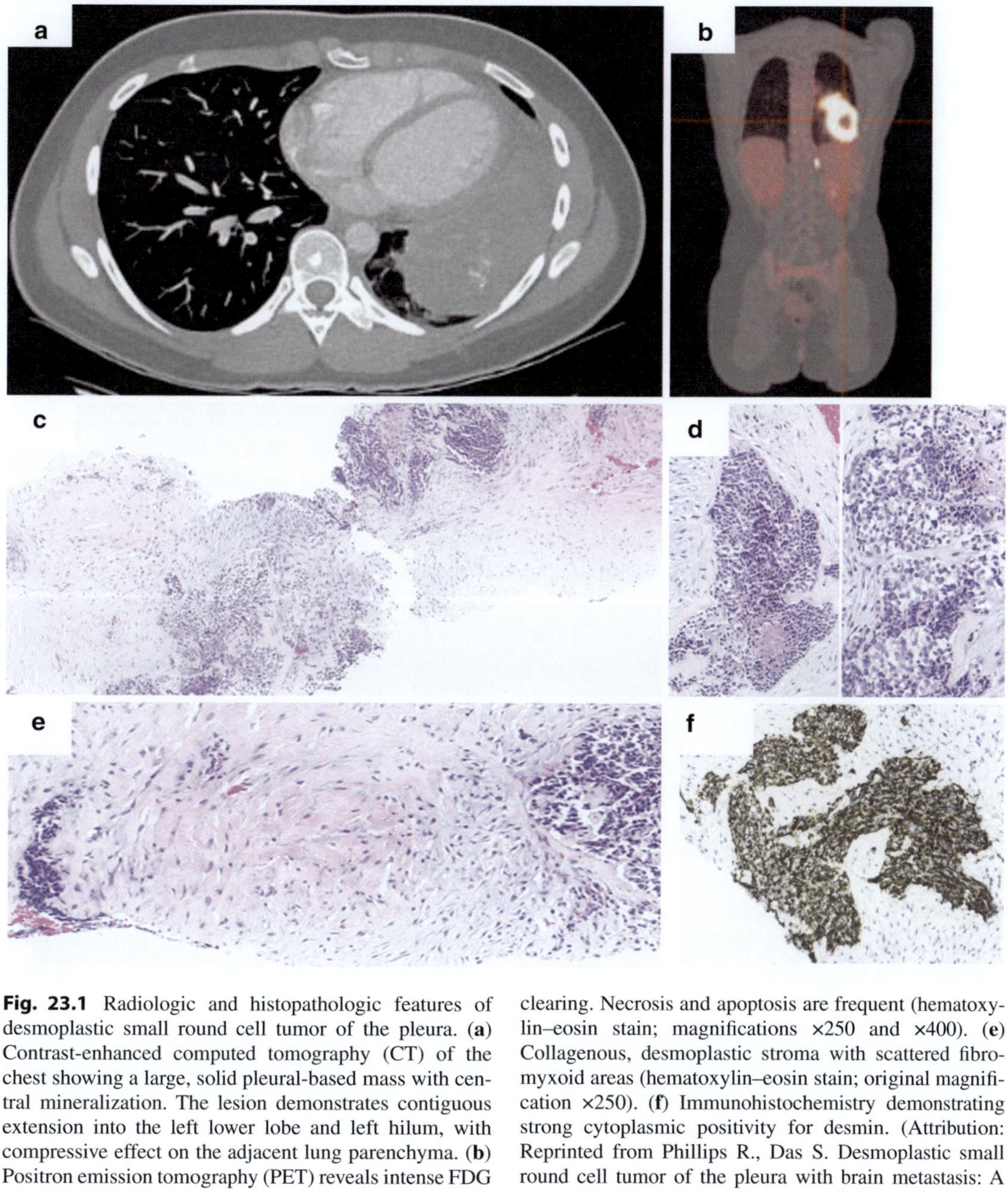

Fig. 23.1 Radiologic and histopathologic features of desmoplastic small round cell tumor of the pleura. (**a**) Contrast-enhanced computed tomography (CT) of the chest showing a large, solid pleural-based mass with central mineralization. The lesion demonstrates contiguous extension into the left lower lobe and left hilum, with compressive effect on the adjacent lung parenchyma. (**b**) Positron emission tomography (PET) reveals intense FDG uptake within the mass, with central regions of necrosis and calcification. (**c**) Histopathologic section showing densely cellular tumor nests separated by prominent desmoplastic stroma (hematoxylin–eosin stain; original magnification ×100). (**d**) Micronodular nests of round tumor cells with uniform nuclei, evenly dispersed chromatin, and inconspicuous nucleoli; some cells show perinuclear clearing. Necrosis and apoptosis are frequent (hematoxylin–eosin stain; magnifications ×250 and ×400). (**e**) Collagenous, desmoplastic stroma with scattered fibromyxoid areas (hematoxylin–eosin stain; original magnification ×250). (**f**) Immunohistochemistry demonstrating strong cytoplasmic positivity for desmin. (Attribution: Reprinted from Phillips R., Das S. Desmoplastic small round cell tumor of the pleura with brain metastasis: A case report and literature review. J Case Rep Images Pathol. 2023; 9(2): 5–12. © 2023 Rebecca Phillips et al. This article is distributed under the terms of the Creative Commons Attribution License, which permits unrestricted use, distribution, and reproduction in any medium, provided the original author(s) and publisher are properly credited)

phase contrast-enhanced CT is recommended, as the involved pleura demonstrates moderate enhancement, with Hounsfield unit (HU) values rising from 28 HU to 38 HU [26].

Gadolinium-enhanced magnetic resonance imaging (MRI) may reveal heterogeneous enhancement on T2-weighted scans, occasionally with central necrosis [30]. Although MRI can assist in differentiating sarcomas, including DSRCT, from cystic lesions or tumors of neural origin, such as schwannomas, it offers minimal additional diagnostic value compared with CT and is not recommended for routine evaluation of pleural DSRCT [31].

Like most sarcomas, DSRCT exhibits strong avidity for fluorodeoxyglucose on positron emission tomography (PET-FDG) in both thoracic and extra-thoracic disease sites (Fig. 23.1b) [32–34]. However, other neoplasms with pleural metastasis and malignant mesothelioma are also PET-FDG avid, which limits specificity [32]. The National Comprehensive Cancer Network (NCCN) Soft Tissue Sarcoma Guidelines recommend that staging evaluation prior to surgery should include PET-CT to define the full extent of disease involvement [35]. Routine brain imaging is not required, as brain metastases have not been reported in DSRCT and are exceedingly rare in other soft tissue sarcomas [36, 37]. However, currently, there is no universally accepted staging system for DSRCT in general, especially for pleural DSRCT.

Since radiologic features are insufficient for diagnosis, tissue sampling with histopathologic examination is required. Historically, pleural DSRCT was diagnosed primarily through surgical pleural biopsy and, in some cases, by transcutaneous fine-needle biopsy (FNB) [4]. However, the scarcity of cases makes it difficult to determine the sensitivity and specificity of pleural effusion sampling in this disease, and there are no published reports regarding the ability to detect the t(11;22)(p13;q12) translocation in pleural fluid [4].

In the past, a large surgical biopsy was often required for diagnosis; however, with advances in diagnostic techniques, fine-needle aspiration (FNA) has increasingly been shown to provide adequate material for diagnosis in many cases [23, 44]. In one series of patients with soft tissue sarcomas (STS), FNA demonstrated a sensitivity of 89% when compared with core needle biopsy (CNB) [44]. Surgical biopsies have since fallen out of favor, as several studies have reported high sensitivity rates of 85–97% for CNB in STS, comparable to those achieved with surgical biopsy [46, 48].

Concerns have been raised regarding the possibility of tumor seeding along the tract of a transcutaneous CNB. This phenomenon has been documented in other types of STS [45, 46], but it has not been shown to increase recurrence rates when compared with incisional biopsy [47]. Current NCCN guidelines do not specify a single preferred modality, but emphasize the importance of obtaining an adequate tissue sample. They recommend CNB or incisional, nonsurgical biopsy over surgical biopsy in cases where FNA is nondiagnostic or anticipated to yield insufficient material [39].

Pathology

Histologically, DSRST is characterized by a nest of poorly differentiated, round tumor cells, surrounded by an abundant, dense desmoplastic stroma (Fig. 23.1c–e). Neoplastic mimickers include other round cell sarcomas, small cell neuroendocrine tumors, and lymphoblastic lymphoma [38, 39]. Histopathological differentiation can be challenging to achieve due to the poorly differentiated morphology of the cells. Immunohistochemical staining and genetic evaluation are necessary for a definitive diagnosis [38, 40]. The tumor cells stain positively for various mesenchymal and neuroendocrine markers, namely vimentin, desmin, and neuron-specific enolase (NSE) (Fig. 23.1f). Negative stains include cytokeratins 7,8, and 20 [23]. The detection of the t(11;22)(p13;q12) translocation with *an EWSRI-WT1 gene fusion can be performed using fluorescence* in situ *hybridization (FISH)* and is unique for DSRCT. Cytology from a pleural effusion may show abnormally appearing small round cells, which stain positively for the nonspecific neoplastic marker desmin and vimentin [27, 41].

Treatment

Owing to the rarity of pleural DSRCT, no standardized treatment guidelines have been established. Therapeutic approaches have been documented in only ten reported cases. In nearly all instances, neoadjuvant chemotherapy served as the initial modality, typically administered for six cycles unless radiographic progression was observed during this interval. The most frequently utilized regimens were P6 (cyclophosphamide, doxorubicin, vincristine, ifosfamide, and etoposide) and Vincristine, Dactinomycin (Actinomycin D), Ifosfamide, and Doxorubicin (Adriamycin) (VAIA), both of which were adapted from established sarcoma treatment protocols. Surgical resection following neoadjuvant chemotherapy was performed in seven patients, although details regarding the surgical technique and extent of resection were not consistently provided. Radiation therapy was administered in five cases; however, information concerning total dose and treatment duration was not specified. Given the paucity of data, current management strategies are primarily extrapolated from therapeutic principles applied to peritoneal DSRCT and pleural malignancies, such as mesothelioma. It has been proposed that treatment strategies developed for abdominal DSRCT may also be reasonably extended to pleural presentations of the disease [42].

The authors recommend that the initial step entail classifying the disease as either limited or metastatic. In cases confined to the pleura and adjacent lung, where complete surgical resection is feasible, neoadjuvant chemotherapy should be administered. The chemotherapeutic agents employed are extrapolated from treatment regimens used in Ewing sarcoma (ES) and may include the P6 protocol or the VAIA regimen [43, 44]. These regimens are also endorsed by the National Comprehensive Cancer Network guidelines [35]. Response to neoadjuvant chemotherapy occurred in approximately 40–50% of patients with abdominal DSRCT [42, 44].

In cases demonstrating a favorable response to neoadjuvant chemotherapy, complete cytoreductive surgery (CCS) should be undertaken. In abdominal diseases, CCS is considered successful when no macroscopic tumor remains at the completion of surgery or when residual tumor implants measure less than 2.5 mm [42]. Successful cytoreduction has been shown to improve overall survival and progression-free survival compared with less extensive resections, with several studies reporting a hazard ratio for mortality of 0.6 [42, 45–47]. Although some degree of selection bias is inherent in these studies, achieving complete resection (R0 or R1) independently probably improves survival, rather than serving merely as a marker of less aggressive disease. Therefore, complete resection should be regarded as a primary therapeutic objective. To date, only seven cases of surgical management for pleural DSRCT have been published, and none has provided detailed descriptions of the surgical technique employed [4, 11, 26, 27, 29].

Given the aggressive nature of DSRCT, micrometastatic spread is considered virtually inevitable, as reflected by the high recurrence rate. This has prompted the use of consolidative treatment strategies, most commonly hyperthermic intraperitoneal chemotherapy (HIPEC) and postoperative whole-abdomen radiotherapy (WAR). HIPEC involves the instillation of heated chemotherapeutic agents into the serosal cavity, allowing for uniform distribution across the serosal surface and penetration to a depth of 1–3 mm while minimizing systemic absorption and associated toxicity [48, 49]. The most frequently used agent for abdominal DSRCT is cisplatin [43, 50, 51]. To date, no studies or case reports have described the application of HIPEC in the pleural setting (termed hyperthermic intrathoracic chemotherapy, HITHOC) for pleural DSRCT. Technical feasibility has been demonstrated in malignant mesothelioma, where HITHOC has shown acceptable safety and low complication rates; however, results are inconsistent, and no survival benefit has been demonstrated [52, 53]. A more detailed description of the technique and associated toxicities is available elsewhere [54]. In selected patients with abdominal DSRCT limited to the peritoneal cavity, without hepatic or distant metastases, and in whom R0 or R1 cytoreduction has been achieved,

HIPEC has been shown to more than double progression-free survival [47, 55]. Although current evidence does not support the use of HITHOC in pleural DSRCT, the approach appears biologically plausible and potentially justified, particularly as the unfavorable results in mesothelioma likely reflect the inherent chemoresistance of that tumor type [56]. Patients with abdominal DSRCT who develop pleural metastases should be considered inoperable, and management of such cases is addressed separately below.

Whole-abdomen radiotherapy has been used extensively in the management of abdominal DSRCT. However, no standardized guidelines exist regarding its precise application. Most centers recommend administering postoperative WAR within 2 months following cytoreductive surgery and HIPEC, likely to exploit the radiosensitizing effect of chemotherapy [57, 58]. As with HIPEC, WAR is not advised in cases of extra-peritoneal metastases [57, 58]. Current protocols generally prescribe a total dose of 30 Gy delivered in 20 fractions, with an additional boost of 6–24 Gy to areas of residual disease following incomplete resection (R1 or R2) [57–60]. Patients with disease involving both the abdomen and pleura should be regarded as inoperable and managed with systemic therapy alone, without radiotherapy. To date, only three cases of pleural DSRCT treated with radiotherapy have been reported, and none provided detailed information on dosage or technique. Given the radiosensitivity of DSRCT, adjuvant radiotherapy may improve outcomes in cases of fully resected pleural disease and can be administered at doses up to 54 Gy, although the risk of radiation pneumonitis must be carefully considered [61–63]. As in peritoneal DSRCT, radiotherapy in pleural DSRCT should ideally be delivered within 2 months of completing chemotherapy.

Metastatic or unresectable disease should initially be managed with first-line chemotherapy, most commonly the P6 or VAIA protocol. After an initial treatment course, typically 6 months in duration, patients should undergo reevaluation. If the disease remains unresectable or the patient is deemed unfit for surgery, second-line chemotherapy is indicated. Recommended regimens include temozolomide/irinotecan, cyclophosphamide/topotecan, and high-dose ifosfamide. A similar approach is advised when disease progression occurs during first-line therapy [64–67]. Non-chemotherapeutic agents have primarily been employed as salvage therapy or in patients with contraindications to standard agents. Pazopanib, a tyrosine kinase inhibitor targeting angiogenesis, has been reported to achieve disease control in a case of postsurgical recurrence of pleural DSRCT, as well as in a cohort of 29 patients with abdominal disease [11, 68]. Notable toxicities include leukopenia, thrombocytopenia, and renal impairment [68, 69]. The NCCN guidelines recommend pazopanib as an alternative first-line therapy for soft tissue sarcomas and as a second-line or salvage option for metastatic disease [35]. Autologous hematopoietic stem cell transplantation has been investigated as an adjunctive consolidative strategy, in combination with HIPEC and/or WAR, for abdominal DSRCT. However, studies have not demonstrated a significant survival benefit, and its role remains unproven [70, 71].

Prognosis

Abdominal DSRCT carries a poor prognosis, with reported 5-year overall survival (OS) rates ranging between 10% and 35% [42, 51, 59, 64]. Pleural DSRCT demonstrates similarly unfavorable outcomes, with an estimated 5-year OS of approximately 13% [4]. The precise impact of chemotherapy on survival remains difficult to quantify in the absence of controlled clinical trials; however, recurrence rates are high, and a substantial proportion of patients exhibit primary resistance to treatment.

The principal risk factors for mortality include unresectability at presentation due to extensive locally advanced or metastatic disease (hazard ratio [HR] = 5–7.8) and failure to achieve complete surgical resection (HR = 5.3) [72]. Additional poor prognostic indicators include elevated C-reactive protein and the presence of paraneoplastic thrombosis (Trousseau's syndrome) [44]. To date, individual patient characteristics have not been consistently shown to predict mortality reliably.

Future Directions

The poor outcomes associated with DSRCT highlight an unmet need for more effective therapeutic strategies, with particular emphasis on systemic therapy. The universal presence of the EWS–WT1 gene rearrangement in DSRCT suggests that candidate therapies may include agents targeting proteins within its downstream signaling cascade. Notable examples include T-cell acute lymphoblastic leukemia–associated antigen 1 (TALLA-1), which influences cell migration and metastasis, and equilibrative nucleoside transporter 4 (ENT4) [73, 74]. Experimental silencing of EWS–WT1 has been shown to induce tumor cell death, representing a promising therapeutic avenue [75].

An alternative strategy to direct gene targeting is the repurposing of drugs. In this context, biologic agents directed against tumor angiogenesis, as well as agents modulating pathways such as mTOR and DNA damage repair, have demonstrated encouraging in vitro activity, although in vivo validation is required [76, 77]. Several tyrosine kinase inhibitors (TKIs) beyond pazopanib, specifically those targeting VEGF, VEGFR, and PDGFRα, have also been explored clinically, with positive responses reported in individual case reports [78, 79].

References

1. Gerald WL, Rosai J. Case 2. Desmoplastic small cell tumor with divergent differentiation. Pediatr Pathol. 1989;9(2):177–83.
2. de Pinieux G, Karanian M, Le Loarer F, Le Guellec S, Chabaud S, Terrier P, et al. Nationwide incidence of sarcomas and connective tissue tumors of intermediate malignancy over four years using an expert pathology review network. PLoS One. 2021;16(2):e0246958.
3. Lettieri CK, Garcia-Filion P, Hingorani P. Incidence and outcomes of desmoplastic small round cell tumor: results from the surveillance, epidemiology, and end results database. J Cancer Epidemiol. 2014;2014:1–5.
4. Fois AG, Pirina P, Arcadu A, Becciu F, Manca S, Marras V, et al. Desmoplastic small round cell tumors of the pleura: a review of the clinical literature. Multidiscip Respir Med. 2017;12:22.
5. Kretschmar CS, Colbach C, Bhan I, Crombleholme TM. Desmoplastic small cell tumor: a report of three cases and a review of the literature. J Pediatr Hematol Oncol. 1996;18(3):293–8.
6. Sun M, Shao M, Jiang X, Yin T, Wang Q, Zhao L, et al. Desmoplastic small round cell tumor of the head and neck: a clinicopathological, immunohistochemical and molecular analysis of three cases with literature review. Int J Surg Pathol. 2023;31(5):742–50.
7. Galliani CA, Bisceglia M, Del Giudice A, Cretì G. Desmoplastic small round cell tumor of the kidney: report of a case, literature review, and comprehensive discussion of the distinctive morphologic, immunohistochemical, and molecular features in the differential diagnosis of small round cell tumors affecting the kidney. Adv Anat Pathol. 2020;27(6):408–21.
8. Muramatsu T, Shimamura M, Furuichi M, Nishii T, Takeshita S, Shiono M. Desmoplastic small round cell tumor of the lung. Ann Thorac Surg. 2010;90(6):e86–7.
9. Hayes-Jordan A, Anderson PM. The diagnosis and management of desmoplastic small round cell tumor: a review. Curr Opin Oncol. 2011;23(4):385–9.
10. Ouarssani A, Atoini F, Ait Lhou F, Rguibi Idrissi M. Desmoplastic small round cell tumor of the pleura. Thorac Cancer. 2011;2(3):117–9.
11. Ikeue T, Ohi I, Noguchi S, Fukao A, Terashita S, Horikawa S, et al. Desmoplastic small round cell tumor of the pleura successfully treated with a lower dose of pazopanib. Intern Med. 2016;55(17):2463–7.
12. Sawyer JR, Tryka AF, Lewis JM. A novel reciprocal chromosome translocation t(11,22)(p13;q12) in an intraabdominal desmoplastic small round-cell tumor. Am J Surg Pathol. 1992;16(4):411–6.
13. Rodriguez E, Sreekantaiah C, Gerald W, Reuter VE, Motzer RJ, Chaganti RSK. A recurring translocation, t(11;22)(p13;q11.2), characterizes intra-abdominal desmoplastic small round-cell tumors. Cancer Genet Cytogenet. 1993;69(1):17–21.
14. Lee SB, Kolquist KA, Nichols K, Englert C, Maheswaran S, Ladanyi M, et al. The EWS-WT1 translocation product induces PDGFA in desmoplastic small round-cell tumour. Nat Genet. 1997;17(3):309–13.
15. Wong JC, Lee SB, Bell MD, Reynolds PA, Fiore E, Stamenkovic I, et al. Induction of the interleukin-2/15 receptor beta-chain by the EWS-WT1 translocation product. Oncogene. 2002;21(13):2009–19.
16. Ramsay CH, Bodin NO, Hansson E. Absorption, distribution, biotransformation, and excretion of azidocillin, a new semi-synthetic penicillin, in mice, rats and dogs. Arzneimittelforschung. 1972;22(11):1962–70.
17. Worley BS, van den Broeke LT, Goletz TJ, Pendleton CD, Daschbach EM, Thomas EK, et al. Antigenicity of fusion proteins from sarcoma-

associated chromosomal translocations. Cancer Res. 2001;61(18):6868–75.
18. Devecchi A, De Cecco L, Dugo M, Penso D, Dagrada G, Brich S, et al. The genomics of desmoplastic small round cell tumor reveals the deregulation of genes related to DNA damage response, epithelial–mesenchymal transition, and immune response. Cancer Commun. 2018;38(1):1–14.
19. Shukla N, Ameur N, Yilmaz I, Nafa K, Lau CY, Marchetti A, et al. Oncogene mutation profiling of pediatric solid tumors reveals significant subsets of embryonal rhabdomyosarcoma and neuroblastoma with mutated genes in growth signaling pathways. Clin Cancer Res. 2012;18(3):748–57.
20. Ferreira EN, Barros BDF, de Souza JE, Almeida RV, Torrezan GT, Garcia S, et al. A genomic case study of desmoplastic small round cell tumor: comprehensive analysis reveals insights into potential therapeutic targets and development of a monitoring tool for a rare and aggressive disease. Hum Genomics. 2016;10(1):36.
21. La Starza R, Barba G, Nofrini V, Pierini T, Pierini V, Marcomigni L, et al. Multiple EWSR1-WT1 and WT1-EWSR1 copies in two cases of desmoplastic round cell tumor. Cancer Genet. 2013;206(11):387–92.
22. Silva JG, Corrales-Medina FF, Maher OM, Tannir N, Huh WW, Rytting ME, et al. Clinical next generation sequencing of pediatric-type malignancies in adult patients identifies novel somatic aberrations. Oncoscience. 2015;2(2):187–92.
23. Granja NM, Begnami MD, Bortolan J, Filho AL, Schmitt FC. Desmoplastic small round cell tumour: cytological and immunocytochemical features. Cytojournal. 2005;2(1):6.
24. Ostoros G, Orosz Z, Kovács G, Soltész I. Desmoplastic small round cell tumour of the pleura: a case report with unusual follow-up. Lung Cancer. 2002;36(3):333–6.
25. Jian Z, Shaohong H, Wenzhao Z, Lijia G. Misdiagnosed desmoplastic small round cell tumor of the pleura: case report and literature review. J Formos Med Assoc. 2014;113(1):60–1.
26. Cao Y, Chen Y, Yang LI, Qian ZH, Han SG, Li QH, et al. Desmoplastic small round cell tumor: a case report of a rare differential diagnosis of solid tumors of the pleura. Oncol Lett. 2015;10(5):2991–5.
27. Bian Y, Jordan AG, Rupp M, Cohn H, McLaughlin CJ, Miettinen M. Effusion cytology of desmoplastic small round cell tumor of the pleura. A case report. Acta Cytol. 1993;37(1):77–82.
28. Hou W, Dai J, Tian R. Metastatic pulmonary desmoplastic small round cell tumor on FDG PET/CT. Clin Nucl Med. 2023;48(9):828–9.
29. Parkash V, Gerald WL, Parma A, Miettinen M, Rosai J. Desmoplastic small round cell tumor of the pleura. Am J Surg Pathol. 1995;19(6):659–65.
30. Kis B, O'Regan KN, Agoston A, Javery O, Jagannathan J, Ramaiya NH. Imaging of desmoplastic small round cell tumour in adults. Br J Radiol. 2012;85(1010):187–92.
31. Zöllner SK, Amatruda JF, Bauer S, Collaud S, de Álava E, DuBois SG, et al. Ewing sarcoma-diagnosis, treatment, clinical challenges and future perspectives. J Clin Med. 2021;10(8):1685.
32. Dubreuil J, Giammarile F, Rousset P, Rubello D, Colletti PM, Glehen O, et al. 18F-FDG-PET/CT of peritoneal tumors: a pictorial essay. Nucl Med Commun. 2017;38(1):1–9.
33. Magnan H, Abramson SJ, Price AP, Grewal RK, Merchant MS, LaQuaglia MP, et al. Positron emission tomography for response assessment in desmoplastic small round cell tumor. J Pediatr Hematol Oncol. 2013;35(5):e190–3.
34. Ostermeier A, McCarville MB, Navid F, Snyder SE, Shulkin BL. FDG PET/CT imaging of desmoplastic small round cell tumor: findings at staging, during treatment and at follow-up. Pediatr Radiol. 2015;45(9):1308–15.
35. von Mehren M, et al. Soft tissue sarcoma, version 2.2022. J Natl Compr Canc Netw. 2022;20(7):815–33. https://doi.org/10.6004/jnccn.2022.0035.
36. Ogose A, Morita T, Hotta T, Kobayashi H, Otsuka H, Hirata Y, et al. Brain metastases in musculoskeletal sarcomas. Jpn J Clin Oncol. 1999;29(5):245–7.
37. Poh JZ. Secondary brain metastases of Ewing's sarcoma presenting with collapse after 6 years of complete remission. Clin Case Reports. 2021;9(1):560–5.
38. Domanski HA. The small round cell sarcomas complexities and desmoplastic presentation. Acta Cytol. 2022;66(4):279–94.
39. Wang LL, Ji ZH, Gao Y, Chang H, Sun PP, Li Y. Clinicopathological features of desmoplastic small round cell tumors: clinical series and literature review. World J Surg Oncol. 2021;19(1):193.
40. Sbaraglia M, Righi A, Gambarotti M, Dei Tos AP. Ewing sarcoma and Ewing-like tumors. Virchows Arch Int J Pathol. 2020;476(1):109–19.
41. Choi JK, van Hoeven K, Brooks JJ, Gupta PK. Desmoplastic small round cell tumor presenting in pleural fluid and accompanied by desmin-positive mesothelial cells. Acta Cytol. 1995;39(2):377–8.
42. Subbiah V, Lamhamedi-Cherradi SE, Cuglievan B, Menegaz BA, Camacho P, Huh W, et al. Multimodality treatment of desmoplastic small round cell tumor: chemotherapy and complete cytoreductive surgery improve patient survival. Clin Cancer Res. 2018;24(19):4865–73.
43. Reijers SJM, Siew CCH, Kok NFM, Honoré C, van Houdt WJ. Intra-abdominal desmoplastic small round cell tumor (DSRCT) and the role of hyperthermic intraperitoneal chemotherapy (HIPEC): a review. Curr Oncol Tor Ont. 2023;30(4):3951–63.
44. Scheer M, Vokuhl C, Blank B, Hallmen E, von Kalle T, Münter M, et al. Desmoplastic small round cell tumors: multimodality treatment and new risk factors. Cancer Med. 2019;8(2):527–42.
45. Lal DR, Su WT, Wolden SL, Loh KC, Modak S, La Quaglia MP. Results of multimodal treatment for desmoplastic small round cell tumors. J Pediatr Surg. 2005;40(1):251–5.

46. Zhang S, Zhang Y, Yu YH, Li J. Results of multimodal treatment for desmoplastic small round cell tumor of the abdomen and pelvis. Int J Clin Exp Med. 2015;8(6):9658–66.
47. Hayes-Jordan A, Green HL, Lin H, Owusu-Agyemang P, Fitzgerald N, Arunkumar R, et al. Complete cytoreduction and HIPEC improves survival in desmoplastic small round cell tumor. Ann Surg Oncol. 2014;21(1):220–4.
48. Kusamura S, Dominique E, Baratti D, Younan R, Deraco M. Drugs, carrier solutions and temperature in hyperthermic intraperitoneal chemotherapy. J Surg Oncol. 2008;98(4):247–52.
49. Sugarbaker PH, Van der Speeten K. Surgical technology and pharmacology of hyperthermic perioperative chemotherapy. J Gastrointest Oncol. 2016;7(1):29–44.
50. Sjoberg Bexelius T, Chisholm JC, Okoye B, Cecil T, Angelini P, Dayal S. Hyperthermic intraperitoneal chemotherapy (HIPEC) as another treatment modality for desmoplastic round cell tumour patients: first paediatric experience from UK. BMJ Case Rep. 2021;14(1):e234876.
51. Campos F, Coutinho DL, Silva MLG, Lopes A, Nascimento A, Aguiar Júnior S, et al. Clinical characteristics, management, and outcomes of 19 nonpediatric patients with desmoplastic small round cell tumor: a cohort of Brazilian patients. Sarcoma. 2020;2020:8713165.
52. Zhou H, Wu W, Tang X, Zhou J, Shen Y. Effect of hyperthermic intrathoracic chemotherapy (HITHOC) on the malignant pleural effusion: a systematic review and meta-analysis. Medicine (Baltimore). 2017;96(1):e5532.
53. Järvinen T, Paajanen J, Ilonen I, Räsänen J. Hyperthermic intrathoracic chemoperfusion for malignant pleural mesothelioma: systematic review and meta-analysis. Cancer. 2021;13(14):3637.
54. Campany ME, Reck Dos Santos PA, Donato BB, Alwardt CM, Ernani V, D'Cunha J, et al. Hyperthermic intrapleural chemotherapy: an update. J Thorac Dis. 2023;15(9):5064–73.
55. Hayes-Jordan AA, Coakley BA, Green HL, Xiao L, Fournier KF, Herzog CE, et al. Desmoplastic small round cell tumor treated with cytoreductive surgery and hyperthermic intraperitoneal chemotherapy: results of a phase 2 trial. Ann Surg Oncol. 2018;25(4):872–7.
56. Terenziani R, Zoppi S, Fumarola C, Alfieri R, Bonelli M. Immunotherapeutic approaches in malignant pleural mesothelioma. Cancer. 2021;13(11):2793.
57. Osborne EM, Briere TM, Hayes-Jordan A, Levy LB, Huh WW, Mahajan A, et al. Survival and toxicity following sequential multimodality treatment including whole abdominopelvic radiotherapy for patients with desmoplastic small round cell tumor. Radiother Oncol. 2016;119(1):40–4.
58. Bronshteĭn IE, Korenkov IP, Liberman AN, Orobeĭ VV, Shurupov SB. Radiation safety in using current x-ray analytical devices. Gig Tr Prof Zabol. 1990;7:51–3.
59. Honoré C, Amroun K, Vilcot L, Mir O, Domont J, Terrier P, et al. Abdominal desmoplastic small round cell tumor: multimodal treatment combining chemotherapy, surgery, and radiotherapy is the best option. Ann Surg Oncol. 2015;22(4):1073–9.
60. Desai NB, Stein NF, LaQuaglia MP, Alektiar KM, Kushner BH, Modak S, et al. Reduced toxicity with intensity modulated radiation therapy (IMRT) for desmoplastic small round cell tumor (DSRCT): an update on the whole abdominopelvic radiation therapy (WAP-RT) experience. Int J Radiat Oncol Biol Phys. 2013;85(1):e67–72.
61. Giraud P, Sylvestre A, Zefkili S, Lisbona A, Bonnette P, Le Pimpec Barthes F, et al. Helical tomotherapy for resected malignant pleural mesothelioma: dosimetric evaluation and toxicity. Radiother Oncol J Eur Soc Ther Radiol Oncol. 2011;101(2):303–6.
62. Alley EW, Katz SI, Cengel KA, Simone CB. Immunotherapy and radiation therapy for malignant pleural mesothelioma. Transl Lung Cancer Res. 2017;6(2):212–9.
63. Rosenzweig KE, Zauderer MG, Laser B, Krug LM, Yorke E, Sima CS, et al. Pleural intensity-modulated radiotherapy for malignant pleural mesothelioma. Int J Radiat Oncol Biol Phys. 2012;83(4):1278–83.
64. Hayes-Jordan A, LaQuaglia MP, Modak S. Management of desmoplastic small round cell tumor. Semin Pediatr Surg. 2016;25(5):299–304.
65. Kushner BH, LaQuaglia MP, Wollner N, Meyers PA, Lindsley KL, Ghavimi F, et al. Desmoplastic small round-cell tumor: prolonged progression-free survival with aggressive multimodality therapy. J Clin Oncol. 1996;14(5):1526–31.
66. Meyer-Burg J, Mielke F, Arbeiter G. Peritoneoscopic and morphological aspects of the surface lymphatic vessels of the liver (author's transl). Leber Magen Darm. 1974;4(6):280–91.
67. Chicago Consensus Working Group. The Chicago consensus on peritoneal surface malignancies: management of desmoplastic small round cell tumor, breast, and gastrointestinal stromal tumors. Ann Surg Oncol. 2020;27(6):1793–7.
68. Menegaz BA, Cuglievan B, Benson J, Camacho P, Lamhamedi-Cherradi SE, Leung CH, et al. Clinical activity of pazopanib in patients with advanced desmoplastic small round cell tumor. Oncologist. 2018;23(3):360–6.
69. Frezza AM, Benson C, Judson IR, Litiere S, Marreaud S, Sleijfer S, et al. Pazopanib in advanced desmoplastic small round cell tumours: a multi-institutional experience. Clin Sarcoma Res. 2014;4:7.
70. Siddiqui A, Pinto N, Applebaum MA, Mak GZ, Cunningham JM, LaBelle JL, et al. The addition of autologous stem cell transplantation to neoadjuvant chemotherapy, radiation, and HIPEC for patients with unresectable desmoplastic small round cell tumor: a single center case series. Int J Surg Oncol. 2020;5(6):e95.

71. Bailey K, Roth M, Weiser D, Gill J. High-dose chemotherapy with stem cell rescue in desmoplastic small round cell tumor: a single-institution experience and review of the literature. Sarcoma. 2018;2018:1948093.
72. Stiles ZE, Dickson PV, Glazer ES, Murphy AJ, Davidoff AM, Behrman SW, et al. Desmoplastic small round cell tumor: a nationwide study of a rare sarcoma. J Surg Oncol. 2018;117(8):1759–67.
73. Ito E, Honma R, Imai J i, Azuma S, Kanno T, Mori S, et al. A tetraspanin-family protein, T-cell acute lymphoblastic leukemia-associated antigen 1, is induced by the Ewing's sarcoma-Wilms' tumor 1 fusion protein of desmoplastic small round-cell tumor. Am J Pathol. 2003;163(6):2165–72.
74. Li H, Smolen GA, Beers LF, Xia L, Gerald W, Wang J, et al. Adenosine transporter ENT4 is a direct target of EWS/WT1 translocation product and is highly expressed in desmoplastic small round cell tumor. PLoS One. 2008;3(6):e2353.
75. Gedminas JM, Chasse MH, McBrairty M, Beddows I, Kitchen-Goosen SM, Grohar PJ. Desmoplastic small round cell tumor is dependent on the EWS-WT1 transcription factor. Oncogene. 2020;9(4):41.
76. Subbiah V, Brown RE, Jiang Y, Buryanek J, Hayes-Jordan A, Kurzrock R, et al. Morphoproteomic profiling of the mammalian target of rapamycin (mTOR) signaling pathway in desmoplastic small round cell tumor (EWS/WT1), Ewing's sarcoma (EWS/FLI1) and Wilms' tumor(WT1). PLoS One. 2013;8(7):e68985.
77. Magnan HD, Price A, Chou AJ, Riedel E, Wexler LH, Ambati SR, et al. A pilot trial of irinotecan, temozolomide and bevacizumab (ITB) for treatment of newly diagnosed patients with desmoplastic small round cell tumor (DSRCT). J Clin Oncol. 2017;35(15_suppl):11050.
78. Bétrian S, Bergeron C, Blay JY, Bompas E, Cassier PA, Chevallier L, et al. Antiangiogenic effects in patients with progressive desmoplastic small round cell tumor: data from the French national registry dedicated to the use of off-labeled targeted therapy in sarcoma (OUTC'S). Clin Sarcoma Res. 2017;7:10.
79. Shi C, Feng Y, Zhang LC, Ding DY, Yan MY, Pan L. Effective treatment of apatinib in desmoplastic small round cell tumor: a case report and literature review. BMC Cancer. 2018;18(1):338.

Pleuropulmonary Erdheim-Chester Disease

24

Steven Tessier, Ronald S. Go, and Jay H. Ryu

Introduction

Erdheim-Chester disease (ECD) was first documented in 1930 by the American physician William Chester (1903–1974), a fellowship trainee of the pathologist Jakob Erdheim (1874–1937) at the University of Vienna [1]. Chester's paper, written in German, described two cases involving a unique form of "lipoid-granulomatosis" he considered distinct from Hand-Schüller-Christian disease (now known as Langerhans cell histiocytosis (LCH)) [2]. Thirty-four years later, the Norwegian physician Sörenson published a similar unusual case, which, upon review by Jaffe for his book on diseases of bones and joints in 1972, inspired the view that these cases collectively represented the same disease [3, 4]. Jaffe's book included an additional case and was enriched by numerous pathological specimens from Erdheim's collection [4]. Paying homage to its discoverers, Jaffe coined the eponym Erdheim-Chester disease (ECD).

For many years, ECD remained an obscure entity, overlooked by its rarity and diverse clinical manifestations. Its cause was unknown. Leading pathogenetic hypotheses included lipid storage and inflammatory disease [5–7]. An underlying immunopathogenesis was supported by the discovery of elevated cytokine-chemokine networks in patients with ECD, akin to profiles reported in rheumatologic diseases [8–11]. Advances in molecular-genetic research later revealed that ECD is a myeloid neoplasm arising from the monocytic lineage [12, 13]. The narrative of ECD is thus historical and contemporary; inflammatory and neoplastic. Treatment options were initially limited in their focus on modulating inflammation (i.e., steroids, interferon [IFN]-α, cytokine blockade). Today, a variety of targeted and systemic therapies are used with increasing success.

S. Tessier (✉)
Department of Internal Medicine, Mayo Clinic, Rochester, MN, USA
e-mail: Tessier.Steven@mayo.edu

R. S. Go
Division of Hematology, Department of Internal Medicine, Mayo Clinic, Rochester, MN, USA
e-mail: Go.Ronald@mayo.edu

J. H. Ryu
Division of Pulmonary and Critical Care Medicine, Department of Internal Medicine, Mayo Clinic, Rochester, MN, USA
e-mail: Ryu.Jay@mayo.edu

Origins and Pathophysiology

ECD is caused by multiorgan accumulation and infiltration of clonal non-Langerhans histiocytes. Clonality is typically driven by gain-of-function somatic mutations in proto-oncogenes within the MAPK-ERK or PI3K-AKT pathways (Fig. 24.1), which are key in the regulation of various cellular processes including growth, survival, differ-

F. Ido (ed.), *Rare Pleural Diseases*, https://doi.org/10.1007/978-3-032-14873-5_24

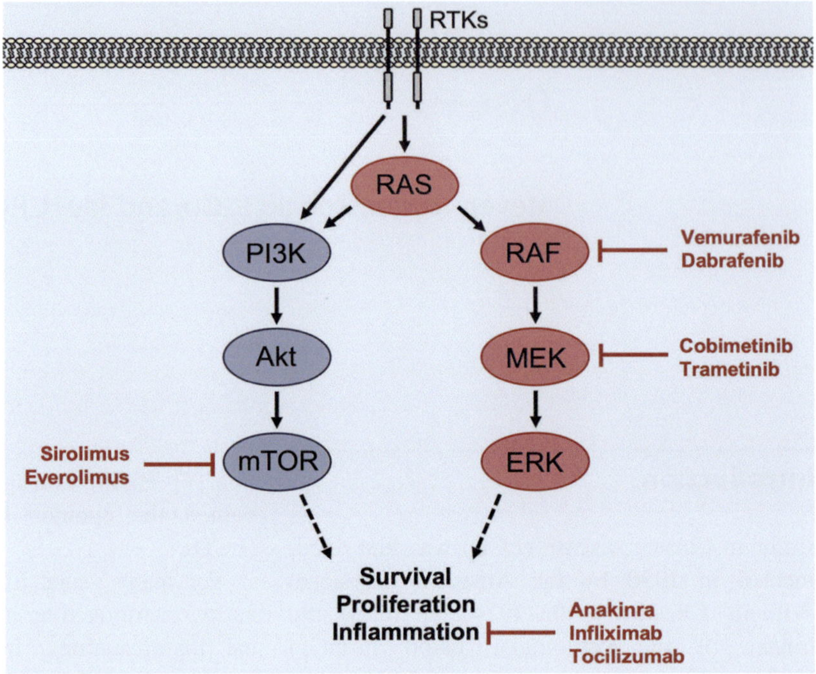

Fig. 24.1 Schematic showing the molecular basis of ECD and the established treatment targets of the MAPK-ERK and PI3K-AKT pathways. (Attribution: Original image courtesy of *Dr. Steven Tessier*. This figure has not been previously published and are reproduced here with permission of the author)

entiation, and metabolism. *BRAF*^{V600E} is the most common mutation (approximately 50-60%), affecting more than half of patients with ECD [14]. The BRAF mutation often occurs with a very low variant allele frequency (VAF) [15]. BRAF is an intracellular serine-threonine kinase involved in the MAPK signaling cascade. This signal transduction pathway is activated by growth factor stimulation of membrane tyrosine kinase receptors. *BRAF*^{V600E} results in constitutive activation of RAS, which in turn activates the downstream MEK-ERK pathway independent of MAPK, promoting cell proliferation and survival. Other pathogenic mutations have been reported in *MAP2K1*, *KRAS*, *NRAS*, *ARAF*, *PIK3CA*, and *CSF1R* (macrophage colony-stimulating factor receptor), all of which are implicated in the MAPK-ERK or PI3K-AKT pathways (CSF1R can activate both pathways through its receptor activity) [12, 16]. Translocations involving *BRAF*, *ALK*, and *NTRK1* are also rarely implicated [12]. The oncogenic mutations that drive ECD likely originate in the bone marrow hematopoietic stem cells [17, 18]. There is also evidence that ECD involvement of the central nervous system derives from the yolk sac erythro-myeloid progenitors of microglia [19].

The paradigms of oncogenesis and immunopathogenesis in ECD may be unified by an intrinsic cellular response called the oncogene-induced senescence (OIS) program [23]. In OIS, upon detection of oncogenic signaling, the cell compensates by increasing tumor-suppressor genes such as P16^{Ink4a} (cell cycle inhibitor), thereby entering a state of senescence. P16^{Ink4a} is a strong inducer of pro-inflammatory genes. Cells with the *BRAF*^{V600E} mutation have been shown to produce a wide variety of cytokines (i.e., interleukin [IL]-1β, IL-6, tumor necrosis factor [TNF]-α, IFN-γ, C-C motif chemokine ligand 2 [CCL2], CCL4, C-X-C motif chemokine ligand 8 [CXCL8], CXCL10); likewise, patients with ECD are known to have elevated levels of inflammatory markers such as C-reactive protein (CRP), IL-6, IL-12, IFN-α, and monocyte chemoattractant protein 1 (MCP-1) [10, 11, 20, 21]. In patients with ECD, BRAF^{V600E}-mutated histiocytes are histochemically positive for P16^{Ink4a} [22]. This pro-inflammatory milieu, likely driven by senescent ECD monocytes and histiocytes, may attract circulating inflammatory cells to the locations of disease involvement and sustain the senescent phenotype among infiltrating cells [23]. Such a hypothesis is consistent with the typically slow-growing cadence of ECD.

Epidemiology

ECD is usually diagnosed in adults 40-60 years-of-age with a male predominance (60–75%) [20, 24–26]. Pediatric cases are exceedingly rare [27]. These trends remain true in patients with pleuropulmonary involvement [28, 29]. National registries suggest an incidence rate of 0.9 to 3.5 per 10 million, although this is likely underestimated as the data obtained were primarily from referral centers (thus not including non-referred cases), due to the COVID-19 pandemic, and poor recognition of ECD resulting in undiagnosed cases [26, 30].

Clinical Features

ECD manifests as a wide spectrum of presentations (Fig. 24.2). The most common symptom is bone pain in the arms and legs, as symmetric osteosclerosis of long bones is almost always present (95%) (Fig. 24.2a–c) [24, 25, 31, 32]. Constitutional symptoms include fevers, night sweats, weight loss, and fatigue. Respiratory symptoms may result from pleuropulmonary disease (30–50%) (Fig. 24.3) [24, 25, 28, 32]. Depending on the severity and degree of progression, patients may be asymptomatic or experience chronic dry cough, shortness of breath, and chest tightness. In advanced pleuropulmonary disease, supplemental oxygen for hypoxic respiratory failure may be required [24, 25, 28, 32]. Infiltration of the orbits (30%) (Fig. 24.2d) may cause disturbances in vision, exophthalmos, redness of the eyes, and eye pain [24, 25, 32, 33]. Impaired balance, coordination, speech, and swallowing manifest due to central nervous system involvement (40%), particularly of the cerebellum and brainstem (Fig. 24.2e) [24, 25, 32, 34]. The cerebral white matter, dura, and pituitary stalk can also be affected (Fig. 24.2f, g) [34]. Complaints of polyuria and polydipsia arise from central diabetes insipidus (40%) [24, 25, 32]. Other endocrine abnormalities include panhypopituitarism, hypogonadism (Fig. 24.2q), and adrenal insufficiency [35]. In about 25% of cases, xanthelasma-like and papulonodular skin lesions usually develop around the eyes or on the face, neck, and inguinal folds, although other areas may also be affected (Fig. 24.2h, k) [24, 25, 32, 36]. In rare instances, the breast tissue may be involved (Fig. 24.2n) [37]. Pericardial, myocardial, and right atrial and atrioventricular groove infiltration (40–70%) may present as arrhythmias, valve disease, and heart failure (Fig. 24.2i, j) [24, 25, 32, 38]. Arterial infiltration manifests most characteristically as a "coated aorta" or periaortic thickening, but may also involve the branches of the aortic trunk as well as the coronary and visceral arteries (Fig. 24.2l) [24, 25, 32, 39]. Hypertension due to renal artery stenosis and cardiac ischemia are notable consequences [39]. Within the retroperitoneum (40–50%), "hairy kidneys" or perinephric encasement are conspicuous findings, and obstructive renal disease may develop from invasion of the renal pelvis or ureters (Fig. 24.2m, o) [24, 25, 32, 40]. Hepatomegaly and hepatic infiltration are rare occurrences, although liver decompensation secondary to progressive ECD has been reported (Fig. 24.2p) [24, 41, 42].

Patients with classical bone manifestations tend to have the *BRAF*^{V600E} mutation, whereas patients without these manifestations (non-classical-ECD) tend to have other mutations that affect the MEK-ERK pathway [43]. About 10–15% of patients with ECD have an additional myeloid neoplasm, the most common of which is chronic myelomonocytic leukemia [15, 44]. Indeed, almost half of patients with ECD display evidence of clonal hematopoiesis. The most frequent mutations are strongly implicated in myeloid clonal evolution, including *TET2*, *ASXL1*, *DNMT3A*, and *NRAS* [15].

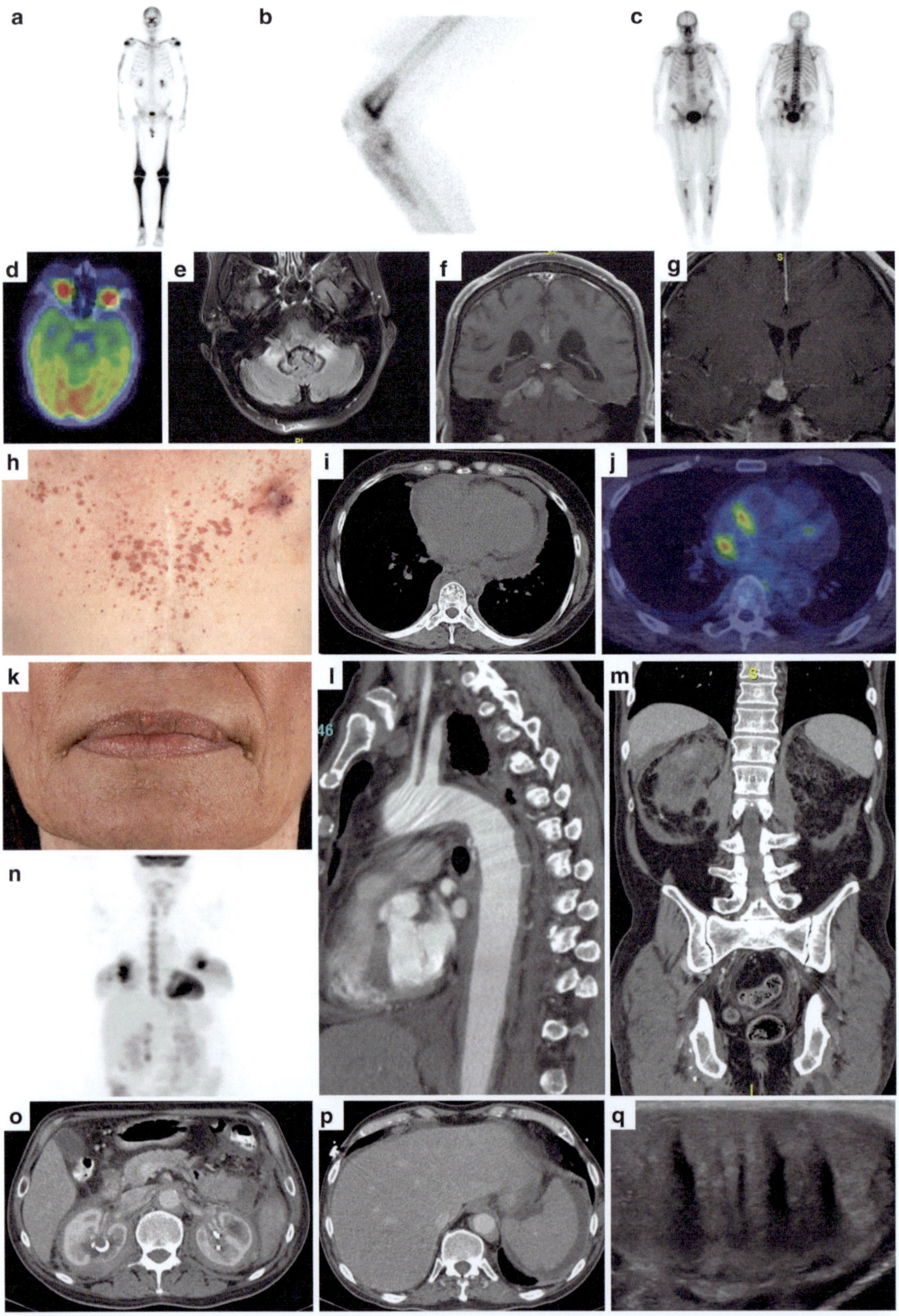

(continued)

Fig. 24.2 (**a, b**) ^{99}Tc bone scans showing classical radiotracer uptake of the distal femur and proximal tibia. (**c**) ^{99}Tc bone scan showing atypical radiotracer uptake of the axial skeleton. (**d**) PET scan showing intense FDG uptake within intraconal soft tissue densities in both orbits. (**e**) Brain MRI of T2 hyperintense signal within both anteromedial cerebellar hemispheres near the bilateral middle cerebellar peduncles. (**f**), T1 brain MRI of nodular enhancing tissue along the free edges of the tentorium. (**g**) T2 brain MRI of an enhancing hypothalamic mass. (**h, k**) Scattered xanthelasma-like and papulonodular skin lesions on the chest and face. (**i**) CT scan showing pericardial thickening and effusion. (**j**) PET scan showing FDG uptake within the right atrium. (**o**) ^{99}Tc uptake in the bilateral breasts. (**l**), CT angiography showing encasement of the aorta and great vessels. (**m**), CT scan showing extensive retroperitoneal fibrosis. (**n**) PET scan showing FDG uptake in the bilateral breasts. (**o**), CT scan showing perinephric fibrosis. (**p**) CT scan showing hepatomegaly and retroperitoneal involvement. (**q**) Ultrasound showing hypoechoic infiltrative process in testes. All images were obtained from patients with biopsy-proven ECD. (Attribution: Original image courtesy of *Dr. Steven Tessier*. This figure has not been previously published and are reproduced here with permission of the author)

Pleural Involvement

Pulmonary parenchymal involvement frequently occurs simultaneously with pleural disease (Fig. 24.3) [28]. However, the true prevalence of pleural disease in ECD is not known. A reasonable estimate based on existing small cohort studies is 30%, with reports as low as 11% and as high as 63% [20, 28, 29, 45, 46]. Pleural effusions are the most common presentation (Fig. 24.3a), occurring unilaterally or bilaterally, and rarely with loculations (Fig. 24.3g) [47, 48]. Pleural thickening usually presents with concurrent pleural effusions, likely due to impaired pleural fluid reabsorption by the affected visceral pleura [47, 48]. Both diffuse thickening and focal pleural lesions have been described (Fig. 24.3b–f). Diffuse thickening typically involves the visceral pleura only, distributed symmetrically and circumferentially, often with extension into the major fissures (Fig. 24.3b–f) [28, 29, 45, 48–50]. Isolated pleural lesions and masses are rare but do occur (Fig. 24.3e, j) [46–48, 51].

Sites such as bone, skin, and the retroperitoneum tend to be preferentially biopsied for diagnostic confirmation of ECD due to their relative ease of access. Therefore, there is a paucity of literature on the histopathology of the affected pleura. The few existing reports and our review of Mayo Clinic cases (Minnesota, Arizona, Florida) suggest that the visceral pleura is thickened by fibrohistiocytic infiltrate with features similar to those described in the lung (Fig. 24.4a, b) [49, 52]. The involved areas tend to lack fibroblast proliferation and are occupied by large foamy histiocytes and multinucleated giant (Touton) cells [49]. These histiocytes are immunohistochemically positive for CD68, CD163, CD14, and factor XIIIa [51]. CD1a and langerin (CD207) are negative, while these markers are positive in LCH [52]. The dendritic cell marker S-100 may be seen in both ECD and LCH, although it is less common in ECD [52, 53]. The areas of fibrohistiocytosis are accompanied by infiltration of additional inflammatory cells, including small lymphocytes, plasma cells, and rare eosinophils [29, 48, 52].

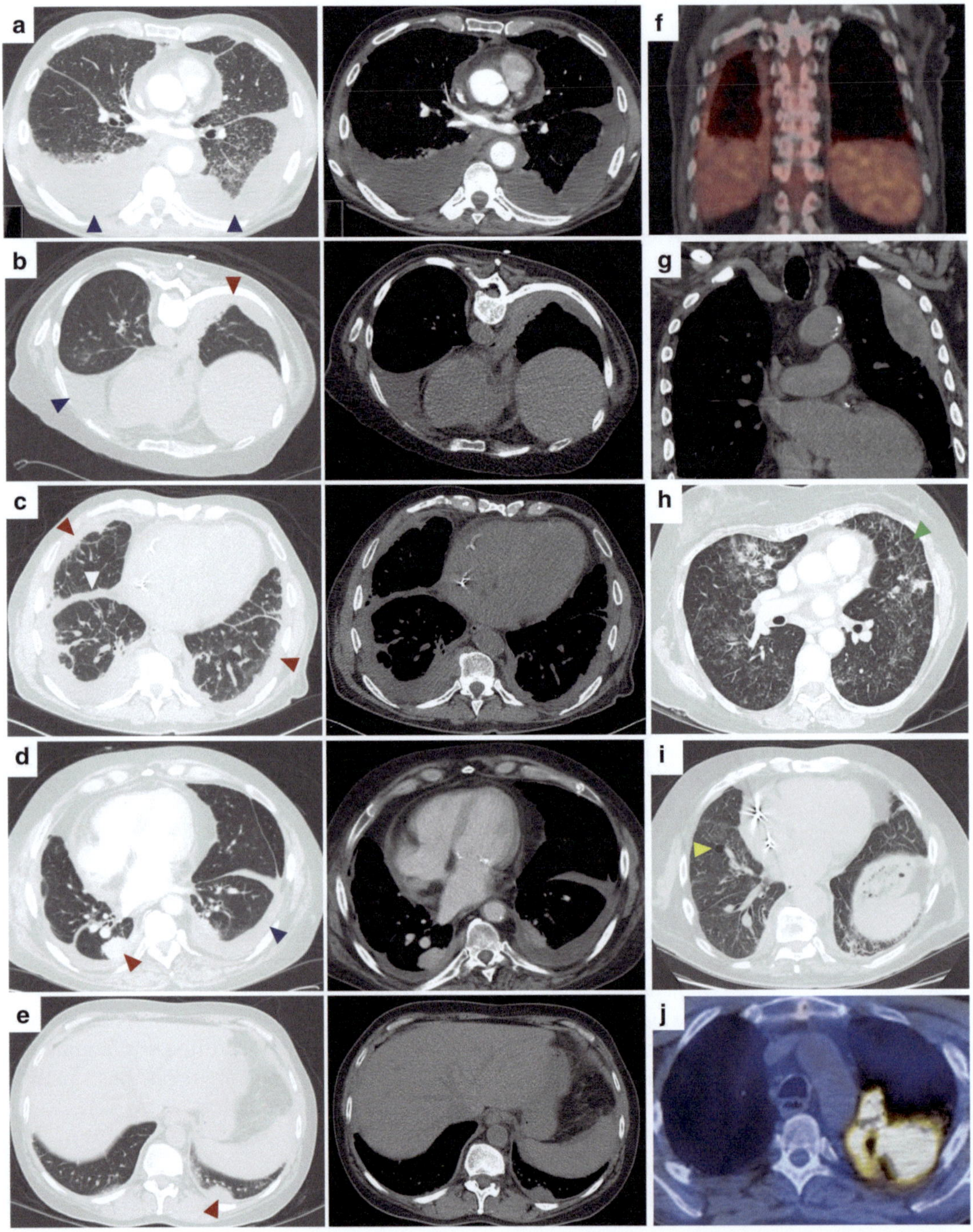

Fig. 24.3 (**a–e**), Chest CT scans showing pleural thickening (red arrowheads), pleural effusions (blue arrowheads), and fissural thickening (white arrowhead) on lung (left column) and mediastinal (right column) windows. (**f**) PET scan diffuse FDG activity in the right thickened pleura. (**g**) CT scan showing a left loculated pleural effusion left upper chest laterally. (**h**) CT scan showing bilateral parenchymal consolidative opacities and interlobular thickening (green arrowhead). (**i**) CT scan showing a thin-walled cyst (yellow arrowhead). (**j**) PET scan showing FDG uptake within a large pulmonary mass. All images were obtained from patients with biopsy-proven ECD. (Attribution: Original image courtesy of *Dr. Steven Tessier*. This figure has not been previously published and are reproduced here with permission of the author)

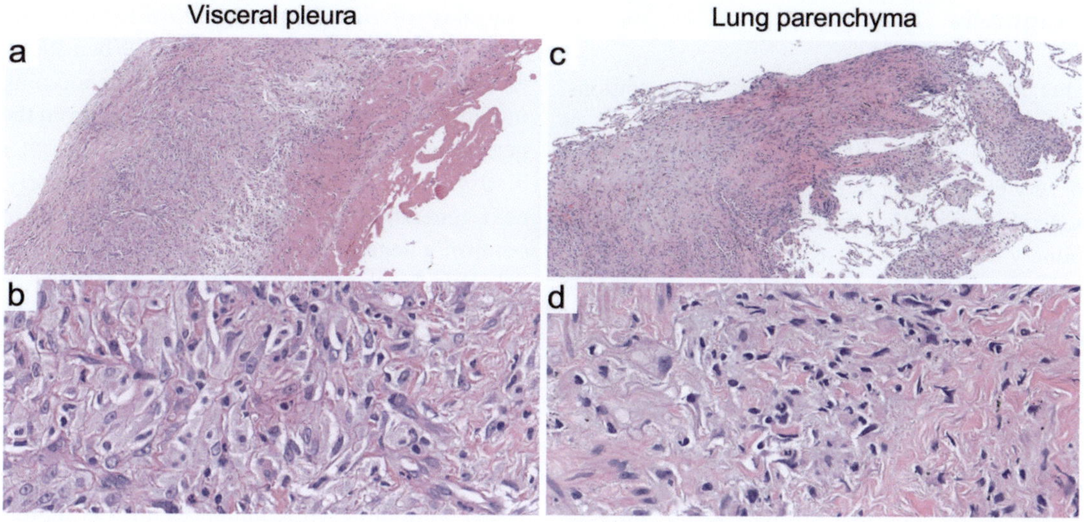

Fig. 24.4 (**a**, **b**) Biopsy of the thickened visceral pleura stained with hematoxylin and eosin showing organizing fibrinous pleuritis and accumulated foamy histiocytes. (**c**, **d**) Wedge biopsy of the lung stained with hematoxylin and eosin showing involvement by atypical histiocytic proliferation. The panels are shown in 5X (**a**, **c**) and 40X (**b**, **d**) magnification. (Attribution: Original image courtesy of *Dr. Steven Tessier*. This figure has not been previously published and are reproduced here with permission of the author)

Pulmonary Involvement

The clinicopathologic presentation of pulmonary disease in ECD is diverse and results from histiocytic infiltration of the lung parenchyma. Pulmonary function testing frequently reveals a restrictive pattern with impaired diffusion capacity, although normal, obstructive, and mixed patterns have been reported [24, 28, 29].

The most common radiologic finding is an interstitial lung disease-like pattern. Involvement is usually bilateral and diffuse, although focally limited disease can occur. Dominant features on chest high-resolution computed tomography (HRCT) include symmetric reticular opacities, smooth thickening of the interlobular septa and fissures, multifocal ground-glass opacities, centrilobular nodular opacities, and traction bronchiectasis [28, 29, 48, 50]. Hilar and mediastinal lymphadenopathy may be observed. Thin-walled cysts are sometimes present, distinguished from Langerhans cell histiocytosis (LCH) by their smaller size and random distribution [29]. Cystic lung disease in ECD is much less likely to be associated with pneumothorax compared to LCH [29]. These radiologic findings correspond with histological fibrohistiocytosis that follows a lymphatic distribution, infiltrates the bronchovascular bundles, and thickens the interlobular septa and fissures (Fig. 24.4c, d) [29, 49, 52].

Mediastinal Involvement

ECD can infiltrate any compartment of the mediastinum, occurring in about 25–60% of cases [24, 45]. Periarortic encasement is a classical presentation. Any aortic segment can be affected, with extension around the supraaortic trunk, its branches, and mediastinal fat, as well as into the retroperitoneum [39, 45, 54]. These lesions display moderate FDG uptake on PET scan and gadolinium enhancement on MRI [55]. Aortic aneurysm and ectasia are seldom complications [39]. Mediastinal lymphadenopathy has been observed in multiple cases, but is a less common finding [29, 30, 51]. Rare presentations include the development of an anterior mediastinal mass, mimicking thymic neoplasia, and infiltration of the pre-vertebral space [56, 57].

Diagnosis

Due to its rarity, heterogeneous presentations, and mimicry of other disease entities such as lymphoma and sarcoidosis, the diagnosis of ECD is very challenging to make. The combination of several diagnostic modalities and multidisciplinary evaluation is usually required. Tissue biopsy confirmation is strongly recommended to establish the diagnosis, rule out other possible diagnoses, and provide tissue for genotyping analysis. Multiple biopsy modalities have been successful, including video-assisted thoracoscopic surgery, CT-guided interventional radiology, thoracotomy, and bronchoscopy; however, it should be recalled that a robust histopathologic diagnosis is more likely to be obtained with a large tissue sample. There is very little data on the utility of bronchoalveolar lavage. When biopsy does not reveal characteristic fibrohistiocytosis, or when *BRAF* mutations are negative, the diagnosis should still be pursued if the clinicoradiologic presentation is highly suggestive of ECD [58].

Full-body (vertex to toe) fluorodeoxyglucose positron emission tomography (FDG PET)-CT is recommended to evaluate organ involvement and characterize disease burden. When PET-CT is not available or feasible, contrast-enhanced CT of the chest, abdomen, and pelvis should be obtained in conjunction with imaging of the lower extremities by CT, magnetic resonance imaging (MRI), or technetium-99 (^{99}Tc) bone scan [96]. Bone lesions are best identified by ^{99}Tc bone scan; however, PET imaging is more useful for surveillance and treatment response assessment [49, 59]. All patients diagnosed with ECD should undergo an MRI of the brain and heart. Select patients should also undergo high-resolution CT of the chest with pulmonary function testing, MRI of the orbits, renal artery ultrasound, and testicular ultrasound [58].

Laboratory testing should include an assessment of kidney function and cytopenias, CRP, and baseline levels of cortisol, GH, prolactin, TSH, LH, and FSH. Bone marrow biopsy should also be considered to evaluate the possibility of an additional myeloid neoplasm [58]. Given the low VAF of *BRAF* mutations, *BRAF* mutation testing is often falsely negative [60]. When *BRAF* testing is negative, an alternative genotyping modality such as cell-free DNA analysis from the peripheral blood and genotyping of another biopsy site should be pursued [58, 61]. Similarly, next-generation sequencing should be used to confirm a negative result by immunohistochemical testing with anti-*BRAF*^{V600E} (VE1) [62].

Treatment

Systemic therapy is needed in the majority of patients with ECD. Targeted therapies include BRAF inhibitors, MEK inhibitors, mTOR inhibitors, tyrosine kinase inhibitors, and immunosuppressive agents (Fig. 24.1). In patients with multisystemic *BRAF*-positive ECD and evidence of organ dysfunction, including pleuropulmonary disease, BRAF inhibition with vemurafenib or dabrafenib is mainstay therapy [63–70]. In certain cases where organ dysfunction is not apparent, it is reasonable to proceed with immunosuppressive or cytotoxic agents, so as to avoid BRAF inhibitor toxicities (skin photosensitivity, hyperkeratosis, other rashes, dysesthesia, joint pain, fatigue, secondary neoplasia, pancreatitis, and sarcoidosis) [71–74]. MEK inhibitors can be used in patients who are *BRAF*-negative and bear mutations in the MEK-ERK pathway, or in combination with BRAF inhibitors in patients who do not fully respond to BRAF inhibition alone [75–77]. Synergistic effects of BRAF-MEK inhibition have been reported; however, the prescribing provider must be wary of toxicity, particularly involving the skin [78, 79].

When first-line targeted therapies are not available, interferon-alpha (IFN-α) is a reasonable option. It should be noted that reports focusing on the ability of IFN-α to improve pleuropulmonary disease are lacking. Response rates appear greatest in CNS and cardiac lesions [80–82]. Intolerable side effects are a notable barrier to IFN-α therapy as patients may experience fatigue, arthralgias, myalgias, and depression with suicidal ideation [83]. The interleukin-1 (IL-1) inhibitor anakinra has demonstrated efficacy in pleural disease and is a viable option, although the limited data show significant variation in responses [84, 85]. Anakinra has also been used to dampen the inflammatory side effects of BRAF and MEK inhibition, enabling retention of first-line therapy [86]. mTOR inhibitors may be considered in patients with refractory ECD. A significant proportion of patients have mutations in *PIK3CA* (15%), which results in the activation of the mTOR pathway [12, 87]. mTOR activation has also been shown in ECD patients who lack *PIK3CA* mutations [88]. The combination of sirolimus and prednisone has demonstrated high overall response rates (without complete response), particularly of retroperitoneal and cardiovascular lesions, and stabilized pulmonary involvement [88]. Other immunosuppressive agents such as TNF-α and IL-6 inhibitors have shown mixed responses [8, 84, 89, 90]. Corticosteroids may be used as adjunctive therapy for the management of acute symptoms. Cytotoxic therapy with cladribine is generally well-tolerated and has demonstrated durable activity in a variety of ECD-infiltrated organs, including the pleura [91, 92].

Due to the systemic nature of ECD with multiorgan involvement, surgery and radiation are generally not recommended. These interventions only provide transient palliation with limited duration; surgery should generally be reserved for diagnostic purposes [93, 94]. Lung transplantation has been successfully performed in one patient with severe pleuropulmonary disease without recurrence at 5-year follow-up [95].

Prognosis

Advances in the treatment of ECD have significantly improved outcomes, and most patients can live with stable chronic disease. In 1996, 5-year overall survival was suggested to be about 43%, with a significant proportion of patients dying within 6 months of diagnosis [96]. The 5-year overall survival is now about 83% [25]. Factors associated with worse prognosis include CNS and retroperitoneum involvement, as well as advanced age [25]. The clinical outcomes of patients with pleuropulmonary involvement are not yet clearly established, although current evidence favors an association with a worse prognosis [20, 25, 28]. Future studies, including larger patient populations, will be required to better define outcomes in patients with histology-proven pleuropulmonary disease.

References

1. Jakob E, Harald K. A case study on Erdheim-Chester disease. Arch Case Rep. 2019;4:001–3.
2. Chester W. Über Lipoidgranulomatose. Virchows Arch Pathol Anat Physiol Klin Med. 1930;279(2):561–602.
3. Sorensen EW. Hyperlipemia. A report of an unusual case complicated by bone lesions, macrocytic anaemia, and leukemoid bone marrow. Acta Med Scand. 1964;175:207–14.
4. Jaffe HL. Metabolic, degenerative, and inflammatory disease of bones and joints. Philadelphia: Lea and Febiger; 1972.
5. Mossetti G, Rendina D, Numis FG, Somma P, Postiglione L, Nunziata V. Biochemical markers of bone turnover, serum levels of interleukin-6/interleukin-6 soluble receptor and bisphosphonate treatment in Erdheim-Chester disease. Clin Exp Rheumatol. 2003;21(2):232–6.
6. Bourke SC, Nicholson AG, Gibson GJ. Erdheim-Chester disease: pulmonary infiltration responding to cyclophosphamide and prednisolone. Thorax. 2003;58(11):1004–5.
7. Farber S, Cohen J, Uzman LL. Lipogranulomatosis: a new lipo-glycoprotein storage disease. J Mt Sinai Hosp N Y. 1957;24(6):816–37.
8. Dagna L, Corti A, Langheim S, Guglielmi B, De Cobelli F, Doglioni C, Fragasso G, Sabbadini MG, Ferrarini M. Tumor necrosis factor α as a master regulator of inflammation in Erdheim-Chester disease: rationale for the treatment of patients with infliximab. J Clin Oncol. 2012;30(28):e286–90.
9. Dagna L, Girlanda S, Langheim S, Rizzo N, Bozzolo EP, Sabbadini MG, Ferrarini M. Erdheim-Chester disease: report on a case and new insights on its immunopathogenesis. Rheumatology (Oxford). 2010;49(6):1203–6.
10. Arnaud L, Gorochov G, Charlotte F, Lvovschi V, Parizot C, Larsen M, Ghillani-Dalbin P, Hervier B, Kahn JE, Deback C, Musset L, Amoura Z, Haroche J. Systemic perturbation of cytokine and chemokine networks in Erdheim-Chester disease: a single-center series of 37 patients. Blood. 2011;117(10):2783–90.
11. Stoppacciaro A, Ferrarini M, Salmaggi C, Colarossi C, Praderio L, Tresoldi M, Beretta AA, Sabbadini MG. Immunohistochemical evidence of a cyto-

kine and chemokine network in three patients with Erdheim-Chester disease: implications for pathogenesis. Arthritis Rheum. 2006;54(12):4018–22.
12. Diamond EL, Durham BH, Haroche J, Yao Z, Ma J, Parikh SA, Wang Z, Choi J, Kim E, Cohen-Aubart F, Lee SC, Gao Y, Micol JB, Campbell P, Walsh MP, Sylvester B, Dolgalev I, Aminova O, Heguy A, Zappile P, Nakitandwe J, Ganzel C, Dalton JD, Ellison DW, Estrada-Veras J, Lacouture M, Gahl WA, Stephens PJ, Miller VA, Ross JS, Ali SM, Briggs SR, Fasan O, Block J, Héritier S, Donadieu J, Solit DB, Hyman DM, Baselga J, Janku F, Taylor BS, Park CY, Amoura Z, Dogan A, Emile JF, Rosen N, Gruber TA, Abdel-Wahab O. Diverse and targetable kinase alterations drive histiocytic neoplasms. Cancer Discov. 2016;6(2):154–65.
13. Badalian-Very G, Vergilio JA, Degar BA, MacConaill LE, Brandner B, Calicchio ML, Kuo FC, Ligon AH, Stevenson KE, Kehoe SM, Garraway LA, Hahn WC, Meyerson M, Fleming MD, Rollins BJ. Recurrent BRAF mutations in Langerhans cell histiocytosis. Blood. 2010;116(11):1919–23. https://doi.org/10.1182/blood-2010-04-279083.
14. Haroche J, Charlotte F, Arnaud L, von Deimling A, Hélias-Rodzewicz Z, Hervier B, Cohen-Aubart F, Launay D, Lesot A, Mokhtari K, Canioni D, Galmiche L, Rose C, Schmalzing M, Croockewit S, Kambouchner M, Copin MC, Fraitag S, Sahm F, Brousse N, Amoura Z, Donadieu J, Emile JF. High prevalence of BRAF V600E mutations in Erdheim-Chester disease but not in other non-Langerhans cell histiocytoses. Blood. 2012;120(13):2700–3.
15. Cohen Aubart F, Roos-Weil D, Armand M, Marceau-Renaut A, Emile JF, Duployez N, Charlotte F, Poulain S, Lhote R, Hélias-Rodzewicz Z, Della-Valle V, Bernard O, Maloum K, Nguyen-Khac F, Donadieu J, Amoura Z, Abdel-Wahab O, Haroche J. High frequency of clonal hematopoiesis in Erdheim-Chester disease. Blood. 2021;137(4):485–92.
16. Durham BH, Lopez Rodrigo E, Picarsic J, Abramson D, Rotemberg V, De Munck S, Pannecoucke E, Lu SX, Pastore A, Yoshimi A, Mandelker D, Ceyhan-Birsoy O, Ulaner GA, Walsh M, Yabe M, Petrova-Drus K, Arcila ME, Ladanyi M, Solit DB, Berger MF, Hyman DM, Lacouture ME, Erickson C, Saganty R, Ki M, Dunkel IJ, Santa-María López V, Mora J, Haroche J, Emile JF, Decaux O, Geissmann F, Savvides SN, Drilon A, Diamond EL, Abdel-Wahab O. Activating mutations in CSF1R and additional receptor tyrosine kinases in histiocytic neoplasms. Nat Med. 2019;25(12):1839–42. https://doi.org/10.1038/s41591-019-0653-6. Epub 2019 Nov 25. PMID: 31768065; PMCID: PMC6898787.
17. Milne P, Bigley V, Bacon CM, Néel A, McGovern N, Bomken S, Haniffa M, Diamond EL, Durham BH, Visser J, Hunt D, Gunawardena H, Macheta M, McClain KL, Allen C, Abdel-Wahab O, Collin M. Hematopoietic origin of Langerhans cell histiocytosis and Erdheim-Chester disease in adults. Blood. 2017;130(2):167–75.
18. Durham BH, Roos-Weil D, Baillou C, Cohen-Aubart F, Yoshimi A, Miyara M, Papo M, Hélias-Rodzewicz Z, Terrones N, Ozkaya N, Dogan A, Rampal R, Urbain F, Le Fèvre L, Diamond EL, Park CY, Papo T, Charlotte F, Gorochov G, Taly V, Bernard OA, Amoura Z, Abdel-Wahab O, Lemoine FM, Haroche J, Emile JF. Functional evidence for derivation of systemic histiocytic neoplasms from hematopoietic stem/progenitor cells. Blood. 2017;130(2):176–80.
19. Mass E, Jacome-Galarza CE, Blank T, Lazarov T, Durham BH, Ozkaya N, Pastore A, Schwabenland M, Chung YR, Rosenblum MK, Prinz M, Abdel-Wahab O, Geissmann F. A somatic mutation in erythro-myeloid progenitors causes neurodegenerative disease. Nature. 2017;549(7672):389–93.
20. Toya T, Ogura M, Toyama K, Yoshimi A, Shinozaki-Ushiku A, Honda A, Honda K, Hosoya N, Murakami Y, Kawashima H, Nannya Y, Arai S, Nakamura F, Shinoda Y, Nangaku M, Miyagawa K, Fukayama M, Moriya-Saito A, Katayama I, Ogura T, Kurokawa M. Prognostic factors of Erdheim-Chester disease: a nationwide survey in Japan. Haematologica. 2018;103(11):1815–24.
21. Ferrero E, Belloni D, Corti A, Doglioni C, Dagna L, Ferrarini M. TNF-α in Erdheim-Chester disease pericardial effusion promotes endothelial leakage in vitro and is neutralized by infliximab. Rheumatology (Oxford). 2014;53(1):198–200.
22. Cangi MG, Biavasco R, Cavalli G, Grassini G, Dal-Cin E, Campochiaro C, Guglielmi B, Berti A, Lampasona V, von Deimling A, Sabbadini MG, Ferrarini M, Doglioni C, Dagna L. BRAFV600E-mutation is invariably present and associated to oncogene-induced senescence in Erdheim-Chester disease. Ann Rheum Dis. 2015;74(8):1596–602.
23. Cavalli G, Biavasco R, Borgiani B, Dagna L. Oncogene-induced senescence as a new mechanism of disease: the paradigm of Erdheim-Chester disease. Front Immunol. 2014;5:281.
24. Estrada-Veras JI, O'Brien KJ, Boyd LC, Dave RH, Durham B, Xi L, Malayeri AA, Chen MY, Gardner PJ, Alvarado-Enriquez JR, Shah N, Abdel-Wahab O, Gochuico BR, Raffeld M, Jaffe ES, Gahl WA. The clinical spectrum of Erdheim-Chester disease: an observational cohort study. Blood Adv. 2017;1(6):357–66.
25. Cohen-Aubart F, Emile JF, Carrat F, Helias-Rodzewicz Z, Taly V, Charlotte F, Cluzel P, Donadieu J, Idbaih A, Barete S, Amoura Z, Haroche J. Phenotypes and survival in Erdheim-Chester disease: results from a 165-patient cohort. Am J Hematol. 2018;93(5):E114–7.
26. Peyronel F, Haroche J, Campochiaro C, Pegoraro F, Amoura Z, Tomelleri A, Mazzariol M, Papo M, Cavalli G, Benigno GD, Fenaroli P, Grigoratos C, Mengoli MC, Bonometti A, Berti E, Savino G, Cives M, Neri I, Pacinella G, Tuttolomondo A, Marano M, Muratore F, Manfredi A, Broccoli A, Zinzani PL, Didona B, Massaccesi C, Buono A, Ammirati E, Di Lernia V, Dagna L, Vaglio A, Cohen-Aubart F. Epidemiology

and geographic clustering of Erdheim-Chester disease in Italy and France. Blood. 2023;142(24):2119–23.
27. Pegoraro F, Mazzariol M, Trambusti I, Bakhshi S, Mallick S, Dunkel IJ, van den Bos C, Tezol Ö, Shan S, Ocak S, Giordano F, De Fusco C, Gaspari S, Buccoliero AM, Coniglio ML, Buti E, Romagnani P, Picarsic J, Donadieu J, Diamond EL, Emile JF, Sieni E, Haroche J, Vaglio A. Childhood-onset Erdheim-Chester disease in the molecular era: clinical phenotypes and long-term outcomes of 21 patients. Blood. 2023;142(13):1167–71.
28. Arnaud L, Pierre I, Beigelman-Aubry C, Capron F, Brun AL, Rigolet A, Girerd X, Weber N, Piette JC, Grenier PA, Amoura Z, Haroche J. Pulmonary involvement in Erdheim-Chester disease: a single-center study of thirty-four patients and a review of the literature. Arthritis Rheum. 2010;62(11):3504–12.
29. Wang JN, Wang FD, Sun J, Liang ZY, Li J, Zhou DB, Tian X, Cao XX. Pulmonary manifestations of Erdheim-Chester disease: clinical characteristics, outcomes and comparison with Langerhans cell histiocytosis. Br J Haematol. 2021;194(6):1024–33.
30. Tessier S, Abeykoon JP, Ruan G, Bennani NN, Shah MV, Rech KL, Ravindran A, Ryu JH, Vassallo R, Koster MJ, Davidge-Pitts CJ, Gruber LM, Tobin WO, Sartori-Valinotti JC, Hilal T, Jiang J, Mustafa MA, Ahmed AZ, Goyal G, Go RS. Incidence of Erdheim-Chester disease in the United States. Blood. 2024;144:5177.
31. Dion E, Graef C, Miquel A, Haroche J, Wechsler B, Amoura Z, Zeitoun D, Grenier PA, Piette JC, Laredo JD. Bone involvement in Erdheim-Chester disease: imaging findings including periostitis and partial epiphyseal involvement. Radiology. 2006;238(2):632–9.
32. Goyal G, Young JR, Koster MJ, Tobin WO, Vassallo R, Ryu JH, Davidge-Pitts CJ, Hurtado MD, Ravindran A, Sartori Valinotti JC, Bennani NN, Shah MV, Rech KL, Go RS, Mayo Clinic Histiocytosis Working Group. The Mayo Clinic Histiocytosis Working Group consensus statement for the diagnosis and evaluation of adult patients with histiocytic neoplasms: Erdheim-Chester disease, Langerhans cell histiocytosis, and Rosai-Dorfman disease. Mayo Clin Proc. 2019;94(10):2054–71.
33. Haroche J, Gueniche Y, Galanaud D, Cohen-Aubart F, Dormont D, Rousseau T, Amoura Z, Touitou V, Shor N. Erdheim-Chester disease: look it in the eye. An orbital magnetic resonance imaging study. Haematologica. 2022;107(11):2667–74.
34. Boyd LC, O'Brien KJ, Ozkaya N, Lehky T, Meoded A, Gochuico BR, Hannah-Shmouni F, Nath A, Toro C, Gahl WA, Estrada-Veras JI, Dave RH. Neurological manifestations of Erdheim-Chester disease. Ann Clin Transl Neurol. 2020;7(4):497–506.
35. Manaka K, Sato J, Makita N. Neuroendocrine manifestations of Erdheim-Chester disease. Handb Clin Neurol. 2021;181:137–47.
36. Chasset F, Barete S, Charlotte F, Cohen-Aubart F, Arnaud L, Le Pelletier F, Emile JF, Francès C, Amoura Z, Haroche J. Cutaneous manifestations of Erdheim-Chester disease (ECD): clinical, pathological, and molecular features in a monocentric series of 40 patients. J Am Acad Dermatol. 2016;74(3):513–20.
37. Guo S, Yan Q, Rohr J, Wang Y, Fan L, Wang Z, Erdheim-Chester disease involving the breast—a rare but important differential diagnosis. Hum Pathol. 2015;46(1):159–64.
38. Das JP, Xie L, Riedl CC, Hayes SA, Ginsberg MS, Halpenny DF. Cardiothoracic manifestations of Erdheim-Chester disease. Br J Radiol. 2019;92(1104):20190473.
39. Villatoro-Villar M, Bold MS, Warrington KJ, Crowson CS, Goyal G, Shah M, Go RS, Koster MJ. Arterial involvement in Erdheim-Chester disease: a retrospective cohort study. Medicine (Baltimore). 2018;97(49):e13452.
40. Chazal T, Pegoraro F, Manari G, Bettiol A, Maniscalco V, Gelain E, Charlotte F, Mazor RD, Renard-Penna R, Amoura Z, Cohen-Aubart F, Haroche J, Izzedine H, Vaglio A. Clinical phenotypes and long-term outcome of kidney involvement in Erdheim-Chester histiocytosis. Kidney Int. 2023;103(1):177–86.
41. Ivan D, Neto A, Lemos L, Gupta A. Erdheim-Chester disease: a unique presentation with liver involvement and vertebral osteolytic lesions. Arch Pathol Lab Med. 2003;127(8):e337–9.
42. Balasubramanian G, Modiri A, Affi M, Hagen CE, Batdorf B, Oshima K, Michaelis L, Saeian K. A fatal case of Erdheim-Chester disease with hepatic involvement. ACG Case Rep J. 2017;4:e95.
43. Hazim AZ, Acosta-Medina AA, Young JR, Ruan GJ, Abeykoon JP, Ravindran A, Vassallo R, Ryu JH, Tobin WO, Koster MJ, Bennani NN, Rech KL, Shah MV, Witzig TE, Goyal G, Go RS, Mayo Clinic-University of Alabama at Birmingham Histiocytosis Working Group. Classical and non-classical phenotypes of Erdheim-Chester disease: correlating clinical, radiographic and genotypic findings. Br J Haematol. 2022;199(3):454–7.
44. Papo M, Diamond EL, Cohen-Aubart F, Emile JF, Roos-Weil D, Gupta N, Durham BH, Ozkaya N, Dogan A, Ulaner GA, Rampal R, Kahn JE, Sené T, Charlotte F, Hervier B, Besnard C, Bernard OA, Settegrana C, Droin N, Hélias-Rodzewicz Z, Amoura Z, Abdel-Wahab O, Haroche J. High prevalence of myeloid neoplasms in adults with non-Langerhans cell histiocytosis. Blood. 2017;130(8):1007–13.
45. Mirmomen SM, Sirajuddin A, Nikpanah M, Symons R, Paschall AK, Papageorgiou I, Gahl WA, O'Brien K, Estrada-Veras JI, Malayeri AA. Thoracic involvement in Erdheim-Chester disease: computed tomography imaging findings and their association with the $BRAF^{V600E}$ mutation. Eur Radiol. 2018;28(11):4635–42.
46. Wang F, Cao X, Niu N, Zhang Y, Wang Y, Feng F, Jin Z. Multisystemic imaging findings in Chinese patients with Erdheim-Chester disease. AJR Am J Roentgenol. 2019;213(6):1179–86.

47. Mazor RD, Manevich-Mazor M, Kesler A, Aizenstein O, Eshed I, Jaffe R, Pessach Y, Goldberg I, Sprecher E, Yaish I, Gural A, Ganzel C, Shoenfeld Y. Clinical considerations and key issues in the management of patients with Erdheim-Chester disease: a seven case series. BMC Med. 2014;12:221.
48. Wittenberg KH, Swensen SJ, Myers JL. Pulmonary involvement with Erdheim-Chester disease: radiographic and CT findings. AJR Am J Roentgenol. 2000;174(5):1327–31.
49. Egan AJ, Boardman LA, Tazelaar HD, Swensen SJ, Jett JR, Yousem SA, Myers JL. Erdheim-Chester disease: clinical, radiologic, and histopathologic findings in five patients with interstitial lung disease. Am J Surg Pathol. 1999;23(1):17–26.
50. Brun AL, Touitou-Gottenberg D, Haroche J, Toledano D, Cluzel P, Beigelman-Aubry C, Piette JC, Amoura Z, Grenier PA. Erdheim-Chester disease: CT findings of thoracic involvement. Eur Radiol. 2010;20(11):2579–87.
51. Sung YE, Lee YS, Lee J, Lee KY. Erdheim-Chester disease involving lymph nodes and liver clinically mimicking lymphoma: a case report. J Pathol Transl Med. 2018;52(3):183–90.
52. Rush WL, Andriko JA, Galateau-Salle F, Brambilla E, Brambilla C, Ziany-bey I, Rosado-de-Christenson ML, Travis WD. Pulmonary pathology of Erdheim-Chester disease. Mod Pathol. 2000;13(7):747–54.
53. El Demellawy D, Young JL, de Nanassy J, Chernetsova E, Nasr A. Langerhans cell histiocytosis: a comprehensive review. Pathology. 2015;47(4):294–301.
54. Dion E, Graef C, Haroche J, Renard-Penna R, Cluzel P, Wechsler B, Piette JC, Grenier PA. Imaging of thoracoabdominal involvement in Erdheim-Chester disease. AJR Am J Roentgenol. 2004;183(5):1253–60.
55. Young JR, Johnson GB, Murphy RC, Go RS, Broski SM. ^{18}F-FDG PET/CT in Erdheim-Chester disease: imaging findings and potential BRAF mutation biomarker. J Nucl Med. 2018;59(5):774–9.
56. Massaccesi C, Colella S, Fioretti F, D'Emilio V, Panella G, Primomo G, Barbisan F, Pela R, Poletti V. An unusual thoracic localizations of Erdheim-Chester disease: a case report. Respir Med Case Rep. 2017;20:116–9.
57. Lee K, Kim HR, Roh J, Ok YJ, Jeon BB, Kim YW. Erdheim-Chester disease presenting as an anterior mediastinal tumor without skeletal involvement. Korean J Thorac Cardiovasc Surg. 2018;51(3):223–6.
58. Goyal G, Heaney ML, Collin M, Cohen-Aubart F, Vaglio A, Durham BH, Hershkovitz-Rokah O, Girschikofsky M, Jacobsen ED, Toyama K, Goodman AM, Hendrie P, Cao XX, Estrada-Veras JI, Shpilberg O, Abdo A, Kurokawa M, Dagna L, McClain KL, Mazor RD, Picarsic J, Janku F, Go RS, Haroche J, Diamond EL. Erdheim-Chester disease: consensus recommendations for evaluation, diagnosis, and treatment in the molecular era. Blood. 2020;135(22):1929–45.
59. García-Gómez FJ, Acevedo-Báñez I, Martínez-Castillo R, Tirado-Hospital JL, Cuenca-Cuenca JI, Pachón-Garrudo VM, Álvarez-Pérez RM, García-Jiménez R, Rivas-Infante E, García-Morillo JS, Borrego-Dorado I. The role of 18FDG, 18FDOPA PET/CT and 99mTc bone scintigraphy imaging in Erdheim-Chester disease. Eur J Radiol. 2015;84(8):1586–92.
60. Diamond EL, Dagna L, Hyman DM, Cavalli G, Janku F, Estrada-Veras J, Ferrarini M, Abdel-Wahab O, Heaney ML, Scheel PJ, Feeley NK, Ferrero E, McClain KL, Vaglio A, Colby T, Arnaud L, Haroche J. Consensus guidelines for the diagnosis and clinical management of Erdheim-Chester disease. Blood. 2014;124(4):483–92.
61. Melloul S, Hélias-Rodzewicz Z, Cohen-Aubart F, Charlotte F, Fraitag S, Terrones N, Riller Q, Chazal T, Héritier S, Moreau A, Kambouchner M, Copin MC, Donadieu J, Taly V, Amoura Z, Haroche J, Emile JF. Highly sensitive methods are required to detect mutations in histiocytoses. Haematologica. 2019;104(3):e97–9.
62. Janku F, Diamond EL, Goodman AM, Raghavan VK, Barnes TG, Kato S, Abdel-Wahab O, Durham BH, Meric-Bernstam F, Kurzrock R. Molecular profiling of tumor tissue and plasma cell-free DNA from patients with non-Langerhans cell histiocytosis. Mol Cancer Ther. 2019;18(6):1149–57.
63. Oneal PA, Kwitkowski V, Luo L, Shen YL, Subramaniam S, Shord S, Goldberg KB, McKee AE, Kaminskas E, Farrell A, Pazdur R. FDA approval summary: vemurafenib for the treatment of patients with Erdheim-Chester disease with the *BRAF*V600 mutation. Oncologist. 2018;23(12):1520–4.
64. Diamond EL, Subbiah V, Lockhart AC, Blay JY, Puzanov I, Chau I, Raje NS, Wolf J, Erinjeri JP, Torrisi J, Lacouture M, Elez E, Martínez-Valle F, Durham B, Arcila ME, Ulaner G, Abdel-Wahab O, Pitcher B, Makrutzki M, Riehl T, Baselga J, Hyman DM. Vemurafenib for BRAF V600-mutant Erdheim-Chester disease and Langerhans cell histiocytosis: analysis of data from the histology-independent, phase 2, Open-label VE-BASKET study. JAMA Oncol. 2018;4(3):384–8. https://doi.org/10.1001/jamaoncol.2017.5029. Erratum in: JAMA Oncol. 2019;5(1):122.
65. Ruan GJ, Hazim A, Abeykoon JP, Scheckel C, Vassallo R, Ryu JH, Tobin WO, Koster MJ, Bennani NN, Rech KL, Young JR, Shah MV, Goyal G, Go RS. Low-dose vemurafenib monotherapy in *BRAFV600E* -mutated Erdheim-Chester disease. Leuk Lymphoma. 2020;61(11):2733–7.
66. Bhatia A, Ulaner G, Rampal R, Hyman DM, Abdel-Wahab O, Durham BH, Dogan A, Ozkaya N, Lacouture ME, Hajdenberg J, Ganzel C, Diamond EL. Single-agent dabrafenib for *BRAF*^{V600E}-mutated histiocytosis. Haematologica. 2018;103(4):e177–80.
67. Haroche J, Cohen-Aubart F, Emile JF, Maksud P, Drier A, Tolédano D, Barete S, Charlotte F, Cluzel P, Donadieu J, Benameur N, Grenier PA, Besnard S, Ory JP, Lifermann F, Idbaih A, Granel B, Graffin

B, Hervier B, Arnaud L, Amoura Z. Reproducible and sustained efficacy of targeted therapy with vemurafenib in patients with BRAF(V600E)-mutated Erdheim-Chester disease. J Clin Oncol. 2015;33(5):411–8.
68. Haroche J, Cohen-Aubart F, Emile JF, Arnaud L, Maksud P, Charlotte F, Cluzel P, Drier A, Hervier B, Benameur N, Besnard S, Donadieu J, Amoura Z. Dramatic efficacy of vemurafenib in both multisystemic and refractory Erdheim-Chester disease and Langerhans cell histiocytosis harboring the BRAF V600E mutation. Blood. 2013;121(9):1495–500.
69. Borys D, Nystrom L, Song A, Lomasney LM. Erdheim Chester disease with appendicular skeletal, renal and pleural involvement responding to Zelboraf (BRAF inhibitor) treatment: case report. Skeletal Radiol. 2016;45(10):1397–402.
70. Shen KN, Chang L, Niu N, Li J, Cao XX. Pulmonary Erdheim-Chester disease successfully treated with vemurafenib. Ann Hematol. 2024;103(2):673–5.
71. Garutti M, Bergnach M, Polesel J, Palmero L, Pizzichetta MA, Puglisi F. BRAF and MEK inhibitors and their toxicities: a meta-analysis. Cancers (Basel). 2022;15(1):141.
72. Ruan GJ, Goyal G, Shah MV, Cohen-Aubart F, Amoura Z, Straetmans N, Benameur N, Haroche J, Go RS, Mayo Clinic Histiocytosis Working Group. Acute pancreatitis from treatment with BRAF inhibitors in Erdheim-Chester disease: a report from 2 tertiary referral centers. Pancreas. 2021;50(1):e6–8.
73. Amoura A, Haroche J, Emile JF, Barete S, Helias-Rodzewicz Z, Charlotte F, Maisonobe T, Amoura Z, Cohen Aubart F. Sarcoidosis occurring during BRAF/MEK inhibitors is associated with paradoxical ERK activation in Erdheim-Chester patients. J Eur Acad Dermatol Venereol. 2019;33(10):e348–50.
74. Callahan MK, Rampal R, Harding JJ, Klimek VM, Chung YR, Merghoub T, Wolchok JD, Solit DB, Rosen N, Abdel-Wahab O, Levine RL, Chapman PB. Progression of RAS-mutant leukemia during RAF inhibitor treatment. N Engl J Med. 2012;367(24):2316–21.
75. Diamond EL, Durham BH, Ulaner GA, Drill E, Buthorn J, Ki M, Bitner L, Cho H, Young RJ, Francis JH, Rampal R, Lacouture M, Brody LA, Ozkaya N, Dogan A, Rosen N, Iasonos A, Abdel-Wahab O, Hyman DM. Efficacy of MEK inhibition in patients with histiocytic neoplasms. Nature. 2019;567(7749):521–4.
76. Cohen Aubart F, Emile JF, Maksud P, Galanaud D, Cluzel P, Benameur N, Aumaitre O, Amoura Z, Haroche J. Efficacy of the MEK inhibitor cobimetinib for wild-type BRAF Erdheim-Chester disease. Br J Haematol. 2018;180(1):150–3.
77. Acosta Medina AA, Zanwar S, Ruan G, Abeykoon JP, Rech K, Ravindran A, Bennani NN, Davidge-Pitts CJ, Koster M, Ryu J, Shah MV, Tobin OW, Vassallo R, Young JR, Goyal G, Ronald G. Efficacy of MEK inhibitors in Erdheim Chester disease. Blood. 2022;140(Supplement 1):9733–4.
78. Nordmann TM, Juengling FD, Recher M, Berger CT, Kalbermatten D, Wicki A, Paasinen-Sohns A, Cathomas G, Tzankov A, Daikeler T. Trametinib after disease reactivation under dabrafenib in Erdheim-Chester disease with both *BRAF* and *KRAS* mutations. Blood. 2017;129(7):879–82.
79. Mazor RD, Weissman R, Luckman J, Domachevsky L, Diamond EL, Abdel-Wahab O, Shapira S, Hershkovitz-Rokah O, Groshar D, Shpilberg O. Dual BRAF/MEK blockade restores CNS responses in BRAF-mutant Erdheim-Chester disease patients following BRAF inhibitor monotherapy. Neurooncol Adv. 2020;2(1):vdaa024.
80. Hervier B, Arnaud L, Charlotte F, Wechsler B, Piette JC, Amoura Z, Haroche J. Treatment of Erdheim-Chester disease with long-term high-dose interferon-α. Semin Arthritis Rheum. 2012;41(6):907–13.
81. Cao XX, Niu N, Sun J, Cai H, Wang FD, Wang YN, Duan MH, Zhou DB, Li J. Clinical and positron emission tomography responses to long-term high-dose interferon-α treatment among patients with Erdheim-Chester disease. Orphanet J Rare Dis. 2019;14(1):11.
82. Haroche J, Amoura Z, Trad SG, Wechsler B, Cluzel P, Grenier PA, Piette JC. Variability in the efficacy of interferon-alpha in Erdheim-Chester disease by patient and site of involvement: results in eight patients. Arthritis Rheum. 2006;54(10):3330–6.
83. Sleijfer S, Bannink M, Van Gool AR, Kruit WH, Stoter G. Side effects of interferon-alpha therapy. Pharm World Sci. 2005;27(6):423–31.
84. Goyal G, Shah MV, Call TG, Litzow MR, Wolanskyj-Spinner AP, Koster MJ, Tobin WO, Vassallo R, Ryu JH, Hook CC, Hogan WJ, Go RS. Efficacy of biological agents in the treatment of Erdheim-Chester disease. Br J Haematol. 2018;183(3):520–4.
85. Cohen-Aubart F, Maksud P, Saadoun D, Drier A, Charlotte F, Cluzel P, Amoura Z, Haroche J. Variability in the efficacy of the IL1 receptor antagonist anakinra for treating Erdheim-Chester disease. Blood. 2016;127(11):1509–12.
86. Campochiaro C, Cavalli G, Farina N, Tomelleri A, De Luca G, Dagna L. Efficacy and improved tolerability of combination therapy with interleukin-1 blockade and MAPK pathway inhibitors for the treatment of Erdheim-Chester disease. Ann Rheum Dis. 2022;81(1):e11.
87. Emile JF, Diamond EL, Hélias-Rodzewicz Z, Cohen-Aubart F, Charlotte F, Hyman DM, Kim E, Rampal R, Patel M, Ganzel C, Aumann S, Faucher G, Le Gall C, Leroy K, Colombat M, Kahn JE, Trad S, Nizard P, Donadieu J, Taly V, Amoura Z, Abdel-Wahab O, Haroche J. Recurrent RAS and PIK3CA mutations in Erdheim-Chester disease. Blood. 2014;124(19):3016–9.
88. Gianfreda D, Nicastro M, Galetti M, Alberici F, Corradi D, Becchi G, Baldari G, De Filippo M, Ferretti S, Moroni G, Foti R, Di Gangi M, Jeannin G, Saffroy R, Emile JF, Buzio C, Vaglio A. Sirolimus plus prednisone for Erdheim-Chester disease: an open-label trial. Blood. 2015;126(10):1163–71.

89. Berti A, Cavalli G, Guglielmi B, Biavasco R, Campochiaro C, Tomelleri A, Nicoletti R, Panzacchi A, Ferrarini M, Dagna L. Tocilizumab in patients with multisystem Erdheim-Chester disease. Onco Targets Ther. 2017;6(6):e1318237.
90. Cohen-Aubart F, Maksud P, Emile JF, Benameur N, Charlotte F, Cluzel P, Amoura Z, Haroche J. Efficacy of infliximab in the treatment of Erdheim-Chester disease. Ann Rheum Dis. 2018;77(9):1387–90.
91. Azadeh N, Tazelaar HD, Gotway MB, Mookadam F, Fonseca R. Erdheim Chester disease treated successfully with cladribine. Respir Med Case Rep. 2016;18:37–40.
92. Goyal G, Shah MV, Call TG, Litzow MR, Hogan WJ, Go RS. Clinical and radiologic responses to cladribine for the treatment of Erdheim-Chester disease. JAMA Oncol. 2017;3(9):1253–6.
93. Miller RC, Villà S, Kamer S, Pasquier D, Poortmans P, Micke O, Call TG. Palliative treatment of Erdheim-Chester disease with radiotherapy: a rare cancer network study. Radiother Oncol. 2006;80(3):323–6.
94. Alfieri A, Gazzeri R, Galarza M, Neroni M. Surgical treatment of intracranial Erdheim-Chester disease. J Clin Neurosci. 2010;17(12):1489–92.
95. Hashimoto K, Miyoshi K, Mizutani H, Otani S, Sugimoto S, Yamane M, Oto T. Successful lung transplantation for pulmonary disease associated with Erdheim-Chester disease. Ann Thorac Surg. 2017;104(1):e13–5.
96. Veyssier-Belot C, Cacoub P, Caparros-Lefebvre D, Wechsler J, Brun B, Remy M, Wallaert B, Petit H, Grimaldi A, Wechsler B, Godeau P, Erdheim-Chester disease. Clinical and radiologic characteristics of 59 cases. Medicine (Baltimore). 1996;75(3):157–69.

Index

F. Ido (ed.), *Rare Pleural Diseases*, https://doi.org/10.1007/978-3-032-14873-5